W9-BKP-109

Complications of Interventional Procedures

TOPICS IN CLINICAL CARDIOLOGY

Series Editor: J. WILLIS HURST, M.D.

New Types of Cardiovascular Disease
J. Willis Hurst, M.D.

Complications of Interventional Procedures
Jerre F. Lutz, M.D.

TOPICS IN CLINICAL CARDIOLOGY

Complications of Interventional Procedures

Jerre Lutz, M.D.

Assistant Professor of Medicine (Cardiology)
Division of Cardiology
Department of Medicine
Emory University Hospital
Atlanta, Georgia

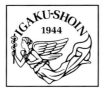

IGAKU-SHOIN   New York   •   Tokyo

Published and distributed by

IGAKU-SHOIN Medical Publishers, Inc.
One Madison Avenue, New York, New York 10010

IGAKU-SHOIN Ltd.,
5-24-3 Hongo, Bunkyo-ku, Tokyo 113-91

Copyright © 1995 by IGAKU-SHOIN Medical Publishers, Inc.
All rights reserved. No part of this book may be translated or reproduced in any form by print,
photo-print, microfilm or any other means without written permission from the publisher.

Library of Congress Cataloging-in-Publication Data

Complications of interventional procedures / [edited by] Jerre Lutz.
    p.   cm. — (Topics in clinical cardiology)
  Includes bibliographical references and index.
   1. Heart—Diseases—Treatment—Complications. 2. Heart—Surgery—
Complications. I. Lutz, Jerre F. II. Series.
  [DNLM: 1. Heart Function Tests—adverse effects. 2. Heart
Diseases—therapy. 3. Intraoperative Complications. WG 141 C7375
1995]
RC683.8.C65 1995
616.1'2—dc20
DNLM/DLC
for Library of Congress   94-46842
                                                CIP

ISBN: 0-89640-260-6 (New York)
ISBN: 4-260-14260-7 (Tokyo)

Printed and bound in the U.S.A.

10 9 8 7 6 5 4 3 2 1

Preface

For years, Dr. J. Willis Hurst has preached to attendings, cardiology fellows, and younger trainees that the value of a procedure cannot be measured without knowing both the good and the harm that can accompany that procedure. "Were there any problems yesterday?", he queried on at least a daily basis. Dr. Hurst emphasized that a practicing physician needed to know not only the morbidity and mortality of a procedure in the most expert hands but the success and failure rates at one's own hospital. If there were choices concerning which procedure to perform, perhaps one's own institution had excellent results with a particular procedure but less admirable results with an alternative. A discerning patient wants to know complication figures in the hands of the doctor to whom he has entrusted his care. The best possible results and average national results are merely benchmarks against which to compare the results of the individual who is proposing to perform the procedure. "Suppose it was your mother. What would you recommend?" Dr. Hurst retorted.

Cardiology has exploded in its breadth and depth since the 1960s. The ability to diagnose and treat heart disease has blossomed to such a degree that physicians now have to choose which procedure is best to treat the individual patient. Life was much simpler when there was only medical therapy (and few choices there also).

Each chapter in this volume begins with a description of the evolution of the procedure. Historical perspectives are followed by a brief discussion of indications and contraindications for the procedure. Legal ramifications as well as patients' unhappiness increase incrementally with failure to take appropriate precautions. Dr. Hurst would caution, "Never get involved with any mess you can't get out of or shouldn't have been involved with in the first place." The next section provides a description of complications, including expected frequencies. Where possible, our authors have included clues on how to avoid problems or, in the event of a misadventure, how to correct the situation and achieve the greatest chance of a favorable outcome for both the doctor and the patient.

In closing, remember the words of Dr. Andreas Gruentzig: "It is easy to be a hero when the procedure goes well. The mark of a really good doctor is how he handles a situation in which he is *not* the hero."

Jerre F. Lutz, M.D.

DEDICATION

To Carlin DeMore Lutz—my wife, my friend, and my advocate.

Contributors

George S. Abela, M.D.
Co-Director, Institute for the Prevention of Cardiovascular Disease
New England Deaconess Hospital
Associate Professor of Medicine
Harvard Medical School
Boston, Massachusetts

Kenneth L. Baughman, M.D.
Professor of Medicine
Chief, Division of Cardiology
Johns Hopkins Hospital
Baltimore, Maryland

John A. Bittl, M.D.
Director of Interventional Cardiology
Brigham and Women's Hospital
Associate Professor of Medicine
Harvard Medical School
Boston, Massachusetts

Peter C. Block, M.D.
Associate Director
The Heart Institute of St. Vincent
Hospital and Medical Center
Portland, Oregon

M. Erick Burton, M.D.
Fellow in Medicine (Cardiology) 1990–1994
Emory University School of Medicine
Southwest Florida Heart Group
Fort Myers, Florida

David S. Caras, M.D.
Former Fellow in Medicine (Cardiology) 1991–1994
Emory University School of Medicine
Atlanta, Georgia
Staff Cardiologist—Cardiovascular Medicine
Marietta, Georgia

Stephen D. Clements, Jr., M.D.
Professor of Medicine (Cardiology)
Emory University School of Medicine
Atlanta, Georgia

David A. Cutler, M.D.
Assistant Professor
Division of Cardiology
University of Texas Medical Branch
Galveston, Texas

John S. Douglas, Jr., M.D.
Associate Professor of Medicine
Emory University School of Medicine
Co-Director, Cardiovascular Laboratory
Emory University Hospital
Atlanta, Georgia

Stephen G. Ellis, M.D.
Professor of Medicine
Ohio State University
Director—Cardiac Catheterization Laboratory
The Cleveland Clinic Foundation
Cleveland, Ohio

Pedro Estella, M.D.
Research Fellow
Brigham and Women's Hospital
Harvard Medical School
Boston, Massachusetts

Robert S. Fishel, M.D.
Fellow in Cardiology
Division of Cardiology
Emory University School of Medicine
Atlanta, Georgia

Gerald F. Fletcher, M.D.
Professor and Chairman
Department of Rehabilitation Medicine
Professor of Medicine (Cardiology)
Emory University School of Medicine
Medical Director
Emory Health Enhancement Program
Atlanta, Georgia

Ziyad Ghazzal, M.D.
Assistant Professor of Medicine (Cardiology)
Emory University School of Medicine
Atlanta, Georgia

Edward K. Kasper, M.D.
Assistant Professor of Medicine
Director, Johns Hopkins Cardiomyopathy and Heart Transplant Service
Baltimore, Maryland

Paul E. Kazanjian, M.D.
Former Fellow in Cardiothoracic Anesthesiology and Critical Care
Emory University School of Medicine
Atlanta, Georgia
Lecturer of Anesthesiology
University of Michigan Medical School
Ann Arbor, Michigan

Spencer B. King, M.D.
Director, Andreas Gruentzig Cardiovascular Center
Professor of Medicine (Cardiology) and Radiology
Emory University School of Medicine
Atlanta, Georgia

Jonathan Langberg, M.D.
Professor of Medicine (Cardiology)
Emory University School of Medicine
Director, Cardiac Electrophysiology Laboratories
Emory University Hospital
Atlanta, Georgia

Angel R. Leon, M.D.
Assistant Professor of Cardiology (Medicine)
Emory University School of Medicine
Director, Cardiac Electrophysiology and Arrhythmia Center
Emory/Crawford Long Hospital
Atlanta, Georgia

Jerre F. Lutz, M.D.
Assistant Professor of Medicine (Cardiology)
Division of Cardiology
Department of Medicine
Emory University Hospital
Atlanta, Georgia

Randolph P. Martin, M.D.
Professor of Medicine (Cardiology)
Director of Non Invasive Cardiology
Emory University School of Medicine
Atlanta, Georgia

Terrence P. May, M.D.
Fellow in Electrophysiology
Division of Cardiology
Department of Medicine
Emory University School of Medicine
Atlanta, Georgia

Nowamagbe A. Omoigui, M.D., M.P.H.
Former Fellow, Cleveland Clinic Foundation
Associate Professor
Director, Division of Cardiology
University of South Carolina
Columbia, South Carolina

Albert E. Raizner, M.D.
Professor of Clinical Medicine
Baylor College of Medicine
Director, Cardiac Catheterization Laboratories
The Methodist Hospital
Houston, Texas

James G. Ramsay, M.D.
Associate Professor of Anesthesiology
Emory University School of Medicine
Atlanta, Georgia

Marschall S. Runge, M.D., Ph.D.
Chief, Division of Cardiology
University of Texas Medical Branch
Galveston, Texas

Vipul Shah, M.D.
Former Fellow in Cardiology 1992–1994
Division of Cardiology
Emory University Hospital

Atlanta, Georgia
Assistant Professor of Medicine (Cardiology)
Director of Echocardiography
Medical College of Georgia
Augusta, Georgia

Andrew L. Smith, M.D.
Assistant Professor of Medicine
Division of Cardiology
Department of Medicine
Emory University School of Medicine
Atlanta, Georgia

Laurence S. Sperling, M.D.
Fellow in Medicine (Cardiology)
Division of Cardiology
Emory University
Atlanta, Georgia

Cyril B. Tawa, M.D.
Fellow in Cardiology
Baylor College of Medicine
Houston, Texas

John P. Vansant, M.D.
Assistant Professor of Radiology and Internal Medicine
Director, Clinical Cardiac Imaging
Division of Nuclear Medicine
Department of Radiology
Emory University School of Medicine
Atlanta, Georgia

Brent Videau, M.D.
Former Fellow in Cardiology (Medicine) 1991–1994
Emory University School of Medicine
Cardiology Consultants
Pensacola, Florida

Paul F. Walter, M.D.
Professor of Medicine (Cardiology)
Emory University School of Medicine
Atlanta, Georgia

Patrick L. Whitlow, M.D.
Director Interventional Cardiology
Cleveland Clinic Foundation
Cleveland, Ohio

Contents

—1—

Complications of Exercise Testing

Gerald F. Fletcher, M.D.

DESCRIPTION OF PROCEDURE

Exercise testing involves subjecting an individual to an acute exercise "stress" in order to evaluate the physiologic, electrocardiographic, and metabolic responses to a given intensity of exercise. This procedure is particularly valuable and useful in assessing the response of the cardiovascular system. The test usually comprises a progressive graduated exercise stress beginning at low level with increasing increments of workload every two to three minutes. Exercise tests are usually done on a motorized treadmill or bicycle ergometer. Ideally, the upright treadmill should be utilized if at all possible, as this enables a subject to achieve a higher maximum oxygen consumption compared to other types of exercise. The seated bicycle test is, however, weight independent; therefore the workload can be transposed to metabolic equivalents (METs) in ml/kg/min directly regardless of body weight. Exercise testing is done under the supervision of a physician—often with a nurse or exercise specialist actually doing the testing. The blood pressure, heart rate and rhythm, and electrocardiogram are monitored throughout the test while the patient has constant dialogue with staff regarding symptoms. Tests are often also performed using metabolic studies that determine carbon dioxide and oxygen contents in expired air to assess the level of oxygen consumption or work capacity.[1]

HISTORY OF THE PROCEDURE

Exercise testing has been done for many years and began in the early 1900s with the simple step test. This method entailed a subject's repeatedly stepping up and

1

down on a small, two-level step bench. Electrocardiographic monitoring could be done effectively; however, blood pressure recording was difficult during the "stepping." In recent times, treadmill exercise using upright walking has become the most popular method of exercise testing, although cycle ergometry and, to some extent, arm ergometry are also used. These systems permit easy recordings of blood pressure during exercise and in addition metabolic studies when appropriate.

Exercise testing is most often done to evaluate subjects with recognized or suspected coronary artery disease to determine the degree and manifestations of myocardial ischemia. Stress testing may also be used to assess the cardiovascular functional capacity in patients with valvular or primary myocardial heart disease. The procedure is done quite frequently—as often as seven or eight tests being done in one day in a physician's office as part of routine outpatient care.

INDICATIONS FOR THE TEST

The exercise test is appropriately used in a cardiovascular evaluation as the first diagnostic procedure after the history, physical examination and the basic laboratory work which includes a chest x-ray and a 12 lead-ECG. It can be done effectively and safely as an outpatient procedure and is generally a more cost-effective screening test than certain more involved interventional evaluations. Table 1.1 reveals general indications for exercise testing.[2]

CONTRAINDICATIONS

Contraindications to exercise are limited to those that are potentially harmful to the subject's current medical stability or that might aggravate an existing medical condition. Absolute and related contraindications to testing are cited in Table 1.2.[2]

SAFETY MEASURES FOR EXERCISE TESTING

There should be a definite plan of emergency action for an exercise test including the duties of each member of the team. In addition to direct patient care, the plan should include notification of appropriate individuals and providing other necessities for patient transfer and prompt admission to an intensive cardiac care unit if need be. All members of the team should be trained in cardiopulmonary resuscitation. A defibrillator should be within cable reach of the treadmill, turned on and charged (200 J). An emergency drug kit should be available with intravenous solutions, administration sets, needles and syringes. An oropharyngeal airway, laryngoscope, endotracheal tubes, ventilation bag, and suction machine with equipment for the administration of oxygen should be available.[3,4–6]

TABLE 1.1. General Indications for Exercise Testing

Conditions for which there is general agreement that exercise testing is justified.

To assess functional capacity and aid in assessing the prognosis of subjects with known coronary artery disease (CAD)

To evaluate the prognosis and functional capacity of patients with CAD after a myocardial infarction, coronary artery bypass surgery, or coronary angioplasty

To evaluate subjects with symptoms consistent with exercise-induced cardiac arrhythmias

To evaluate the functional capacity of certain patients with congenital heart disease

To evaluate patients with rate-responsive pacemakers

Conditions for which exercise testing is frequently performed but in which there is a divergence of opinion with respect to its value and appropriateness

To evaluate asymptomatic subjects over the age of 40 with special occupations (pilots, air traffic controllers, fire fighters, police officers, bus or truck drivers, and railroad engineers)

To evaluate asymptomatic subjects over the age of 40 with two or more risk factors for CAD

To evaluate sedentary subjects over the age of 40 years who plan to enter a vigorous exercise program

To assist in the diagnosis of CAD in women with a history of chest pain

To assist in the diagnosis of CAD in subjects who are taking digitalis or who have complete right bundle branch block

To evaluate the functional capacity and response to therapy with cardiovascular drugs in patients with CAD or heart failure

To evaluate subjects with variant angina

To follow-up serially (at 1-year intervals or longer) patients with known CAD

To evaluate on a routine, yearly basis patients who remain asymptomatic after a revascularization procedure

To evaluate the functional capacity of selected patients with valvular heart disease

To evaluate the blood pressure response of patients being treated for systemic arterial hypertension

With modification from Schlant RC, Blomqvist CG, Brandenburg RO, DeBusk R, Ellestad MH, Fletcher GF, et al. Special report. In: Guidelines for exercise testing. A report of the Joint American College of Cardiology/American Heart Association Task Force on Assessment of Cardiovascular Procedures (Subcommittee on Exercise Testing). *Circulation.* 74:653A–667A, 1986. Reproduced with permission.

COMPLICATIONS OF EXERCISE TESTING

Complications of exercise testing—especially of critical degree—occur infrequently. There are, however, reports of infarction and death related to the procedure in the range of 10 per 10000 tests.[1] Such events occur in patients who are post–cardiac event or those being evaluated for high-grade ventricular arrhythmias. Table 1.3 outlines the basic complications of exercise testing. Bradyarrhythmias are generally treated with atropine, intravenous fluid and leg elevation to increase venous return. atrioventricular block if not responsive to atropine may require temporary transcuta-

TABLE 1.2. Contraindications to Exercise Testing

Absolute	Relative*
Acute myocardial infarction or recent change on resting ECG	Less serious noncardiac disorder
Unstable angina	Significant arterial or pulmonary hypertension
Serious cardiac arrhythmias	Tachyarrhythmias or bradyarrhythmias
Acute pericarditis	Moderate valvular heart disease
Endocarditis	Drug effect or electrolyte abnormalities
Severe aortic stenosis	Left main coronary obstruction or its equivalent
Severe left ventricular dysfunction	Hypertrophic cardiomyopathy
Acute pulmonary embolus or pulmonary infarction	Psychiatric disease
Acute or serious noncardiac disorder	
Severe physical disability	

*Under certain circumstances and with appropriate precautions, relative contraindications can be superseded.

With modification from Schlant RC, Blomqvist CG, Brandenburg RO, DeBusk R, Ellestad MH, Fletcher GF, et al. Special report. In: Guidelines for exercise testing. A report of the Joint American College of Cardiology/American Heart Association Task Force on Assessment of Cardiovascular Procedures (Subcommittee on Exercise Testing). *Circulation.* 74:653A–667A, 1986. Reproduced with permission.

neous or transvenous pacing. Asystole and ventricular tachycardia/fibrillation are treated by following advanced cardiac life support guidelines. Myocardial infarction requires rapid mobilization to the previously defined support facility for institution of lytic therapy or more invasive procedures where appropriate.

As cited in Table 1.3, "psychological" complications of the test should be considered. These complications include anxiety that a subject may have about a test. Such may occur secondary to a subject's anticipation of having an abnormal test or simply to the testing technique itself and may at times manifest as hyperventilation or a vasovagal reaction. Careful attention to the subject by experienced staff will usually prevent such reactions or decrease their magnitude. Musculoskeletal problems are also rare, but may occur when subjects fall from the treadmill or have a hand or extremity caught beneath the "belt" of the treadmill. In such situations, contusions or fractures may occur. "Technical" accidents such as initiating the motion of the belt when a subject is sitting on the treadmill and complications of placing electrodes with regard to skin burns, allergy, and other skin reactions occur rarely. As aforementioned, the most common complications (when they do occur) are those relative to the cardiovascular system. High-grade arrhythmias, myocardial infarction, and sudden death are the most critical. Others include abnormal increases in blood pressure and, with left ventricular dysfunction, lack of a normal increase. Variable types of high-grade heart block may occur in the form of 2:1 and complete atrioventricular block. In accord with this, it shall be emphasized that careful assessment of the subject's clinical state before the exercise test will usually alert the testing staff to the likelihood

TABLE 1.3. Complications of Exercise Testing

CARDIAC	

Bradyarrhythmias
  Sinus
  Atrioventricular junctional
  Ventricular
  Atrioventricular block
  Asystole
	Sudden death (ventricular tachycardia/fibrillation)
	Myocardial infarction
	Heart failure
	Hypotension and shock

NONCARDIAC
Musculoskeletal trauma, Psychological-Anxiety Reactions

MISCELLANEOUS
Severe fatigue, dizziness, fainting, general malaise, "body aches," and fatigue, sometimes persisting for days

With modification from Fletcher GF, Froelicher VF, Hartley LH, Haskell WL, Pollock ML. Exercise standards: a statement for health professionals from the American Heart Association. *Circulation.* 82:2286–2322, 1990. Reproduced with permission.

of the occurrence of such complications. In such instances, testing staff can intervene quickly if complications occur.

SUMMARY

Complications of exercise testing are relatively rare. These can usually be prevented and controlled by proper evaluation of the subject before the test and proper medical staff supervision of testing procedures. It must be understood that this is one of the few tests in the practice of medicine in which a patient is asked to exercise vigorously. Such exercise must be done with proper clothing, proper shoes, and without the intake of solid food within an hour before the test. As mentioned before, with preventative measures and proper instructions about the test, complications are rarely seen and usually can be controlled without difficulty.

REFERENCES

1. Fletcher GF, Froelicher VF, Hartley H, et al. Exercise standards: a statement for health professionals from the American Heart Association. *Circulation.* 82:2286–2322, 1990.
2. Schlant RC, Blomqvist CG, Brandenburg RO, DeBusk R, Ellestad MH, Fletcher GF, et al. Special report. In: Guidelines for exercise testing: a report of the joint American College of Cardiology/American Heart Association Task Force on Assessment of Cardiovascular Procedures (Subcommittee on Exercise Testing). *Circulation.* 74:653A–667A, 1986.

3. Fletcher GF, ed. *Exercise in the Practice of Medicine.* 2nd ed. Mt Kisco, NY: Futura, 1988.

4. Sheffield LT, Haskell W, Heiss G, et al. Safety of exercise testing volunteer subjects: the Lipid Research Clinics' Prevalence Study. *J Cardiopulm Rehab.* 2:395–400, 1982.

5. Young DZ, Lampert S, Graboys TB, et al. Safety of maximal exercise stress testing in patients at high risk for ventricular arrhythmia. *Circulation.* 70:184–191, 1984.

6. Gibbons LW, Blair SN, Kohl HW, III, et al. The safety of maximal exercise testing. *Circulation.* 80:846–852, 1989.

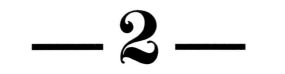

Complications of Dobutamine Stress Echocardiography

David S. Caras, M.D.
Vipul Shah, M.D.
Brent Videau, M.D.
Randolph P Martin, M.D.

Dobutamine stress echocardiography (DSE) is one of many ways to assess coronary atherosclerotic heart disease in patients who can not exercise. Its main advantage over pharmacological stress with dipyridamole or adenosine is that it mimics exercise, increasing heart rate, systolic blood pressure, and rate-pressure product.

HISTORY OF THE PROCEDURE

Since 1986, when DSE was first used to evaluate multivessel coronary artery disease by Berthe,[1] its use for preoperative risk assessment, diagnosis of coronary artery disease and assessment of known coronary artery lesions has become routine at many centers. At Emory University the use of DSE has seen dramatic growth, from just a handful of studies five years ago to well over 700 studies last year.

INDICATIONS AND CONTRAINDICATIONS

With increased experience, the indications for DSE have increased while the lists of absolute contraindications have decreased. Initially DSE was used only for patients

TABLE 2.1.   Indications for Dobutamine Stress Echo

Preoperative risk stratification
Detection of functionally significant coronary artery disease
Follow up of cardiac transplant patients
Follow up status-post angioplasty
Evaluation of myocardial viability (low dose)
Evaluation of difficult cases of aortic stenosis
Post myocardial infarction risk stratification

unable to exercise and unable to tolerate dipyridamole thallium imaging. Currently DSE has become the preferred noninvasive test to evaluate coronary artery disease at many centers. Table 2.1 lists the current indications for DSE in patients unable to exercise adequately. During the initial experience at Emory University, abdominal aortic aneurysms (AAA), atrial fibrillation, aortic stenosis, and paroxysmal supraventricular tachycardia (PSVT) were among the absolute contraindications for DSE. However, with increased experience it has become clear that some patients with the preceding problems could tolerate DSE at reduced dosage and with close monitoring of blood pressure, heart rate and ectopy. The physician monitoring these patients should have a low threshold for test termination. Table 2.2 lists the currently accepted contraindications to DSE.

DESCRIPTION OF THE PROCEDURE

The procedure involves obtaining baseline HR, BP, EKG, and Echo images before beginning the intravenous infusion of dobutamine and every three minutes and as needed during the test. The test is initiated at a level of either 5 or 10 micrograms dobutamine per kilogram per minute and increasing the dose in 10 µg/kg/min incre-

TABLE 2.2.   Contraindications for Dobutamine Stress Echo

Hypertrophic cardiomyopathy with outflow obstruction
Known severe aortic stenosis
Unstable angina
Severe pulmonary hypertension
Uncontrolled systemic arterial hypertension
Atrial fibrillation or flutter with uncontrolled ventricular response
Paroxysmal ventricular arrhythmias
Pregnancy
Hemodynamic instability
Past adverse reaction to dobutamine
Poor echo images

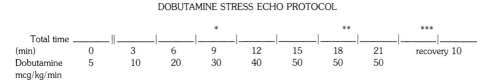

Figure 2.1. Atropine in 0.25-mg increments up to 1 mg usually given beginning at * but can be given beginning at **. Continue dobutamine at maximal dose during atropine administration. β blockers, nitroglycerin, calcium blockers, adenosine given as needed *** in the recovery phase.

ments every three minutes to a maximum dose of 50 μg/kg/min. In addition, atropine 0.25 to 1 mg can be given in the later stages of the test if 85% of the maximum predicted heart rate has not been achieved. Figure 2.1 shows the DSE protocol in timeline form.

Endpoints for termination of the DSE protocol include:

1. Achieving 85% maximum predicted heart rate
2. Achieving maximum dose of dobutamine
3. Intolerable side effects
4. Significant arrhythmias
5. Hypertension
6. Significant fall in systolic blood pressure
7. ST depression greater than or equal to 2 mm
8. Development of regional wall motion abnormalities in at least two segments (16 segment model).

Significant arrhythmias include ventricular tachycardia, atrial fibrillation or flutter, and supraventricular tachycardia. Other arrhythmias such as frequent premature ventricular contractions (PVCs), couplets, triplets, and so on may also constitute an endpoint, but the exact cutoff depends on the judgment of the supervising cardiologist. Exact levels of systolic or diastolic blood pressure that would cause test termination are also subject to physician discretion but a recommended maximum level of 240 mm Hg for systolic and greater than 120 mm Hg for diastolic pressure would seem prudent. A fall in systolic blood pressure greater than 40 mm Hg or an absolute systolic pressure less than 85 mm Hg is the usual guideline for test termination in asymptomatic patients, but the exact level must be determined on an individual basis.

COMPLICATIONS OF THE PROCEDURE

If the preceding endpoints are followed, DSE is a very safe procedure. Table 2.3 describes the complications of DSE. In a study involving 1118 patients Mertes et al[2] found no deaths, myocardial infarctions, syncope, or sustained ventricular tachycardia. Likewise, in a study involving 906 patients, Table 2.4, Hendrix and Gordon[3] also found no deaths, myocardial infarctions, or serious ventricular arrhythmias.

TABLE 2.3.   Complications of Dobutamine Stress Echo

Ventricular arrhythmias
Atrial fibrillation or flutter
Supraventricular tachycardia
Prolonged angina
Dynamic left ventricular outflow tract obstruction
Severe hypertension
Hypotension
AV block (transient)

The study by Mertes et al,[2] despite finding no deaths, myocardial infarctions, syncope, or sustained ventricular tachycardia, did report a significant number of less serious side effects. Nonsustained ventricular tachycardia (NSVT) occurred in 40 (3.6%) patients. Of note, the longest duration was 20 seconds, most runs constituted less than 10 beats and all were asymptomatic. Only one patient received lidocaine. No relationship of the NSVT to the induction of ischemia was noted, nor was there an increased incidence in the 189 patients tested within six weeks of a myocardial infarction. The addition of atropine also had no effect on the frequency of NSVT. Frequent PVCs (>6/min) occurred in 15.3% of patients.

In the group studied by Mertes et al[2] atrial arrhythmias occurred in 12% of patients and included premature atrial contractions, (>6/min) in 7.7%, atrial fibrillation in 0.6%, atrial flutter in 0.1% and supraventricular tachycardia (SVT) in 3.4%. Other arrhythmias included junctional tachycardia in 2.5% and transient second-degree AV block in 0.6%. The incidence of arrhythmias in this study was higher in the patients given the high dose protocol (50 μg/kg/min) vs the lower dose protocol (30 μg/kg/min). Overall arrhythmias occurred in 37% of those given the high dose vs 24% of those given the lower dose. This was also true for all subsets of arrhythmias: NSVT 4.2% vs 0, SVT 3.1% vs 1.45%, and PACs 7% vs 3.7%.

In the group evaluated by Mertes et al[2] cardiovascular symptoms occurred in approximately one third of patients: angina in 19%, dyspnea in 5% and atypical chest pain in 8%. No patient required IV nitroglycerin or emergent cardiac cath, although 37% of patients with angina received β-blockers and or sublingual nitroglycerin. Non-cardiac side effects occurred in 26% of patients and included nausea (8%), anxiety (6%), headache (4%), tremor (3.7%) and urgency (1%). Most symptoms were well tolerated and required termination in only 3% of cases.

Lalka et al[4] used dobutamine up to 50 μg/kg/min and atropine up to 1 mg (as needed) to screen 60 patients before aortic surgery. Using this protocol, two patients had significant arrhythmias: one with supraventricular tachycardia and the other a 15-beat run of ventricular tachycardia associated with hypotension. Both arrhythmias converted spontaneously and occurred only after diagnostic wall motion information had been obtained. Angina occurred in 6.7% of patients. Minor side effects occurred in 20% of patients and included nausea, shortness of breath, headache, tremor, palpitations, and dizziness but in no case did these symptoms necessitate premature termination of the DSE protocol.

TABLE 2.4. Complications of Dobutamine Infusion

	Mertes (2)	Hendrix (3)	Lalka (4)	Poldermans (5)	Davila-Roman (6)	Pennell (7)	Hays (8)	Eichelberger (9)	McNeil (10)
N	1118	906	60	626	93	30	144	75	80
Death or MI	0	0	0	0	0	0	0	0	0
VF	0	0	0	1	0	0	0	0	0
Sustained VT	0	0	0	3	0	0	0	0	0
NSVT	40 (3.6%)	—	1	12	1	1	4	0	3
PVCs	171 (15.3%)	NR	NR	64	6	12	72	NR	0
Atrial Fibrillation Flutter	8 (.7%)	NR	0	8	0	0	1	1	0
SVT	38 (3.4%)	NR	1	0	2	0	2	0	0
Severe Hypertension	0	NR	0	1	3	0	2	3	0
Significant Hypotension	36 (3.2%)	NR	2	4	0	0	0	9	0
Chest pain	301 (27%)	NR	4	145	3	20	44	9	21

In a study involving 652 DSE examinations in 626 consecutive patients, Poldermans et al[5] reported on the safety of dobutamine (maximum dose 40 μg/kg/min) and atropine. No deaths or myocardial infarctions occurred. One patient developed ventricular fibrillation but was successfully defibrillated (it is unclear if this is the same patient reported on in their earlier study). Three patients developed sustained ventricular tachycardia and 12 had nonsustained ventricular tachycardia. These episodes reverted spontaneously or with intravenous metoprolol. Atrial fibrillation occurred in eight patients. The development of ventricular arrhythmias appeared to have a strong relation to a previous history of ventricular arrhythmias. Significant hypertension (SBP ≥ 220 mm Hg) occurred in one patient and hypotension (>40 mm Hg decline compared to baseline) occurred in four. Chest pain occurred in 145 (22%) patients and chills occurred in six. Other side effects were not reported. Atropine, which was given to 239 patients, did not change the incidence of any arrhythmias or any side effects.

Davila-Roman et al[6] studied 93 patients undergoing vascular surgery (60% for abdominal or thoracoabdominal aortic aneurysms) using up to 40 μg/kg/min of dobutamine and atropine up to 2 mg beginning at dobutamine levels of 30 μg/kg/min if the heart rate response was inadequate. No patient had a major adverse effect defined as myocardial infarction, intractable arrhythmia, or death. Three patients developed marked hypertension (SBP ≥ 240 mm Hg, DBP ≥ 120 mm Hg). One patient developed short runs of nonsustained ventricular tachycardia, and six patients developed frequent premature ventricular contractions requiring test termination in one. Supraventricular tachycardia developed in two patients and frequent premature atrial contractions in three. Three patients developed chest pain with new wall motion abnormalities and EKG changes in two of the three. Minor side effects including nausea, headache, tingling, and palpitations occurred in eleven patients.

Pennel, Underwood and Ell et al[7] used dobutamine to a dose of 40 μg/kg/min as the stress agent for 30 patients with asthma undergoing thallium scintigraphy. One patient had a six-beat run of ventricular tachycardia, two had ventricular couplets, and 10 had premature ventricular contractions. Twenty patients developed chest pain and eight developed dyspnea. Twenty-three patients had minor side effects including shaking, pounding, tingling, flushing, headache, lightheadedness, and nausea.

Hays et al[8] used dobutamine (up to 40 μg/kg/min) without atropine in 144 patients undergoing thallium scintigraphy. No deaths, myocardial infarctions, or episodes of sustained ventricular tachycardia occurred. Nonsustained ventricular tachycardia occurred in 4 patients, 9 patients had couplets, and 63 had premature ventricular contractions. Ventricular ectopy was mostly dose related and in all cases resolved spontaneously with termination of the dobutamine infusion. One patient developed paroxysmal atrial fibrillation and another supraventricular tachycardia; both resolved with termination of the infusion. Side effects were common, occurring in 75% of patients and included angina (26%), atypical chest pain (5%), and palpitations (29%). Flushing, headache, and dyspnea each occurred in 14%. Other side effects including paresthesias, nausea, and dizziness were less common. All side effects were transient, resolving within several minutes of test completion.

Eichelberger et al[9] used DSE (maximum dose dobutamine 40/μg/kg/min and atropine up to 1 mg beginning at 15 μg/kg/min of dobutamine) to study 75 patients before vascular surgery. Nine patients developed hypotension, defined as a drop in systolic pressure > 20 mm Hg or an absolute systolic pressure of < 85 mm Hg, requiring discontinuation of the dobutamine. Only one patient was symptomatic, and all episodes resolved promptly with test termination. Seven additional patients required discontinuation of the dobutamine infusion: one patient developed significant left ventricular outflow tract gradient, three developed systolic blood pressure >240 mm Hg, one developed atrial fibrillation, and two because of patient discomfort. No ventricular arrhythmias were reported.

McNeill et al[10] systematically studied the effect of the addition of up to 1 mg of atropine to 40 μg/kg/min of dobutamine. Forty-nine out of a total of 80 patients required atropine to achieve the goal heart rate. The test was found to be equally safe in those patients tested with or without atropine. No serious complications occurred in either group. Minor arrhythmias were seen in five patients: three with three-beat runs of ventricular tachycardia, one each with atrial ectopics and nodal rhythm. Twenty-one patients developed chest pain requiring metoprolol: equally distributed between those tested with or without atropine.

Summarizing the preceding data, clearly demonstrates that dobutamine stress echocardiography is a safe test. In testing involving 3132 patients, no deaths or myocardial infarctions have occurred (Table 2.5). Ventricular ectopic activity is common, occurring in up to 50% of patients in some series although it occurred in only 15.5% of all patients covered in this review. Nonsustained ventricular tachycardia occurred in 62 (2%) of patients tested. Sustained ventricular tachycardia occurred in 3 (0.1%) patients and ventricular fibrillation occurred in 1 (0.03%). The episode of ventricular fibrillation was successfully treated with one defibrillation, and the episodes of sustained ventricular tachycardia resolved spontaneously or with intravenous metoprolol. The frequency of ventricular ectopy appeared to be dose related and occurred more frequently in patients with a previous history of ventricular arrhythmias. Atrial fibrillation or flutter occurred in 0.8% of all patients and supraventricular tachycardia occurred in 1.9%. Severe hypertension occurred during 0.4% of tests and significant hypotension occurred in 2.3%. Each of these arrhythmias were well tolerated and resolved with test termination. Chest pain and other side effects are common, occurring in 24% and 23% respectively. These side effects, although common, are usually well tolerated: causing premature test termination in <5% of cases and resolving with discontinuation of the dobutamine infusion. Chest pain was rarely prolonged

TABLE 2.5. Complications of Dobutamine Infusion (Pooled Data from 10 Studies)

Event	No. of Pts	%
Death or MI	0/3132	0
VF	1-2/3132	0.03%
SVT	3/3132	0.1%
NSVT	62/3132	2% (1.1% to 3.7%)
PVCs	325/2091	15.5% (0% to 50%)
Afib/flutter	18/2226	0.8% (0% to 1.3%)
SVT	43/2226	1.9% (0% to 3.4%)
Severe hypertension	9/2226	0.4% (0% to 4%)
Sign. hypotension	51/2226	2.3% (0% to 12%)
Chest pain	560/2362	23.7% (3% to 66%)

and resolved with test termination in the vast majority of cases. Chest pain occasionally required intravenous metoprolol or sublingual nitroglycerin for relief.

Thus, the safety and side-effect profile of dobutamine stress echocardiography is comparable to other pharmacological stress protocols. To maintain the good safety record already established, it is imperative that all echocardiography laboratories have a defibrillator on site along with intravenous β-blockers, adenosine, lidocaine, and sublingual nitroglycerin. With this preparation, appropriate attention to contraindications, and the thoughtful application of study endpoints, dobutamine stress echocardiography will continue to be a safe and useful test.

REFERENCES

1. Berthe C, Pierard La, Hiernaux M, et al. Predicting the extent and location of coronary artery disease in acute myocardial infarction by echocardiography during dobutamine infusion. *Am J Cardiol.* 58:1167–1177, 1986.
2. Mertes H, Sawada S, Ryan T, et al. Symptoms, adverse effects, and complications associated with dobutamine stress echocardiography experience with 1118 patients. *Circulation.* 88:15–19, 1993.
3. Hendrix G, Gordon L. Sensitivity and safety of dobutamine stress thallium in detection of significant coronary artery disease. *Circulation.* Abstract. 84(suppl 2): 576, 1991.
4. Lalka S, Sanada S, Dalsing M, et al. Dobutamine stress echocardiography as a predictor of cardiac events associated with aortic surgery. *J Vasc Surg.* 15:831–842, 1992.
5. Poldermans D, Fioretti P, Boersma E, et al. Safety of dobutamine-atropine stress echocardiography in patients with suspected or proven coronary artery disease. *Am Cardiol.* 73:456–459, 1994.
6. Davila-Roman V, Waggoner A, Sicard G, et al. Dobutamine stress echocardiography predicts surgical outcome in patients with aortic aneurysm and peripheral vascular disease. *J Am Coll Cardiol.* 21:957–963, 1993.
7. Pennell D, Underwood R, Ell P. Safety of dobutamine stress for thallium-201 myocardial perfusion tomography in patients with asthma. *Am J Cardiol.* 71:1346–1350, 1993.
8. Hays J, Mahmariam J, Cochran A, et al. Dobutamine thallium 201-tomography for evaluating patients with suspected coronary artery disease unable to undergo exercise or vasodilator pharmacologic stress testing. *J Am Coll Cardiol.* 21:1583–1590, 1993.
9. Eichelberger J, Schwarz K, Black E, et al. Predictive value of dobutamine echocardiography just before noncardiac vascular surgery. *Am J Cardiol.* 72:602–607, 1993.
10. McNeill A, Fioretti P, El-Said M, et al: Enhanced sensitivity for detection of coronary artery disease by addition of atropine to dobutamine stress echocardiography. *Am J Cardiol.* 70:41–46, 1992.

ADDITIONAL READING

Bach DS, Armstrong WF. Dobutamine stress echocardiography. *Am J Cardiol.* 69:90H–96H, 1992.

Cigarroa CG, deFillip, Shristopher R, Brickner E, et al. Dobutamine stress echocardiography identifies hibernating myocardium and predicts recovery of left ventricular function after coronary revascularization. *Circulation.* 88:430–436, 1993.

Elliot BM, Robison JG, Zellner JL, et al. Dobutamine 201-T1 imaging: assessing cardiac risks associated with vascular surgery. *Circulation.* 84(suppl 3): III 54–III 60, 1991.

Martin TW, Seaworth JF, Johns JP, et al. Comparison of adenosine, dipyridamole, and dobutamine in stress echocardiography. *Ann Intern Med.* 116(3):190–196, 1992.

Pennell DJ, Underwood SR, Swanton RH, et al. Dobutamine thallium myocardial perfusion tomography. *J Am Coll Cardiol.* 18:1471–1479, 1991.

Poldermans D, Fioretti P, Forster T, et al. Dobutamine stress echocardiography for assessment of perioperative cardiac risk in patients undergoing major vascular surgery. *Circulation.* 87:1506–1512, 1993.

Rosamond TL, Vacek JL, Hurwitz A, et al. Hypotension during dobutamine stress echocardiography: initial description and clinical relevance. *Am Heart J.* 123:403–407, 1992.

Rugge FP Van, Wall EE Van der, Bruschke AVG: New developments in pharmacologic stress imaging. *Am Heart J.* 124(2):468–485, 1992.

Smart SC, Sawada S, Ryan T, et al. Low-dose dobutamine echocardiography detect reversible dysfunction after thrombolytic therapy of acute myocardial infarction. *Circulation.* 88:405–415, 1993.

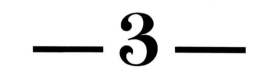

— 3 —

Complications of Myocardial Perfusion Imaging

John P. Vansant, M.D.

EXERCISE AND PHARMACOLOGICAL STRESS TESTING

Myocardial perfusion imaging is typically performed in conjunction with graded tread-mill exercise, which provides additional clinical information in regard to the patient's cardiac functional capacities and ECG evidence of ischemia. With exercise, coronary blood flow may increase in normal vessels from 2 to 2.5 times the resting level. In stenosed vessels, flow fails to increase adequately with exercise, and myocardium supplied by such vessels appears as regional areas of relative hypoperfusion, demonstrating decreased counts of the perfusion tracer.

The diagnostic utility and potential complications of exercise testing are well established. The sensitivity of diagnostic ST segment changes for ischemia on exercise ECG is a function of effort. Similarly, the sensitivity of initial defect detection by thallium-201 scintigraphy increases at high work loads.[1] Many patients in whom a noninvasive diagnosis of coronary artery disease is desirable cannot achieve an adequate level of exercise to provide for the optimal test sensitivity for disease detection. This patient population is extensive and may account for as much as 50% of the diagnostic studies performed in some nuclear cardiology laboratories. Such patient subsets would include individuals with neurologic or orthopedic debilities, patients unaccustomed to exercise because of sedentary lifestyle, or individuals incapable of

Acknowledgment. The author would like to express his appreciation to Mr. Jerry Byrd for secretarial services, Ms. Margie Jones CNMT and Mr. Russell Folks CNMT for technical assistance, and Dr. Elizabeth Krawczynska for providing a resource for various case illustrations.

adequate exercise because of underlying chronic illness. A growing population of patients includes those for preoperative evaluation with intermediate probability of coronary artery disease. In addition, patients taking negative chronotropic agents, such as β-blockers and calcium-channel blockers, cannot usually achieve adequate heart rate response with exercise. The indications and contraindications to exercise stress testing were covered in Chapter 1.

Pharmacologic coronary vasodilatation, with either intravenous dipyridamole or adenosine as a diagnostic alternative to exercise, is currently widely practiced and the diagnostic accuracy is well established.[2] A growing interest has developed in the use of dobutamine to adequately simulate myocardial stress in myocardial perfusion imaging.[3–4] It is critical for the examining physician to understand the pharmacology, methodology, complications, and potential side effects of these pharmacological agents.

DIPYRIDAMOLE AND ADENOSINE

Pharmacology

Dipyridamole and adenosine are potent coronary vasodilators capable of increasing myocardial blood flow three to five times the resting level in myocardial regions supplied by normal coronary vessels. The pharmacological effect of dipyridamole is due to the potentiation of endogenous adenosine by blockade of adenosine receptors. Adenosine is a direct coronary vasodilator and activates the adenosine A_2 receptors in the coronary arterial wall. This leads to increased adenosine cyclase and C-AMP levels, decreased transmembrane calcium uptake and, thus, coronary vasodilatation.[5] In myocardial territories supplied by diseased coronary vessels, the hyperemic response is attenuated, causing flow inhomogeneity and, thus, abnormal tracer distribution. In some situations myocardial perfusion may actually decrease below the resting level in regions supplied by stenosed coronary arteries, resulting in the phenomenon of "coronary steal."[6–7]

Maximal vasodilatory effect of dipyridamole occurs approximately five minutes following administration and persists for at least 30 minutes postinfusion.[8] In contrast to dipyridamole, intravenous adenosine has a direct, immediate effect with maximal coronary vasodilatation occurring within two minutes following infusion with up to fourfold increase in coronary flow.[9] The serum half-life is approximately 10 seconds or less,[10] thereby providing immediate reversibility of its effect by terminating the infusion.

Dipyridamole and adenosine are generally used to stress patients incapable of diagnostic exercise testing because of low heart rate response or concomitant illnesses such as orthopedic problems.

Complications

Complications from pharmacologic vasodilatation in myocardial perfusion imaging using dipyridamole or adenosine would best be addressed relative to the patient's preexisting illness(es), methodology of administration, concurrent medications, and potential adverse effects on image quality based upon augmented splanchnic blood flow.

Contraindications to coronary vasodilator infusion include patients with bronchospastic lung disease, unstable angina, acute-phase myocardial infarction, critical aortic stenosis, hypertrophic cardiomyopathy, and hypotension (systolic blood pressure less than 90 mm Hg). Since aminophylline is the drug of choice in reversing adverse effects of dipyridamole or adenosine, care must be taken to identify and exclude patients with known allergy to aminophylline. Because of the short half-life of adenosine, discontinuing infusion is typically adequate in reversing any side effects. However, bronchospasm may be histamine-mediated and aminophylline administration may be necessary. In treating dipyridamole-induced adverse reactions with intravenous aminophylline, an intravenous loading dose of 50 to 75 mg is typically administered followed by a continuous intravenous infusion of 200 to 250 mg over a 20-minute period. It is critical to recall that dipyridamole has a sustained mechanism of action, and adverse reactions may be delayed up to 20 minutes following infusion. It is for this reason that aminophylline must be given over a sustained period of time because of its comparably short half-life. Although some centers routinely administer aminophylline prophylactically following injection of the perfusion agent, care must be taken to withhold aminophylline administration for a minimum of one minute following the tracer administration to negate the possibility of a false-negative study due to inhibition of adequate vasodilatory response. Similarly, care must be taken to discontinue other xanthine derivatives, such as theophylline, at least 24 hours before examination. Caffeine intake can result in inadequate coronary vasodilatation with dipyridamole.[11] The biologic half-life of caffeine may be up to 8.5 hours. Therefore, caffeinated beverages should ideally be withheld for 24 hours before testing. However, pentoxifylline (Trental), a methylxanthine used in the treatment of intermittent cladication, does not inhibit dipyridamole-induced vasodilatation.[12]

Finally, some investigators feel it preferable to have the patient perform low level exercise following pharmacological stress testing when using vasodilatory agents to further augment coronary blood flow.[13] Moreover, limited exercise decreases splanchnic blood flow, thereby decreasing liver and bowel activity, which may adversely affect scan interpretation because of unusually close proximity of these structures to the myocardium in many patients.

Side Effects

The occurrence and types of side effects of intravenous dipyridamole have been reported in approximately 4000 patients from 64 individual investigators with an adverse reaction occurring in approximately 47% of patients studied. The following adverse reactions were observed: chest pain (angina) 20%, headache 12%, dizziness 12%, ECG ST segment changes 8%, ventricular extrasystoles 5%, hypotension 5%, and nausea 5%. Severe reactions occurred in less than 1%, including fatal and nonfatal myocardial infarction (0.1%) and severe bronchospasm (0.2%).[14] A recent review of the safety profile of dipyridamole reported the incidence of cardiac death to be 1 per 10000 studies.[15]

The side effects of adenosine are more frequent than those with dipyridamole and reported to occur in over 85% of patients studied. A recent review of over 9000 patients reported: flushing 37%, chest pain 35%, shortness of breath 35%, headaches and/or lightheadedness 23%, ECG changes and/or arrhythmias 9%, and AV block 8%.[16] By a currently undefined mechanism, adenosine produces varying degrees of block at the level of the AV node. This effect is used therapeutically in the treatment of supraventricular tachycardias. Adenosine is currently under FDA phase-three clinical trial for pharmacological stress testing. When using adenosine as a diagnostic pharmacologic stress agent, patients with first- or second-degree heart block should be excluded. Infranodal block, such as bundle branch block, is not influenced by adenosine and is not a contraindication to its use. A high incidence (11%) of transient high-grade AV block has been reported with rapid thallium-201 infusion through the same IV access used for adenosine infusion.[17] Therefore, to avoid a bolus injection of adenosine, it is recommended that patients undergoing myocardial perfusion imaging with adenosine have two separate IV sites for study purposes. Despite the relatively high occurrence of side effects with over 10000 patient studies reported, no patient has suffered a cardiac death.

DOBUTAMINE

On occasions, a patient is referred for myocardial perfusion imaging unable to exercise while additionally having significant bronchospastic lung disease, in which case the use of either dipyridamole or adenosine is contraindicated. It is in this patient subset that the recent use and growing interest in dobutamine myocardial perfusion imaging has developed.[18–19] Dobutamine acts as a sympatheticomimetic agent to increase myocardial oxygen consumption by increasing heart rate, contractility, and arterial blood pressure.

Contraindications to the use of dobutamine include patients with hypertension (BP $\geq$ 180/110), atrial fibrillation/flutter with rapid ventricular response, significant left ventricular outflow obstruction, unstable angina, acute or recent myocardial infarction (within five days), supraventricular tachycardia or recurrent ventricular tachycardia. The routine discontinuation of β-blockers before study is advised because of their antagonistic action on dobutamine beta receptor stimulation. However, a recent report found similar sensitivity for detecting coronary artery disease in a group of patients evaluated with and without β-blockers.[20]

Methodology

Methodology of dobutamine administration has varied throughout the literature. The current method employed at Emory University is, in part, described by Hayes et al.[20] Dobutamine is administered at incremental doses of 5, 10, 20, 30, and up to 40 μg/kg/min at 3-minute intervals. If at maximal dose an end point is not obtained and the heart rate response is less than 85% of maximum predicted heart rate, atropine at 0.25 mg is administered up to a total maximum dose of 0.75 mg in an attempt to approximate a similar degree of myocardial oxygen demand as provided for in exercise testing. End points include a decrease in systolic blood pressure greater than 10 to 20 mm Hg, moderate to severe angina, ST segment depression greater than 2 mm, and significant dysrhythmias. After one minute of maximal dose infusion, the perfusion tracer is administered through a second IV access and infusion continued for an additional two minutes. With thallium-201, tomographic images are performed 5 to 10 minutes following termination of infusion and again three to four hours later.

Side Effects

Reported side effects in over 1300 patients studied occurred in approximately 75% of patients and included the following: chest pain 45%, flushing 10%, headache 7%, dyspnea 3%, supraventricular tachycardia/atrial fibrillation 2%, hypotension 1%, and AV block 0.4%. There are no currently reported cardiac deaths when using dobutamine for pharmacological stress myocardial perfusion imaging.[20–22]

Because of its short half-life of 120 seconds, treatment of adverse reactions to dobutamine is typically accomplished by simply discontinuing the infusion. However, if necessary, a short-acting cardioselective β-blocker, such as esmolol (Brevibloc) may be administered. Additionally, in this situation aminophylline should be readily available if the patient has known or suspected underlying lung disease. Thus, dobutamine stress when used with myocardial perfusion agents is both a reliable and safe method of assessing patients at risk for coronary disease.

DIAGNOSING CORONARY ARTERY DISEASE

In this era of multiple diagnostic modalities, it is important to recall that there is no perfect noninvasive test to diagnose the presence or absence of coronary artery disease in all patient populations. It is essential to integrate clinical and noninvasive test results to establish a diagnostic probability of disease presence. Bayes' theorem expresses the post-test likelihood of disease as a function of sensitivity and specificity of the test and the prevalence of disease in the patient population being studied. In other words, given the sensitivity and specificity of a diagnostic test and the prevalence of disease in the population under study, one can calculate the likelihood of disease being present on the basis of a normal or abnormal test result.

The sensitivity and specificity of myocardial perfusion imaging is widely recognized. However, when finalizing one's clinical decision regarding the test result, either positive or negative, one must recall that the positive and negative predictive accuracy of perfusion imaging for the presence of coronary artery disease depends on pretest likelihood of angiographically significant coronary artery disease in the patient subset being evaluated.

Much of the original and existing data regarding prevalence of coronary artery disease for different patient populations based on age, sex, and symptoms was provided by Diamond and Forrester.[23] Applications of Bayes' theorem in the relationship between pretest likelihood and posttest likelihood of coronary artery disease for thallium-201 scintigraphy has been demonstrated.[23–25] A positive thallium-201 test in a

TABLE 3.1.   Patients with Intermediate Pretest Likelihood (Prevalence) of Coronary Artery Disease

- A positive exercise ECG in an asymptomatic patient
- A positive, or nondiagnostic, exercise ECG in a patient with nonanginal chest pain
- Most patients with atypical angina

patient with a low likelihood of coronary artery disease does not establish the presence of disease. Likewise, in a patient with a high pretest likelihood of coronary artery disease, a negative thallium-201 test does not rule out the presence of disease. The greatest diagnostic value of the test is in patients with intermediate pretest likelihood of disease (Table 3.1).

COMPLICATIONS IN INTERPRETATION OF MYOCARDIAL PERFUSION IMAGES

Planar vs SPECT Imaging

It is not the purpose of this section to explore and explain in detail all the technical aspects that should be understood and appreciated by the physician interpreting the cardiac perfusion scan. Although some laboratories continue to use the technique of planar imaging, most nuclear cardiology laboratories are now performing tomographic myocardial imaging. Optimal imaging techniques using single-photon-emission computerized tomography (SPECT) demands an understanding of several concepts: (1) the differences between planar and SPECT imaging, (2) basic fundamentals of image acquisition and processing, and (3) the anticipation of various factors (artifacts) that may adversely affect the scan interpretation.

Compared to planar imaging, SPECT provides a more sensitive means of detecting coronary artery disease.[26–28] Tomographic images yield slices of the myocardium without overlapping counts from neighboring slices and background tissue. This attribute provides increased contrast resolution, ie, improved ability to separate differences in tracer concentration of neighboring tissues. Clinically, this translates into an increased sensitivity of less-ischemic perfusion defects and improved identification of individual coronary vascular territories. Additionally, two-dimensional representation of three-dimensional tomographic data using a polar coordinate, or "bullseye" map coupled with existing quantitative techniques, whereby patient data are compared to a gender-matched normal file, provides for improved interobserver variability[29] and compensates for the current lack of scatter correction, variable attenuation, and partial volume effects.[30]

Recent advances of nuclear medicine computer systems coupled with the availability of technetium-99m sestamibi for myocardial perfusion imaging has allowed for the capability of acquiring and reconstructing multigated tomographic studies. This feature provides a mechanism for assessing myocardial global function and assessment of regional viability, and a mechanism for defining fixed defects as attenuation artifacts vs scar.[30–31]

TABLE 3.2. SPECT Artifacts

---

1. **Camera-based factors**
   - Flood-field nonuniformity
   - Center of rotation errors
2. **Technologist-based factors**
   - Processing errors
3. **Patient-dependent factors**
   - Soft tissue attenuation
     Breast
     Diaphragm
     Lateral Chest Wall
   - Patient Motion
   - Overlying visceral activity
   - Myocardial "hot spots"
4. **Noncoronary disease factors**
   - Left bundle branch block
   - Myocardial hypertrophy
   - Cardiomyopathy

FACTORS AFFECTING SPECIFICITY

To receive full advantage offered by SPECT/quantitative techniques in assessing patients with suspected coronary artery disease, one must also accept the increased technical demands requiring strict adherence to quality control factors. Imperfections that go unrecognized in planar imaging may be greatly enhanced in the SPECT reconstruction process, resulting in image artifacts. Common SPECT artifacts have been well described[32] (Table 3.2).

By recognizing such artifacts, the "false-positive" study is minimized, resulting in increased test specificity. Other factors adversely affecting specificity include patient selection bias and angiographic underestimation of the hemodynamic effect of a coronary lesion.[33]

Camera-Based

Correct interpretation of myocardial scans begins with quality control factors of the imaging system. Quality control requirements for SPECT scanning are more stringent than for more conventional planar imaging. Although all aspects of quality control should be well understood by the physician interpreting the scan, the reader should be particularly sensitive to potential scan artifacts and image distortion due to errors related to center of rotation and nonuniformity.

Center of Rotation

Artifacts due to errors in the center of rotation (COR) of the camera are unique to SPECT imaging. The COR is the axis about which the camera rotates. When the camera rotates, the axis of rotation is taken as the origin of the tomographic plane. The center of each projection must be aligned with the same axis. A COR offset parameter is used in the reconstruction process to align the planar projections for correct back-projection. Errors in this process of two pixels or greater result in serious artifacts. However, errors as small as half a pixel (3 mm) may result in image blurring and more subtle artifacts, which are difficult to distinguish as such in the final image interpretation.

Nonuniformity

Today's scintillation cameras correct for differences in energy response from the different photo multiplier tubes. The greatest source of image nonuniformities in SPECT imaging are related to collimator "imperfections." With severe flood-field nonuniformity, one may observe a ringlike artifact in the reconstructed tomographic slices and on the circumferential profile plots. The higher the number of acquired counts for image, the more prominent the artifact. In thallium-201 imaging, where the number of counts per slice is low as compared to statistical noise, minimal nonuniformities may go unrecognized as such while decreasing scan quality and subsequent interpretation.

Technologist-Based

Many aspects of scan processing remain operator dependent. Errors in processing may result in misinterpretation of scan results. It is necessary for the interpreting physician to be able to critique the correctness of various processing parameters, including oblique angle reconstruction, apical/basal slice selection, and the chosen center of the myocardial activity with a defined maximum radius of search. Results of such processing errors are illustrated in Figures 3.1, 3.2 and 3.3, respectively.

Patient-Dependent Factors

The category of patient-dependent factors clearly defines the unconditional and absolute necessity that the dynamic rotating planar projections be assessed as a routine part of the readout session. It is the only resource for observing potential artifacts created by individual variations related to soft tissue attenuation and motion during acquisition. Additionally, these projections provide for a more "complete" assessment of the information available, including supplementary findings, such as lung uptake, left ventricular size, and left ventricular transient dilatation. In the case of thallium-201, the unexpected observation of focal areas of activity within the lung fields, axilla, or breast may hold important serendipitous information as a marker of potential tumor involvement.

Soft-Tissue Attenuation

Decreased myocardial count density is expected in underlying areas of soft tissue thickness. Common soft-tissue attenuators include the female breast, lateral chest

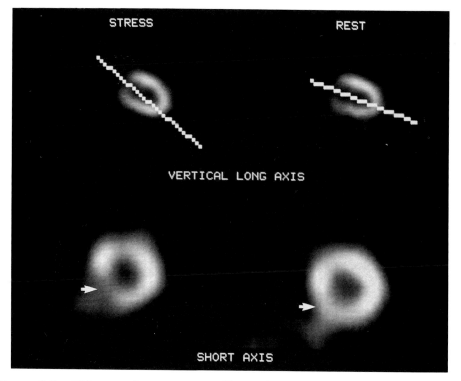

Figure 3.1. Oblique angle reconstruction: The angle of slice orientation chosen from the vertical long axis is incorrectly placed on the stress image, resulting in tomographic short axis images erroneously depicting a reversible inferior septal defect (arrows).

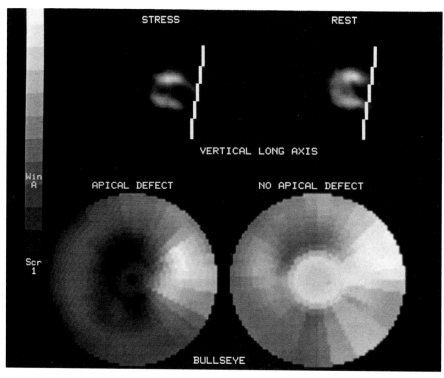

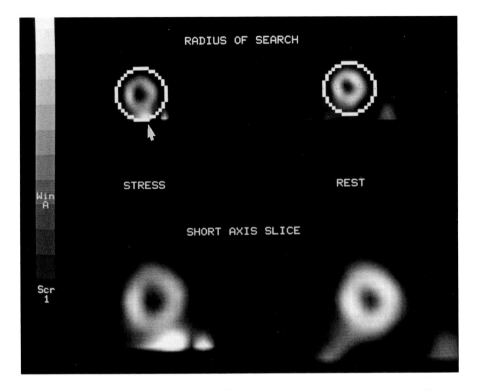

Figure 3.3. Maximum radius of search: Bowel activity on the stress image (arrow) is erroneously included in the radius of search. In such cases where the hottest pixel is due to bowel activity, the computer incorrectly normalizes to the extracardiac activity, causing decreased counts in the myocardial image. The extracardiac activity is not present on delay images. The result of this artifact is a false-positive finding of a reversible defect in the anterior and lateral wall.

wall adipose tissue, and the left hemidiaphragm. The latter two are typically more pronounced in the male patient.

Because of the frequency of wide variations of soft-tissue attenuation among patients, the myocardial count distribution observed on tomographic slices and the quantitative assessment compared to standard normal files often requires one to "read-around" anticipated artifacts. Assuming that patient positioning for immediate and delayed SPECT imaging is identical, all the soft-tissue attenuation artifacts will appear fixed. Thus, the possibility of scar would be suggested. This situation may be further defined with thallium-201 by obtaining an additional planar breast-up image in females with suspected breast artifact and the lateral decubitus image in males

Figure 3.2. Apical slice selection: Incorrect apical slice positioning between stress and rest images in a patient with a fixed apical defect results in an apical "bullseye" artifact, demonstrating apical reversibility. In this patient population the technologist must be consistent in defining the "expected" apical slice. Newer processing programs are being developed to alleviate such errors.

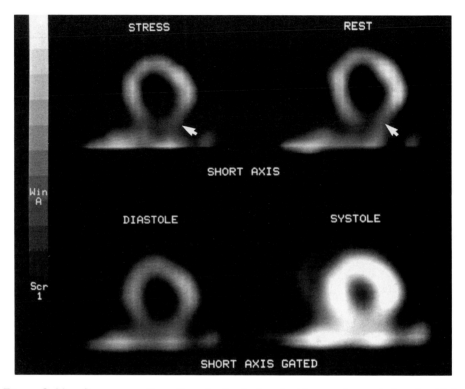

Figure 3.4A. Scar versus attenuation: short axis stress/rest images demonstrate a fixed inferior lateral defect (arrows). This finding is consistent with scar or marked diaphragmatic attenuation. Gated sestamibi images demonstrate myocardial count density change (thickening), clearly defining the inferior-lateral defect as secondary to attenuation artifact and not scar.

when diaphragmatic attenuation is a potential source of error. At Emory University all scans obtained with technetium-99m sestamibi are gated. Therefore, fixed defects secondary to attenuation will demonstrate count density changes (thickening) on the gated image with scar showing no change of count density or thickening[31] (Figure 3.4A, 3.4B).

Patient Motion

Cardiac motion during tomographic imaging is best depicted by observing the multiple planar acquisitions in a dynamic cine format. Patient motion as small as half a pixel (3 mm) can create thallium-201 SPECT image artifacts.[34] The degree of artifact created also depends on factors such as whether the motion is gradual or abrupt, the number and location of frames involved, and whether the heart returns to its original baseline position. In patients who have undergone exercise testing, if image acquisition is begun too early postexercise, a motion artifact resulting from "diaphragmatic creep" may be induced.[35] This artifact is due to increased depth of respiration and diaphragmatic flattening, which occurs immediately postexercise. As image acquisition

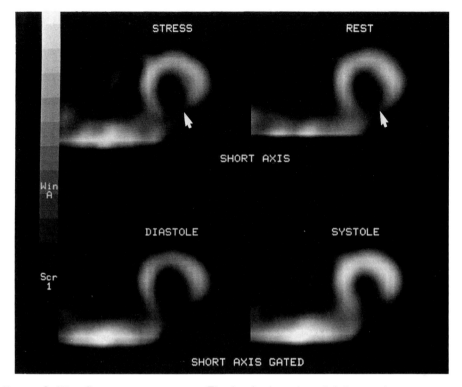

Figure 3.4B. Scar versus attenuation: The fixed inferior-lateral defect on short axis images (arrows) fails to demonstrate "thickening" on gated sestamibi short axis slices. The lack of myocardial wall thickening supports the presence of scar and not attenuation artifact.

proceeds, a slowing and more shallow respiration develops, and the heart gradually "creeps upward." In the reconstructed SPECT images, this "upward creep" appears as an inferior defect on the stress image. Since this artifact does not occur on the delayed images, the inferior defect is no longer present and inferior wall ischemia is suggested. To avoid this phenomenon, it is now universally recommended to delay postexercise image acquisition for 10 to 15 minutes, thus allowing hyperventilation to subside and diaphragmatic stabilization to occur.

Computer algorithms have been developed to automatically detect and correct for patient motion.[36] However, the clinical value of this methodology in eliminating motion artifacts is not currently established (Figure 3.5).

Visceral Activity

The increased use of pharmacological stress imaging coupled with radiopharmaceuticals, such as technetium-99m sestamibi with pronounced hepatobiliary excretion patterns, has resulted in a more frequent occurrence of potential artifacts associated with overlying abdominal visceral activity. The artifact created on tomographic slices and/ or polar coordinate plots may result in at least a suboptimal study and at worst a

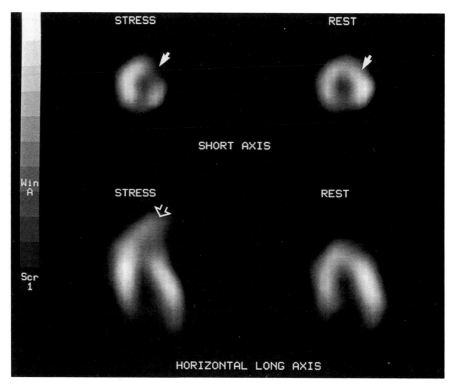

Figure 3.5. Motion artifact: Patient motion during stress acquisition results in an apparent anterior-lateral reversible defect on short axis images (arrows). Anatomical distortion is demonstrated on the horizontal long axis on the stress image (open arrow), alerting the reader to consider artifactual changes.

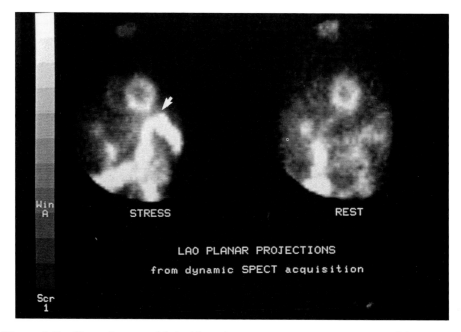

Figure 3.6. Visceral activity: Marked bowel activity in contiguous proximity of the myocardium (arrow) during stress acquisition resulted in the stress image being uninterpretable.

false-positive result, depending on the degree of overlying activity and its occurrence either at stress or delay image acquisition (Figure 3.6).

"Hot Spots"

Focal areas of increased myocardial count density are typically termed "hot spots." Although the specific etiology in many situations is uncertain, the typical pattern of location is felt secondary to variations of myocardial thickness as depicted in regions of the anterior and/or posterior papillary muscles. When tomographic myocardial slices and circumferential polar plots are normalized to the area of greatest count density, these "hot spots" appear as normal with the remaining myocardium appearing as being decreased in count activity. The occurrence of "hot spots" most typically occurs on the immediate postexercise images. However, their occurrence and location are varied and cannot be totally explained by anticipated anatomical markers. The presence of a "hot spot" at stress, which resolves at rest, may cause a perfusion pattern mimicking ischemia.

NONCORONARY DISEASE FACTORS

Left Bundle Branch Block

Noninvasive evaluation of the patient with left bundle branch block (LBBB) for left anterior descending coronary artery disease is problematic. The presence of LBBB precludes meaningful analysis of ST segments during exercise while associated septal wall motion abnormalities prevent conclusive findings by radionuclide ventriculography and/or echocardiography. Additionally, thallium-201 exercise imaging in patients with LBBB has proven to be indeterminate for the detection of left anterior descending coronary disease.[37–38]

Measuring regional myocardial blood flow using radioactive microspheres in dogs with an induced LBBB pattern (Hirzel[39]) demonstrated a 26% reduction in blood flow to the anterior septal wall as compared to the lateral wall. This flow heterogeneity is augmented by exercise and is felt to be the source of low specificity of reversible septal defects found on thallium-201 scintigraphy. Asynchronous septal contraction appears to be the underlying mechanism whereby a "functional" ischemia develops. In LBBB as the heart rate increases, septal asynchrony comprises a greater proportion of the R-R interval, diastolic filling time is reduced, and systolic contraction is augmented, resulting in myocardial septal hypoperfusion.

The specificity of thallium-201 exercise scintigraphy in left anterior descending coronary artery disease in patients with LBBB is reported to range from 10% to 40%, with septal perfusion being most abnormal in patients who achieve high peak heart rates[38] (Figure 3.7).

Pharmacological stress testing with dipyridamole and more recently adenosine has been reported to improve diagnostic accuracy in evaluating patients with LBBB.[40–41] Dipyridamole typically induces only a 20 to 40% increase in heart rate from a baseline state. Predictably, there would be less perfusion abnormality at lower heart rates, because of increased diastolic filling time as compared to exercise testing.

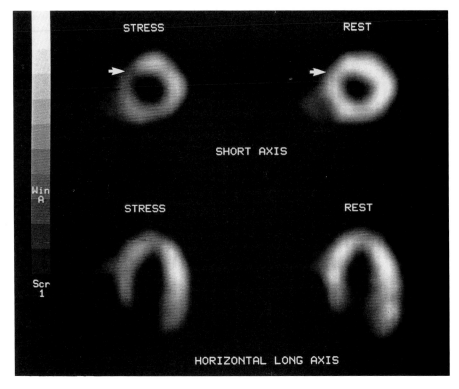

Figure 3.7. Left bundle branch block: Exercise thallium-201 SPECT images of a patient with left bundle branch block. A reversible anteroseptal defect is noted (arrows). Coronary angiography was normal. Reversible septal defects suggesting ischemia in this patient population has decreased specificity.

Burns, et al[40] evaluated patients with LBBB following both exercise and dipyridamole thallium-201 imaging. The specificity for left anterior descending coronary artery disease by visual analysis was 30% with exercise as compared to 80% with dipyridamole. However, the use of pharmacological stress in itself does not totally eliminate the potential for a false-positive study (Figure 3.8). Matzer et al[42] defined a new criterion for defining left anterior descending disease in patients with LBBB based on the associated phenomenon of an apical defect (Figure 3.9).

To optimize diagnostic specificity of myocardial perfusion imaging, it is important that patients with left bundle branch block be selected for pharmacological stress testing and the interpreting physician be attentive to the presence of any associated apical abnormality, giving further evidence of a true-positive vs a false-positive result.

Myocardial Hypertrophy

In myocardial perfusion SPECT imaging, the lateral wall normally has the greatest myocardial count density. A reversal of the normal lateral-to-septal count density ratio

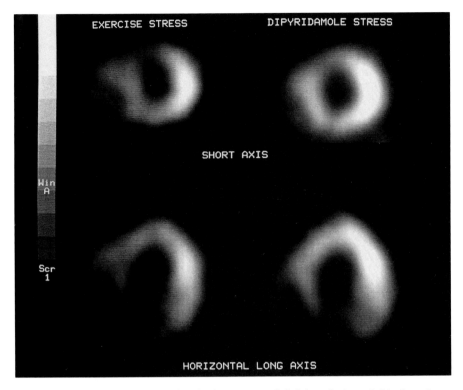

Figure 3.8. Left bundle branch block: A patient with left bundle branch block and angiographic findings of left anterior descending coronary artery disease underwent both exercise and dipyridamole thallium-201 testing. Although in this case the reversible septal defect was a true positive finding for ischemia, note that the severity (extent) of the abnormality is much greater with exercise than with pharmacological testing.

occurring at both stress and delay images (a fixed defect) is anticipated in patients with excessive lateral wall soft-tissue attenuation artifact and in patients with myocardial infarction. Additionally, because of geometric factors affecting photon detection, cardiac dextrorotation and levorotation may cause an apparent decrease in lateral to septal count density. However, a similar pattern has been described in some patients with long-standing hypertension. DePuey et al[43] studied 100 patients with chronic systemic arterial hypertension in a population subset of end-stage renal disease. The authors could not readily explain the decreased lateral wall count density. No positive correlation was demonstrated with electrocardiographic findings nor myocardial wall thickness measured by two-dimensional echocardiography. A possible explanation would be that in a yet undefined subset of patients with left ventricular hypertrophy, altered regional wall motion may exist with concentric myocardial hypertrophy, and both the septum and the lateral wall would possess a greater count density. However, because of the normally decreased septal excursion as compared to the lateral wall, the septum would appear less "blurred" and, hence, appear to possess a higher count density.

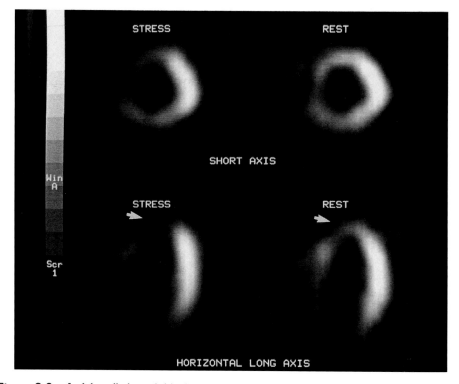

Figure 3.9.   Left bundle branch block: Apical involvement (arrows) in addition to the reversible septal abnormality in this patient with left bundle branch block increased the specificity of the study for left anterior descending coronary artery disease. Subsequent catheterization revealed a significant proximal left anterior descending coronary lesion.

Cardiomyopathy

The ability to differentiate ischemic cardiomyopathy from idiopathic congestive cardiomyopathy (IDC) using planar thallium-201 scintigraphy was explored by Bulkly et al[44] in 1977. Although thallium-201 was superior to technetium-99m gated cardiac blood pool scans in distinguishing the two patient subsets, four of the eight patients with IDC demonstrated segmental defects on thallium-201 imaging, which were greater in size than observed in the normal population. As myocardial infarcts may be both electrocardiographically and symptomatically silent, the absence of such historical evidence for ischemic disease does not exclude an ischemic etiology in patients with congestive cardiomyopathy. Dunn, et al[45] published further evidence against the usefulness of thallium-201 scintigraphy in distinguishing patients with IDC from those with coronary artery disease. Twenty-five patients with severe left ventricular dysfunction and chronic heart failure were studied (10 patients with normal coronary arteries and 15 patients with multivessel disease). All 25 patients had thallium-201 perfusion defects. The number of segments involved, the presence of redistribution on four-hour delay imaging, lung uptake and LV size were similar in both groups. Therefore,

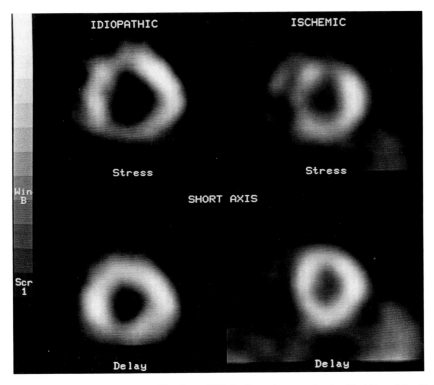

Figure 3.10. Cardiomyopathy: Thallium-201 findings in a patient with idiopathic dilated cardiomyopathy demonstrating a dilated LV and multiple reversible defects is similar to the patient with ischemic cardiomyopathy and multiple-vessel coronary disease. Myocardial perfusion imaging is indeterminate in distinguishing these two patient subsets.

thallium scanning cannot be reliably used in patients with chronic heart failure to distinguish coronary from noncoronary artery disease (Figure 3.10).

REFERENCES

1. McLaughlin PR, Martin RP, Doherty P, Daspit S, Goris M, Haskell W, Lewis S, Kriss JP, Harrison DC. Reproducibility of thallium-201 myocardial imaging. *Circulation.* 55:497–503, 1977.

2. Leppo JA. Dipyridamole-thallium imaging: the lazy man's stress test. *J Nucl Med.* 30:281–287, 1989.

3. Elliott BM, Robison JG, Zellner JL, Hendrix GH. Dobutamine-201-TL imaging: assessing cardiac risks associated with vascular surgery. *Circulation.* 84(suppl 3):III-54–III-60, 1991.

4. Hayes JT, Mahmarian JJ, Cochran AJ, Verani MS. Dobutamine thallium-201 tomography for evaluating patients with suspected coronary artery disease unable to undergo exercise or vasodilator pharmacologic stress testing. *J Am Coll Cardiol.* 21:1583–1590, 1993.

5. Fenton RA, Bruttig SP, Rubio R, et al. Effect of adenosine on calcium uptake by intact and cultured vascular smooth muscle. *Am J Physiol.* 252:H598–H604, 1987.

6. Becker LC. Conditions for vasodilator induced coronary steal in experimental myocardial ischemia. *Circulation.* 57:1103, 1978.

7. Patterson RE, Kirk ES. Coronary steal mechanisms in dogs with one vessel occlusion and other arteries normal. *Circulation.* 67:1009, 1983.

8. Marchante E, Pichard AD, Casanegra P, et al. Effect of intravenous dipyridamole on regional coronary blood flow with 1-vessel coronary artery disease: evidence against coronary steal. *Am J Cardiol.* 53:718–721, 1984.

9. Wilson RF, Wyche K, Christensen BV, et al. Effects of adenosine on human coronary arteries. *Circulation.* 82:1595–1606, 1990.

10. Klabunde RE. Dipyridamole inhibition of adenosine metabolism in human blood. *Eur J Pharmacol.* 93:21–26, 1983.

11. Smits P, Aengevaeren WRM, Corstens FHM, et al. Caffeine reduces dipyridamole-induced myocardial ischemia. *J Nucl Med.* 30:1723–1726, 1989.

12. Brown KA, Slinker BK. Pentoxifylline (Trental) does not inhibit dipyridamole-induced coronary hyperemia: implications for dipyridamole–thallium 201 myocardial imaging. *J Nucl Med.* 31:1020–1024, 1990.

13. Brown BG, Josephson MA, Petersen AB, et al. Intravenous dipyridamole combined with isometric hand grip for near maximal acute increase in coronary flow in patients with coronary artery disease. *Am J Cardiol.* 48:1077–1085, 1981.

14. Ranhosky A, Kempthorne-Rawson J. Intravenous dipyridamole thallium imaging study group: the safety of intravenous dipyridamole thallium myocardial perfusion imaging. *Circulation.* 81:1205–1209, 1990.

15. Lette J, et al. Safety of dipyridamole testing in 64,000 patients: the multicenter dipyridamole safety study. *J Am Coll Cardiol.* 21:207A, 1993; Poster Presentation at the ACC 42nd Annual Scientific Session March 16, 1993.

16. Cerqueira MD, Verani MS, Schwaiger M, Heo J, Iskandrian AS. Safety profile of adenosine stress perfusion imaging: results from the Adenoscan Multicenter Trial Registry. *J Am Coll Cardiol.* 23(2):384–389, 1994 Feb.

17. Ziffer JA, Weintraub WS, Anggelis C, Ike D, Alazraki NP. Risk reduction of severe arrhythmias in adenosine stress thallium-201 myocardial scintigraphy. *J Nucl Med.* 32:978, 1991.

18. Elliott BM, Robinson JG, Zellner JL, Hendrix GH. Dobutamine–201-Tl imaging assessing cardiac risks associated with vascular surgery. *Circulation.* 84(suppl 3):III-54–III-60, 1991.

19. Gunalp B, Dokumaci B, Uyau C, et al. Value of dobutamine technetium-99-m-sestamibi SPECT and echocardiography in the detection of coronary artery disease compared with coronary angiography. *J Nucl Med.* 34:889–894, 1993.

20. Hays JT, Mahmarian JJ, Cochran AJ, Verani MS. Dobutamine thallium-201 tomography for evaluating patients with suspected coronary artery disease unable to undergo exercise or vasodilator pharmacologic stress testing. *J Am Coll Cardiol.* 21:1583–1590, 1993.

21. Marwick T, D'Hondt AM, Daudhuin T, et al. Optimal use of dobutamine stress for the detection and evaluation of coronary artery disease: combination with echocardiography or scintigraphy, or both? *J Am Coll Cardiol.* 22:159–167, 1993.

22. Pennell DJ, Underwood SR, Swanton RH, Walker JM, Ell PJ. Dobutamine thallium myocardial perfusion tomography. *J Am Coll Cardiol.* 18:1471–1479, 1991.

23. Diamond GA, Forrester JS. Analysis of probability as an aid in the clinical diagnosis of coronary artery disease. *N Engl J Med.* 300:1350–1358, 1979.

24. Patterson RE, Horowitz SF, Calvin E, et al. Can exercise electrocardiography and thallium-201 myocardial imaging exclude the diagnosis of coronary artery disease? *Am J Cardiol.* 49:1127–1135, 1982.

25. Weintraub WS, Madeira SW, Bodenheimer MM, et al. Critical analysis of the application

of Bayes' theorem to sequential testing in the noninvasive diagnosis of coronary artery disease. *Am J Cardiol.* 54:43–49, 1984.

26. Caldwell J, Williams D, Harp G, et al. Quantitation of site of relative myocardial perfusion defect by single-photon emission computed tomography. *Circulation.* 70:1048–1056, 1984.

27. Maddahi J, Van Train KF, Wong C, et al. Comparison of thallium-201 SPECT and planar imaging for evaluation of coronary artery disease. *J Nucl Med.* 27:999, 1986. Abstract.

28. De Pasquale EE, Nody AC, DePuey EG, et al. Quantitative rotational thallium-201 tomography for identifying and localizing coronary artery disease. *Circulation.* 77:316–327, 1988.

29. Trobaugh GV, Wackers FJTh, Sokole EB, et al. Thallium-201 myocardial imaging: an interinstitutional study of observer variability. *J Nucl Med.* 19:395, 1978.

30. Marcassa C, Marzullo P, Parodi O, et al. A new method for noninvasive quantitation of segmental myocardial wall thickening using technetium-99m 2-methoxy-isobutylisonitrite scintigraphy—results in normal subjects. *J Nucl Med.* 31:173–177, 1990.

31. Leyendecker J, Vansant J, Pettigrew R. Cine MRI for myocardial scar and viability in the nonacute setting: correlation with SPECT-Sestamibi. Book of abstracts. *Soc Mag Res in Med.* 2507, 1992.

32. DePuey GE, Garcia EV. Optimal specificity of thallium-201 SPECT through recognition of imaging artifacts. *J Nucl Med.* 30:441–449, 1989.

33. Vogel RA. Assessing stenosis significance by coronary arteriography: are the best variables good enough? *J Am Coll Cardiol.* 12:692–693, 1988.

34. Friedman J, Berman DS, Van Train K, et al. Patient motion in thallium-201 myocardial SPECT imaging: an easily identified frequent source of artifactual defect. *Clin Nucl Med.* 13:321–324, 1988.

35. Geckle WJ, Frank TL, Links JM, Becker LC. Correction for patient and organ movement in SPECT: Application to exercise thallium-201 cardiac imaging. *J Nucl Med.* 27:899, 1986. Abstract.

36. Eisner RL, Noever T, Nowak D, et al. Use of cross-correlation function to detect patient motion during SPECT imaging. *J Nucl Med.* 28:97–101, 1987.

37. Huerta EM, Padial LR, Beiras JMC, Illera JP, Cardiel EA. Thallium-201 exercise scintigraphy in patients having complete left bundle branch block with normal coronary arteries. *Int J Cardiol.* 16:43–46, 1987.

38. DePuey EG, Guertler-Krawczynska E, Robbins WL. Thallium-201 SPECT in coronary artery disease patients with left bundle branch block. *J Nucl Med.* 29:1479–1485, 1988.

39. Hirzel HO, Senn M, Nuesch K, et al. Thallium-201 scintigraphy in complete left bundle branch block. *Am J Cardiol.* 53:764–769, 1984.

40. Burns RJ, Galligan L, Wright LM, et al. Improved specificity of myocardial thallium-201 single-photon emission computed tomography in patients with left bundle branch block by dipyridamole. *Am J Cardiol.* 68:504–508, 1991.

41. O'Keefe JH, Bateman TM, Barnhart CS. Adenosine thallium-201 is superior to exercise thallium-201 for detecting coronary artery disease in patients with left bundle branch block. *J Am Coll Cardiol.* 21:1332–1338, 1993.

42. Matzer L, Kiat H, Friedman J, Van Train K, Maddahi J. A new approach to the assessment of tomographic thallium-201 scintigraphy in patients with left bundle branch block. *J Am Coll Cardiol.* 17:1309–1317, 1991.

43. DePuey EG, Buertler-Krawczynska E, Perkins JV, Robbins WL, Whelchel JD, Clements SD. Alterations in myocardial thallium-201 distribution in patients with chronic systemic

hypertension undergoing single-photon emission computed tomography. *Am J Cardiol.* 62:234–238, 1988.

44. Bulkley BH, Hutchins GM, Bailey I, Strauss HW, Pitt B. Thallium-201 imaging and gated cardiac blood pool scans in patients with ischemic and idiopathic cardiomyopathy: a clinical and pathologic study. *Circulation.* 55:753–760, 1977.

45. Dunn RF, Uren RF, Sadick N, et al. Comparison of thallium-201 scanning in idiopathic dilated cardiomyopathy and severe coronary artery disease. *Circulation.* 66:804–810, 1982.

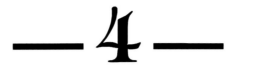

Complications of Central Venous and Arterial Catheterization

Paul E. Kazanjian, M.D.
James G. Ramsay, M.D.

INTRODUCTION

Practitioners who are responsible for the care of critically ill patients are frequently confronted with the need to access the central venous or arterial circulation to obtain hemodynamic measurements, administer medications and parenteral nutrition, or sample blood. The techniques used to catheterize the central veins and peripheral arteries are widely used and familiar to many caregivers. Unfortunately, these techniques carry some risk of complication that may lead to morbidity and mortality. This chapter reviews the various sites available for catheterization and examines some technical aspects of insertion with special emphasis on describing the myriad of potential complications.

Brief History

The history of central venous catheterization and arterial access is more extensively reviewed elsewhere.[1] In 1952, Aubaniac described the infraclavicular route to the central venous system, a technique that he had been using for 10 years. One year later, Seldinger described a technique for percutaneous placement of a catheter using a guidewire which now serves as the basis for a multitude of catheterization procedures.[2] Early use of the femoral vein was associated with a high incidence of complications, especially infection and thrombosis. Wilson reported the use of the subclavian approach for central venous pressure monitoring[3] and later the technique of internal jugular vein cannulation was described.[4] Early enthusiasm for the various techniques of central venous access soon became tempered by numerous reports of complications, some fatal.

The methods used to assess the arterial circulation developed simultaneously with those for venous access. The strain gauge manometer was developed in the late 1940s and allowed mechanical events to be translated to electrical current. Two important advances in percutaneous catheter placement were applied to the arterial circulation. In 1950, the cannula over needle device was introduced for cannulating veins[5] and ten years later this device was applied for use in the radial artery.[6] The aforementioned Seldinger technique proved applicable for arteries as well as veins.

Central venous access was first used to deliver medications and parenteral nutrition. Later, central venous pressure measurement and the flow-directed pulmonary artery catheter were introduced[3,7] and hemodynamic monitoring became an important indication for the placement of a central venous catheter. Likewise, arterial catheterization was, and still is, performed mostly for pressure monitoring and blood sampling.

INDICATIONS, CONTRAINDICATIONS, AND SITE SELECTION

In the emergency room, operating rooms, general care floors and intensive care units central venous access is most often carried out when there is a need to infuse sclerosing or hyperosmolar medications such as norepinephrine, chemotherapy, total parenteral nutrition, or when there is a need for hemodynamic monitoring. Central venous access may be required in patients in whom peripheral access cannot be established either because they are in shock or because their peripheral veins cannot be located.

Occasionally, emergency transvenous pacing or aspiration of venous air is an indication for central venous access. Volume resuscitation alone is never an indication for central venous access (except during some operations such as orthotopic liver transplant or thoracic aortic aneurysm repair) because a short, large-bore peripheral venous catheter provides flow rates comparable or superior to most central venous catheters.

There are no absolute contraindications to central venous catheterization, but some percutaneous sites are relatively contraindicated in certain circumstances. Some sites offer distinct advantages over other sites and these advantages and disadvantages should be taken into consideration when selecting among various sites [Table 4.1]. The five most common sites for central venous access are the internal jugular veins (IJV), the subclavian veins (SV), the femoral veins (FV), the external jugular veins (EJV), and the veins of the antecubital fossa (ACV). Many of these sites offer multiple approaches to the target vessels. In general, the internal jugular, subclavian, and femoral veins are most often used in the clinical setting.

The right internal jugular vein is the preferred route for hemodynamic monitoring, which is most often necessary for patients with cardiogenic shock, septic shock, adult respiratory distress syndrome, pulmonary edema, or congestive heart failure. The right IJV is also the preferred route for transvenous pacing. Other acceptable sites for these indications are, in descending order of preference, the right IJV, the

TABLE 4.1. Relative Rating[a] of Central Venous Access Techniques

	Arm Veins	External Jugular	Internal Jugular	Subclavian	Femoral
Ease of insertion and safety for the inexperienced	1	2	4	5	3
Long term use	4	3	2	1	5
Success rate	5	4	1	3	2
Complications (technique related)	1	2	3	4	3
Ease of PAC[b] insertion	5	2	right = 1, left = 3	right = 4, left = 2	3

[a]In each category: 1 = best, 5 = worst
[b]PAC = pulmonary artery catheter
From: Blitt, CD. *Monitoring in Anesthesia and Critical Care Medicine*, 2nd ed. New York: Churchill Livingstone; 1987:189. Table 9.9, page 189. Used with permission.

left SCV, the left IJV, and the right SCV. The right IJV is popular for perioperative central venous access secondary to the reduced risk of pneumothorax following insertion and the ease of accessibility to the external portion of the catheter while the patient is prepared and draped for operation. Previous carotid endarterectomy, radical neck surgery, or a history of cerebral vascular occlusive disease are relative contraindications to IJV catheterization.

Subclavian lines are desirable for long-term catheterization, as is needed for total parenteral nutrition, because the site is relatively comfortable for the patient and dressings are more easily maintained at this site than at other sites. Percutaneous cannulation of the femoral vessels is a safe and reliable technique that is especially useful for access during cardiopulmonary resuscitation and for use in the anticoagulated patient.

Anticoagulated patients or those patients with a bleeding diathesis are frequently encountered and require special consideration before central venous catheterization due to the risk of hemorrhage and hematoma formation. If the subclavian artery is inadvertently punctured in the patient with a bleeding diathesis a large hemothorax may result because the punctured artery is difficult or impossible to compress directly. Likewise, the close proximity of the common carotid artery to the IJV makes accidental puncture of the artery a frequent complication (4%).[8] Even though the carotid is easily compressed, the consequences of carotid artery puncture in the patient with coagulation problems are significant and some authors suggest that this route be avoided altogether in these patients.[8–10] The EJV, FV, and possibly the ACV are preferred in these patients because arterial and venous bleeding at these sites is less likely to have disastrous consequences and bleeding can be more easily controlled with direct pressure.

GENERAL CONSIDERATIONS AND COMPLICATIONS

Proper education and training along with the development of advanced techniques, materials, and design innovations have made percutaneous vascular catheterization relatively safe.[11,12] Yet, all of these procedures carry a low but significant incidence of morbidity and mortality. The majority of complications due to catheterization of arteries and veins are minor, but major complications, those untoward events that require active treatment, occur also.

Embolism

Embolism of air, catheters, and guidewires can occur during or after central venous or arterial catheterization but should be avoidable with strict adherence to good technique. Catheters and guidewires can be sheared and then embolize when they are withdrawn through or over a needle which is not first or simultaneously withdrawn. Embolized catheters and wires should be snared or removed surgically because of the high incidence of morbidity and mortality associated with conservative management.[13]

Venous air embolism (VAE) can take place in a variety of clinical settings but is most frequently associated with central venous catheterization.[14] VAE may occur during catheterization, but usually occurs afterward due to inadvertent opening of the external tubing system to air through disconnections or open stopcocks.[15] The level of the air-venous blood interface, the right atrial pressure, and the iatrogenic stenting of large vessels with catheters, needles, and dilators are important factors in the development of VAE. Air embolism during insertion can be avoided by careful attention to technique including the use of the Trendelenburg position and the religious occlusion of open needle, catheter, and dilator hubs.[16] Use of secure Luer-Lok connectors at all external connections is recommended.[15]

Vascular Erosions

Large central veins, the right atrium, and the right ventricle are easily perforated with plastic catheters, spring guidewires, and metal wire leads. Erosion of the central veins is a rare (<0.4%) but serious complication appearing one to seven days after catheter insertion.[17,18] Patients with vascular erosions often present with hydrothorax (from the infusion of intravenous fluid into the pleural cavity), sudden onset of shortness of breath, and respiratory insufficiency. Previous chest x-rays do not always demonstrate malposition of the catheter tip. Catheter tip position, catheter stiffness, and the infusion of sclerosing, hyperosmolar solutions may also contribute to vessel damage leading to perforation. A catheter tip is more likely to oppose the vessel wall when placed from the patient's left side (left subclavian or left internal jugular).[18] Correct placement of the catheter tip is crucial in avoiding vascular erosion and pericardial tamponade, and this topic is discussed in the following section.

Pericardial Tamponade

Perforation of the heart leading to pericardial tamponade is a rare but often lethal complication with a mortality between 78% and 95%. Similar to vascular erosion, cardiac perforation often presents several hours, days, or weeks after catheterization. Temporal dissociation between placement of the catheter and cardiovascular decompensation may contribute to failure to recognize and diagnose the problem promptly.

Improper location of the catheter tip occurs following 3% to 4% of line insertions[19] and is the most important factor contributing to cardiac perforation. Transient, overzealous insertion of guidewires, dilators, or catheters may perforate the heart at the time of insertion, or perforation can occur later from a catheter secured with its tip located in an intrapericardial location.[20,21] In addition, catheter tip location can change over time with patient movement and repositioning. Catheter material and the shape of the tip can influence the propensity of the catheter to perforate vital structures but any catheter, no matter how pliable, can perforate the heart if placed too deeply.

In order to assure extrapericardial location of the catheter tip, the tip should rest in the distal innominate vein or the initial segment of the superior vena cava, 3 to 5 cm proximal to the caval-atrial junction. A rough guide to proper tip placement can be made by using the catheter as a ruler to measure the distance from the proposed skin entry site to the supraclavicular notch to the angle of the manubrium. Many catheters and guidewires are manufactured with markings on their surfaces that indicate distance to the tip. In adult patients, central venous catheters, dilators, and guidewires should not be inserted beyond 10 to 15 cm from the right internal jugular and right subclavian positions and not beyond 15 to 18 cm from the left-sided positions.[12,20] Thirty-centimeter catheters should not be used, and the exclusive use of 15- and 16-cm catheters has the potential of reducing right atrial perforations.[22] Finally, a chest roentgenogram is required after successful and failed attempts at catheterization, guidewire exchanges, and other catheter adjustments. A strong index of suspicion for catheter-associated complication should be maintained in any patient with a central line who develops cardiorespiratory embarrassment.

Pneumothorax

Pneumothorax (PTX) can complicate internal jugular approaches but most commonly follows subclavian venous catheterization.[11,19,23] Bilateral PTX have been reported following bilateral and unilateral line insertions. Patients requiring mechanical ventilation, including those ventilated during general anesthesia, are at increased risk of developing a tension pneumothorax.[24] Therefore, the presence of a PTX in a mechanically ventilated patient (no matter how small) requires aspiration, usually using closed chest tube thoracostomy.

Thrombosis

Arterial and venous thrombosis secondary to indwelling catheters occurs frequently but is usually of little clinical significance in nonburned patients.[25–27] Thrombosis appears to be related to the thrombogenicity of the catheters but also may be due to catheter induced injury to the endothelium. Serum proteins are rapidly deposited on artificial material placed in the bloodstream. Protein deposition is followed by platelet activation, platelet adherence, and activation of the intrinsic clotting pathway, leading to the formation of a fibrin sleeve around the artificial material. Venous phlebography has demonstrated the presence of fibrin sleeves around central venous catheters and has even documented embolization of the fibrin sleeve material during withdrawal of catheters.[28,29]

Venography and pathological examination have shown that more extensive thrombotic phenomena, including mural and veno-occlusive thrombi, occur less frequently than fibrin sleeve formation. These larger thrombotic lesions may be due to catheter-induced trauma to the vascular wall which damages the endothelium and endocardium, resulting in the deposition of thrombus on the injured surface.[32] Significant thrombotic events tend to occur in more seriously ill patients and are associated with catheters left in place for longer periods of time.[26,30,32] Symptomatic venous thrombosis and pulmonary embolism are infrequent (0% to 3%).[28,30,31]

Efforts have been made to reduce the thrombogenicity of catheters using techniques to bond heparin to the surface of the catheter. Some studies have suggested that heparin-bonding reduces thrombus formation while others have not.[29,33] In fact, heparin bonding can contribute to low platelet counts and thrombotic complications in patients with heparin-induced thrombocytopenia.[34]

Catheter Associated Infection

The presence of an intravascular cannula may result in local infection, or bloodstream infection. The most likely source is skin flora at the site of insertion. Gram-positive cocci (especially staphylococci) predominate in any study of catheter-related infections, with *Candida albicans* and gram-negative rods occurring less frequently. Many factors may contribute to the development of infection, including insertion technique (adequacy of skin sterilization, sterility of procedure, difficulty in gaining venous access), dressing technique and frequency, and overall duration of catheter residence. Infection due to contamination of IV fluid or contamination of catheter hubs appears to be uncommon. In general, arterial cannulae at any site appear to be at a lower risk of infection than central venous catheters. Of practical importance, it appears that skin preparation with chlorhexidine may be more effective in reducing bacterial counts than povidone-iodine,[35] and that transparent dressings have the potential for moisture buildup and increased skin flora, especially if left for more than two days. Newer, more porous transparent dressings may provide an advantage in this regard.

A contentious issue is the subject of duration of catheter residence, and whether "routine" changes with either a guidewire or new venipuncture should be performed to reduce the risk of infection. There is a large literature on this subject, with few controlled randomized trials. Definitions of infection are also inconsistent, making comparisons of trials complex. For example, "catheter infection" is often defined as simply the finding of significant colonization of the catheter tip. When this definition is used, between 10% and 30% of central venous catheters are "infected," while the incidence of bloodstream infection related to the catheter is usually less than 5%. Two randomized trials published in the last three years have failed to demonstrate that scheduled replacement at three or seven days, either with guidewire exchange or new venipuncture, favorably affected the rate of catheter-related bloodstream infection due to pulmonary artery catheters (PACs) and central venous catheters.[36,37] Both studies suggested that if anything, infection risk and the risk of mechanical complication were *higher* with scheduled replacement.[36,37] In the study by Cobb et al, the incidence of catheter-related bloodstream infection was 2%; the infection rate per catheter inserted ranged from 2% (catheter changed to new site only when clinically indicated; mean catheter residence 6 days) to 10% (routine changes at 3 days over a wire).[37] These studies included 272 patients and 983 catheters. While the Centers for Disease Control has not yet revised its 1982 statement, "the proper frequency for changing [central venous] cannulas that are used for pressure monitoring . . . is not known,"[38] the results of these studies suggest that catheters should stay in place until an indication for their removal exists. If the insertion site appears infected, then a new site should be chosen; if the patient has a fever without an identifiable source, then an acceptable approach that may reduce the incidence of mechanical complications is to replace the catheter over a guidewire. If this is done the old catheter should be cultured and a peripheral blood culture performed as well; if the cultures grow the same organism a new catheter should be placed with a new venipuncture. There are no studies in patients requiring long-term pulmonary artery catheter placement (eg, cardiomyopathy patients awaiting transplantation); while most institutions employ some kind of routine replacement policy, a minimum duration of 7 days appears to be warranted.

Misinterpretation

While a discussion of complications due to indwelling devices usually focuses on morbidity resulting from the insertion or presence of the device, misinterpretation of hemodynamic data from central venous and pulmonary artery catheters has great potential to result in improper diagnosis and therapy. Not only must clinicians fully understand the procedures required for proper insertion of these catheters, they must also be competent to set up, calibrate, and correctly zero the transducers to which they are attached. Location of the transducers at a level only a few centimeters above or below the left atrium can result in a diagnosis that is 100% incorrect. Inability to detect a damped waveform may result in the wrong diagnosis, and failure to recognize abnormal waveforms may result in morbidity. For example, failure to recognize 'v' waves when the balloon of a pulmonary artery catheter is inflated may result in inappropriate advancement of the catheter with the potential for pulmonary infarction, or hemorrhage due to vessel rupture.

Iberti et al assessed the knowledge of 496 clinicians in 13 North American medical facilities in the use and interpretation of PACs.[39] Questions were in the categories of insertion/complications, cardiac physiology, interpretation, and application of data, and clinicians trained in anesthesiology, internal medicine, and surgery were included. Out of a possible score of 31 the mean was 20.7, with the distribution of scores showing a clear relationship between the test result and the level of experience, frequency of use, and nature of the institution; 42% of the variation in test scores was due to these variables. The primary specialty, when adjusted for these variables, did not have a significant effect on the score result. Sixty-one percent of respondents were unable to identify inadvertent arterial cannulation (when given the result of a blood gas), 47% could not determine the pulmonary artery occlusion pressure from a clear tracing, and 44% could not correctly identify the determinants of oxygen delivery.

A common misconception is that the presence of 'v' waves on right or left atrial (ie, pulmonary artery occlusion) pressure tracings means valvular regurgitation. A study by Fuchs et al[40] demonstrated that the size of 'a' and 'v' waves may simply reflect the compliance of the left atrium (and pulmonary veins). In patients with noncompliant or congested left atria large 'v' waves occurred in the absence of mitral regurgitation, and in patients without congestion severe mitral regurgitation could be present in the absence of 'v' waves. Related to this observation is the suggestion that the pulmonary artery catheter can be used as a monitor for myocardial ischemia, in that the development of an elevated PAOP, especially with the appearance of new large 'a' and 'v' waves, suggests an acute reduction in left ventricular compliance. While this is probably true, the majority of episodes of new ST segment depression or new wall motion abnormalities seen on transesophageal echocardiography during general anesthesia are not associated with changes in either the PAOP or the waveform.[41,42] Changes in left ventricular compliance may reduce the utility of pressures as indicators of "preload"; a poor relationship between pressure and volume has been observed in both an ICU setting[43] and after cardiac surgery.[44]

COMPLICATIONS ASSOCIATED WITH SPECIFIC ROUTES OF CENTRAL VENOUS CATHETERIZATION

Antecubital Fossa

The major advantage of using veins in the antecubital fossa for percutaneous access to the central venous circulation is the low incidence of major thoracic complications. The approach is relatively safe in the patient with clotting abnormalities and is suitable for the patient who cannot tolerate the supine or Trendelenburg's position.

The success rate for proper distal placement of the catheter tip is lower with this technique than with other approaches. The position of the catheter tip is difficult to gauge during insertion and despite radiographic confirmation of proper position, the tip can subsequently change position with movement of the patient's arm. As discussed previously, improper location of the catheter tip within vascular or cardiac structures enclosed by the pericardium has the potential of leading to tamponade.

Overall, there is a higher incidence of local site complications such as infection (cellulitis) and thrombophlebitis (16%).[27] Infectious complications occur in 1% to 2% of catheters left in place for less than 72 hours but the incidence increases significantly with catheters left in place longer than 3 days. Clinically significant central venous thrombosis is rare (1% to 2%) but local, sterile phlebitis occurs more frequently and can lead to deep venous thrombosis of the axillary and subclavian veins.[27] Pulmonary embolism occurs less than 0.5% of the time. The brachial artery can be injured during attempts to cannulate the veins of the antecubital fossa.

External Jugular Vein

The external jugular vein is a superficial structure that can usually be found as it courses obliquely over the sternocleidomastoid muscle. The vein has numerous valves and makes a severe, narrow angle at its junction with the subclavian vein, which can make passage of a guidewire or catheter difficult.[45] A guidewire technique increases the rate of successfully placing a catheter in the central venous system and can even be used to place an introducer sheath and pulmonary artery catheter.

In 5% to 15% of patients an EJV cannot be identified and in those patients in whom an EJV can be located, up to 20% of attempted catheterizations fail.[10] Thus, the EJV is not a reliable route for all patients and it is for this reason that catheterization of the EJV is used less frequently. Yet serious complications are extremely rare. Local hematoma occurs in 1% to 5% of patients and can be easily controlled with local pressure that does not risk stimulating a vagal reflex or dislodging a carotid plaque. A hematoma may obscure the anatomy making further line insertion attempts on the same side difficult.

The incidences of infectious, thrombotic and intrathoracic complications are presumed to be similar to the IJV. Pneumothorax is distinctly uncommon, as is inadvertent carotid artery puncture, making this technique a wise first choice in patients who can not tolerate pneumothorax or in patients who have a bleeding diathesis.

Femoral Vein

Femoral venous catheterization is an excellent means of providing short-term venous access for fluid administration especially during cardiopulmonary resuscitation or in patients with hypovolemic shock.[46,47] This technique is also suitable for acute hemodialysis.[48] Femoral venous catheterization is relatively safe in the hands of inexperienced operators and is a reasonable alternative for central venous access in the patient with a bleeding problem.

The inguinal anatomy is fairly constant, assuring a high rate of success (90% to 95%) in cannulating the relatively large femoral vein. The vein is superficial as it crosses the inguinal ligament medial to the femoral artery, which serves as a reliable landmark. If the femoral artery cannot be palpated, however, the location of the femoral vein can be approximated using a blind technique guided by the bony prominences of the pelvis [46]. A line is drawn between the anterior iliac spine and the pubic tubercle. The artery lies beneath the junction of the medial and middle thirds of this line. The vein should be found 1 to 1.5 cm medial to this point.

Femoral venous catheterization is associated with three major groups of complications: thrombosis, arterial hemorrhage, and infection. More recent reports of experience with short-term catheterization for fluid administration and hemodialysis have reported very low rates of thrombosis between 0% to 0.5%.[47–49] The incidence of infection (1% to 2%) and colonization (25% to 30%) due to femoral venous catheters is similar to that for other sites.[12,46,50]

Inadvertent puncture of the femoral artery complicates femoral venous catheterization 5% to 8% of the time.[47,49,51] Arterial puncture can result in hematoma formation in 1.3% while more serious complications such as retroperitoneal hemorrhage,[52] arteriovenous fistula,[53] and pseudoaneurysm formation[54] are fortunately infrequent (<1.0%). Guidewires, dilators, and catheters may perforate or lacerate the inferior vena cava or pelvic veins, resulting in retroperitoneal hematoma.[52] Inadvertent arterial puncture is usually managed easily with 5 to 10 minutes of local pressure. Retroperitoneal hematoma is most reliably diagnosed with computed tomography; conservative treatment is based on removal of the femoral vein catheter, blood volume replacement, and correction of any coagulation defects.[52]

Subclavian Vein

The subclavian route is characterized by identifiable and consistent landmarks that make the technique easy to learn and master. Once mastered, the procedure can be performed quickly with an acceptably low incidence of complications.

The subclavian vein is usually cannulated using the infraclavicular approach; the supraclavicular technique does not offer any clear advantage. Trendelenburg's position helps guard against venous air embolism but it does not distend the vein.[55] After routine preparation, the skin is punctured 2 to 3 cm caudal to the midpoint of the clavicle, and the skin, soft tissues, and periosteum are anesthetized with local anesthetic. The thin-walled needle is directed toward the suprasternal notch or slightly cephalad to the notch. Upon contacting the clavicle, the needle is gently worked under the clavicle until the inferior edge is cleared. It is important to keep the syringe barrel parallel to the skin as the needle is advanced under the clavicle to avoid injuring the pleura. If the first pass does not succeed, subsequent attempts are made with the needle directed in a slightly more cephalad direction.

The subclavian approach is successful 88% to 95% of the time and failure can be due to inability to locate the vein or thread the guidewire (or catheter).[11] Occasionally, the guidewire will pass up the internal jugular vein instead of down the innominate vein toward the heart. If this occurs, the conscious patient may complain of a painful sensation in the ear.

The overall complication rate of central venous access via the SCV varies between 0% and 5%.[11] Factors leading to an increased rate of complication include operator inexperience, an uncooperative or agitated patient, multiple attempts at venipuncture, and catheterization under emergency conditions.[19,56] Pneumothorax and subclavian arterial puncture are the most frequent serious adverse events, accounting for one-fourth to one-half of all complications.[11,23] Experienced operators should have about one-half of the number of complications of operators with less experience.[19] Subclavian artery puncture, occurring 0.5% to 3.1% of the time, is usually benign and self-limited[19] but may lead to the formation of a hemothorax or arteriovenous fistula. Arterial puncture is managed with local pressure for 5 to 10 minutes (which may or may not enhance hemostasis.) Obviously, clotting abnormalities increase the risk of more serious consequences of arterial puncture including hemorrhage and hemothorax. Clinically significant subclavian vein thrombosis may be manifested by arm swelling but its occurrence is distinctly infrequent. As mentioned previously, clinically unapparent mural thrombosis and fibrin sleeve formation probably take place much more often.[28]

Internal Jugular Vein

The internal jugular vein IJV is a popular choice for safe, reliable access to the central venous circulation for a variety of indications. Advantages of this route include a high rate of success, a straight path to the heart and a low incidence of major complications.

The internal jugular vein emerges from the skull at the jugular foramen and passes posterolateral to the internal carotid artery. For the most part, the vein runs beneath the sternocleidomastoid muscle. The IJV is medial to the anterior portion of the sternocleidomastoid muscle in its upper part and runs beneath the triangle formed by the two heads of the sternocleidomastoid muscle as it approaches the sternoclavicular junction. The subclavian vein merges with the IJV behind the sternal part of the clavicle to form the innominate vein.

There are many structures in the neck that can be injured or lacerated by a probing needle or misplaced dilator. A knowledge of the cervical anatomy and location of these structures is vital to understanding the potential for various complications. The stellate ganglion and cervical sympathetic trunk lie posterior to the carotid sheath, and the phrenic and vagus nerves are deep in the root of the neck. On the left side of the neck, the thoracic duct runs behind the left IJV and is much more prominent and easily injured than the corresponding structure on the right.

Because of anatomical considerations, there are several disadvantages to selecting the left IJV over the right. Injury of the thoracic duct may lead to a chylous effusion. The pleural dome is higher on the left and more easily injured. The sharp angle made by the intersection of the left IJV and the left SCV can occasionally make passage of guidewires, dilators, and catheters difficult. In addition, overzealous and inappropriately deep passage of these devices against resistance can tear or lacerate the veins at this point. Finally, vascular erosion and delayed hydrothorax may occur more commonly with catheters placed from the left side.[18]

Each of the three most popular approaches to the IJV, the anterior, central and posterior, are equally reliable and safe. The overall complication rate for the IJV is about 1% to 4%. Operators with more experience tend to have higher success rates and a lower incidence of complications.[19] The most frequent significant complication of IJV catheterization is inadvertent puncture of the carotid artery, occurring 2.8% to 9.9% of the time and accounting for 80% to 90% of all complications.[8,19,57] Other arteries in the neck, including the vertebral artery, can be injured, also.[58,59] The consequences of carotid or vertebral artery puncture depend on the size and nature of the foreign body that injures the vessel and range from a small, limited hematoma to cerebral vascular accident and death. Arterial puncture with a 20- or 22-gauge "finder" needle is usually of no consequence, but arterial placement of an introducer sheath may result in thrombosis of the carotid artery and require operative repair. Hematomas from an arterial or venous puncture can become very large, resulting in damage to local structures, compromise of the airway,[60] or life-threatening hemorrhage.

Many techniques have been described to avoid the disastrous complication of placing a large catheter in the carotid artery. Several authors recommend avoiding the IJV altogether and they first attempt to cannulate the external jugular vein.[10,59] Use of a small-gauge finder needle to first locate the IJV before using a larger needle is recommended but is not foolproof. After locating the IJV with a small needle, we use an 18-gauge "angiocath" in preference to the thin-wall 18-gauge needle for initial cannulation of the vein. After establishing free flow of blood, the small IV catheter can be attached to sterile tubing, allowing one to observe the color and pressure character of the blood in the vessel before introducing a guidewire and larger catheter. Alternatively, the tubing can be attached to a transducer or the blood can be sampled for blood gas analysis (the PaO_2 should not exceed 50). If a large catheter is placed in the carotid artery, it should be left in place and an emergent vascular surgery consultation obtained.[8] Operative exploration and repair of the injured vessel can then be carried out.

Other reported complications include: pneumothorax, thrombosis of the IJV, air embolism, catheter embolism, hydrothorax, pericardial tamponade, cerebral vascular accident, neurologic syndromes, arteriovenous fistula formation, pseudoaneurysm formation, and infection (Table 4.2). Pneumothorax complicates catheterization of the IJV much less frequently than it does for the subclavian vein (0% to 0.2% vs 2% to 4%), and is associated with skin punctures low in the neck close to the clavicle. A misplaced guidewire or dilator may injure the pleura, especially with attempts from the left side.

TABLE 4.2. Complications of Percutaneous Internal Jugular Vein Catheterization

Pneumothorax
Air embolus
Hydrothorax
Hydromediastinum
Thrombophlebitis
Sepsis
Thoracic duct laceration
Horner's syndrome
Bilateral vocal cord paralysis
Brachiocephalic artery pseudoaneurysm
Ascending cervical artery laceration
Hemothorax
Puncture of the aorta
Carotid puncture
Damage to cranial nerves
Hematoma

From reference No. 16. Used with permission.

COMPLICATIONS OF ARTERIAL CATHETERIZATION

More than one-half of patients in ICUs have some type of arterial line placed for hemodynamic monitoring and frequent blood sampling. Placement of an arterial line is easily performed by most operators, is well tolerated by the patient, and involves minimal complications. Rapid beat-to-beat monitoring of arterial blood pressure is a common indication, especially for patients who are acutely hypotensive or hypertensive and those receiving vasoactive medications. Likewise, many patients with serious cardiorespiratory disorders require frequent sampling of arterial blood for blood gas and hematologic or chemical analysis.

Complications common to all sites include thrombosis, cerebral embolism, infection, and miscellaneous mechanical complications such as local tenderness, hematoma, hemorrhage, neuropathies, catheter embolism, and pseudoaneurysm formation (Table 4.3). Arterial thrombosis is the single most common complication of arterial lines; its occurrence varies with the site and duration of cannulation and the size of the catheter. Use of smaller, less thrombogenic catheters along with continuous heparin flush systems has reduced the incidence of thrombotic complications. Arterial thrombosis is most frequently asymptomatic but can lead to digital ischemia signified by decreased temperature and pallor or cyanosis of the skin distal to the catheter.[25,61] Digital ischemia occurs in approximately 4% of catheterizations and is more likely to complicate difficult percutaneous placement or surgical cutdown.[61]

Cerebral air embolization can occur with retrograde passage of air from overly aggressive manual flushing of arterial lines. Cerebral air embolism may be more common with axillary and brachial lines. Catheter-related sepsis is less common with

TABLE 4.3.   Complications Due to Arterial Cannulation and Catheterization

Complications Common to All Sites
Pain and swelling
Thrombosis
Embolization
Hematoma and hemorrhage
Limb ischemia
Peripheral neuropathy and nerve damage
Catheter-related infection
Pseudoaneurysm
Diagnostic blood loss
Complications Associated with Certain Sites
Cerebral embolization: axillary, brachial, radial
Arteriovenous fistula: femoral
Retroperitoneal hemorrhage: femoral
Bowel perforation: femoral

arterial lines than with central venous catheters: colonization occurs 4% to 20% of the time, but catheter-related sepsis is rare (0% to 3%).[25,61,62]

The most common sites for arterial cannulation are the radial, femoral, axillary, brachial, and dorsalis pedis arteries. In most cases, smaller peripheral arteries are cannulated using a 2-inch, 20-gauge, nontapered Teflon catheter over a needle. For larger arteries, we employ the Seldinger technique, using a prepackaged kit containing a 6-inch, 18-gauge Teflon catheter. Larger arteries accommodate larger catheters, which provide more accurate measurement of central pressures. Regardless of the size of the catheter, the arterial pressure waveform varies at different points along the arterial tree. As the pressure wave travels outward from the aorta, it encounters branch points and smaller, less elastic arteries that reflect the wave. The net result is that more peripherally located catheters generate waveforms that have greater amplitudes and upslopes.

The radial artery has three anastomotic connections that provide excellent collateral blood flow to the hand. All anastomotic connections may not be present in all patients, however, and the value of the Allen's test in determining the adequacy of collateral flow is debated. Because of the easy availability of alternative sites, it would seem prudent to avoid the radial artery if an Allen's test suggests insufficient collateral flow.

The dorsalis pedis artery is an uncommon site for arterial line placement because the anatomy is less predictable and success rates are lower. It can be more difficult to adequately secure the line from inadvertent dislodgment.

The brachial artery is less frequently chosen for cannulation owing to concern about a lack of effective collateral circulation. Centers where the brachial artery is used routinely have not reported an increased rate of ischemic complications.[63] The brachial artery is cannulated at or just above the antecubital fossa where it is in close approximation to the median nerve. Needle trauma to the nerve can generate transient paresthesias, and minor bleeding into fascial planes can result in nerve compression and median neuropathy. It is for this reason that brachial artery catheterization is relatively contraindicated in patients with coagulopathy.

The axillary artery is served with an extensive collateral circulation and is often palpable when other peripheral arteries are not. Thus, it serves as an alternate site when the femoral and radial arteries are not available. The optimal site for puncture and catheter placement is at the highest palpable point in the axilla but this leaves the tip of the catheter in a very central location, which increases the risk of cerebral air embolism.

The femoral artery is as safe as other sites for access to the arterial circulation and has a complication rate similar to the radial artery ~7%.[61] Atherosclerosis or previous vascular procedures can make femoral arterial catheterization impossible. Unique complications include retroperitoneal hemorrhage, intra-abdominal hemorrhage and intra-abdominal viscus perforation.

SUMMARY

Catheterization of the central veins and arteries is an indispensable tool of the modern physician. Complications related to the various techniques can lead to an adverse outcome in a certain percentage of patients. Complications can be due to trauma to local structures during insertion or may be secondary to the presence of a foreign body in the vascular tree. The frequency of complications can be reduced by a thorough knowledge of the potential complications, careful attention to insertion guidelines, and clinical experience.

REFERENCES

1. Kalso E. A short history of central venous catheterization. *Acta Anaesth Scand.* 81:7–10, 1985.
2. Seldinger SI. Catheter replacement of the needle in percutaneous arteriography. *Acta Radiol.* 39:368, 1953.
3. Wilson JN, Grow JB, Demong CV, et al. Central venous pressure in optimal blood volume maintenance. *Arch Surg.* 79:238, 1962.
4. English I, Frew RM, Pigott JF, Zaki M. Percutaneous catheterisation of the internal jugular vein. *Anaesthesia.* 24:521, 1969.
5. Massa DJ, Lundy JS, Faulconer, A, Jr, et al. A plastic needle. *Mayo Clin Proc.* 25:413, 1950.
6. Barr PO. Percutaneous puncture of the radial artery with a multi-purpose Teflon catheter for indwelling use. *Acta Physiol Scand.* 51:343–347, 1961.
7. Swan H, Ganz W, Forrester JA, Marcus H, et al. Catheterization of the heart in man with use of a flow-directed balloon-tipped catheter. *N Engl J Med.* 283:447–451, 1970.
8. Schwartz AJ, Jobes DR, Greenhow DE, Stephenson LW, et al. Carotid artery puncture with internal jugular cannulation. *Anesthesiology.* 51:S160, 1980.
9. Klineberg PL, Greenhow DE, Ellison N. Haematoma following internal jugular vein cannulation. *Anaesth Inten Care.* 8:94, 1980.
10. Jobes DR, Schwartz AJ, Greenhow DE, Stephenson LW, et al. Safer jugular vein cannulation: recognition of arterial puncture and preferential use of the external jugular route. *Anesthesiology.* 59:353, 1983.

11. Eerola R, Kaukinen L, Kaukinen S. Analysis of 13800 subclavian catheterizations. *Acta Anaesth Scand.* 29:193, 1985.

12. Seneff MG. Central venous catheterization: a comprehensive review, Part I. *J Inten Care Med.* 2:163–175, 1987.

13. Doering RB, Stemmer EA, Connolly JE. Complications of indwelling venous catheters with particular reference to catheter embolism. *Am J Surg.* 114:259, 1967.

14. Petts JS, Presson RG. A review of the pathophysiology of venous air embolism. *Anesth Rev.* 18:29–37, 1991.

15. Seidelin PH, Stolarek IH, Thompson AM. Central venous catheterization and fatal air embolism. *Br J Hosp Med.* 38:438–439, 1987.

16. McGoon, MD, Benedetto PW, Greene BM. Complications of percutaneous central venous catheterization: a report of two cases and review of the literature. *Johns Hopkins Med J.* 145:1, 1979.

17. Ellis LM, Vogel SB, Copeland EM. Central venous catheter vascular erosions: diagnosis and clinical course. *Ann Surg.* 209:475, 1989.

18. Iberti TJ, Katz LB, Reiner MA, et al. Hydrothorax as a late complication of central venous indwelling catheters. *Surgery.* 94:842, 1983.

19. Sznajder J, Zveibel FR, Bitterman H, et al. Central venous catheterization failure and complication rates by three percutaneous approaches. *Arch Intern Med.* 146:259, 1986.

20. Maschke SP, Rogove HJ. Cardiac tamponade associated with a multilumen central venous catheter. *Crit Care Med.* 12:611–613, 1984.

21. Mitchell MR, Wood DG, Naraghi M, Riopelle JM. Fatal cardiac perforation caused by the dilator of a central venous catheterization kit. *J Clin Monit.* 9:288–291, 1993.

22. McGee WT, Ackerman BL, Rouben LR, Prasad VM, et al. Accurate placement of central venous catheters: a prospective, randomized, multicenter trial. *Crit Care Med.* 21:1118–1123, 1993.

23. Seneff MG. Central venous catheterization: a comprehensive review, Part II. *J Inten Care Med.* 2:218–232, 1987.

24. Cook TL, Dueker CW. Tension pneumothorax following internal jugular cannulation and general anesthesia. *Anesthesiology.* 45:554, 1976.

25. Weiss BM, Gattiker RI. Complications during and following radial artery cannulation: a prospective study. *Inten Care Med.* 12:424–428, 1986.

26. Warden GD, Wilmore DW, Pruitt BA. Central venous thrombosis: a hazard of medical progress. *J Trauma.* 13:620, 1973.

27. Walters MB, Stanger H, Rotem CE. Complications with percutaneous central venous catheters. *JAMA.* 220:1455–1457, 1972.

28. Brismar B, Hardstedt C, Jacobson S. Diagnosis of thrombosis by catheter phlebography after prolonged central venous catheterization. *Ann Surg.* 194:779–783, 1981.

29. Mollenholt P, Eriksson I, Andersson T. Thrombogenicity of pulmonary-artery catheters. *Inten Care Med.* 13:57–59, 1987.

30. Chastre J, Cornud F, Bouchama A, Viau F, et al. Thrombosis as a complication of pulmonary-artery catheterization via the internal jugular vein. *N Engl J Med.* 306:278–281, 1982.

31. Efsing HO, Lindblad B, Mark J, Wolff T. Thromboembolic complications from central venous catheters: a comparison of three catheter materials. *World J Surg.* 7:419, 1983.

32. Connors AF, Castele RJ, Farhat NZ, Tomashefski J, Jr. Complications of right heart catheterization: a prospective autopsy study. *Chest.* 88:567–572, 1985.

33. Hoar PF, Wilson RM, Mangano DT, et al. Heparin bonding reduces thrombogenicity of pulmonary-artery catheters. *N Engl J Med.* 305:993–995, 1981.

34. Laster JL, Nichols WK, Silver D. Thrombocytopenia associated with heparin-coated catheters in patients with heparin-associated antiplatelet antibodies. *Arch Intern Med.* 149:2285, 1989.

35. Maki DG, Alvarado CJ, Ringer M. A prospective, randomized trial of povidone-iodine, alcohol, and chlorhexidine for prevention of infection with central venous and arterial catheters. *Lancet.* 338:339–343, 1991.

36. Eyer S, Brummitt C, Crossley K, Siegel R, et al. Catheter-related sepsis: prospective, randomized study of three methods of long-term catheter maintenance. *Crit Care Med.* 18:1073–1079, 1990.

37. Cobb KD, High KP, Sawyer RG, Sable CA, et al. A controlled trial of scheduled replacement of central venous and pulmonary-artery catheters. *N Engl J Med.* 327:1062–1068, 1992.

38. Simmons BP, Hooton TM, Wong ES, Allen JR. Guidelines for Prevention of Intravascular Infections, 1982. Springfield: National Technical Information Service; 1982.

39. Iberti TJ, Fischer EP, Leibowityz AB, Panacek EA, et al. Pulmonary artery catheter study group: a multicenter study of physicians' knowledge of the pulmonary artery catheter. *JAMA.* 264:2928–2932, 1990.

40. Fuchs RM, Heuser RR, Yin CP, Brinker JA. Limitations of pulmonary v waves in diagnosing mitral regurgitation. *Am J Cardiol.* 49:849–854, 1982.

41. Van Daele ME, Sutherland GR, Mitchell MM, et al. Do changes in the pulmonary capillary wedge pressure adequately reflect myocardial ischemia during anesthesia? *Circulation.* 81:865–871, 1990.

42. Haggmark S, Hohner P, Ostman M, et al. Comparison of hemodynamic, electrocardiographic, mechanical, and metabolic indicators of intraoperative myocardial ischemia in vascular surgical patients with coronary artery disease. *Anesthesiology.* 70:19–25, 1989.

43. Raper R, Sibbald WJ. Misled by the wedge? The Swan-Ganz catheter and left ventricular preload. *Chest.* 89:427–434, 1986.

44. Douglas PS, Edmunds LH, Sutton MS, et al. Unreliability of hemodynamic indexes of left ventricular size during cardiac surgery. *Ann Thorac Surg.* 44:31–34, 1987.

45. Riddell GS, Latto IP, Ng WS. External jugular vein access to the central venous system: a trial of two types of catheter. *Br J Anaesth.* 54:535–537, 1982.

46. Dailey RH. Femoral vein cannulation: a review. *J Emerg Med.* 2:367, 1985.

47. Swanson RS, Uhlig PN, Gross PL, McCabe CJ. Emergency intravenous access through the femoral vein. *Ann Emerg Med.* 13:244, 1984.

48. Kjellstrand CM, Merino GE, Mauer SM, Casali R, et al. Complications of percutaneous femoral vein catheterizations for hemodialysis. *Clin Nephrol.* 4:37–40, 1975.

49. Getzen LC, Pollak EW. Short-term femoral vein catheterization. *Am J Surg.* 138:875, 1979.

50. Collignon P, Suni N, Pearson I, et al. Sepsis associated with central vein catheters in critically ill patients. *Inten Care Med.* 14:227, 1988.

51. Williams JF, Friedman BC, McGrath BJ, et al. The use of femoral venous catheters in critically ill adults: a prospective study. *Crit Care Med.* 17:584, 1989.

52. Sharp KW, Spees EK, Selby LR, Zachary JB, et al. Diagnosis and management of retroperitoneal hematomas after femoral vein cannulation for hemodialysis. *Surgery.* 95:90–95, 1984.

53. Fuller TJ, Mahoney JJ, Juncos LI, Hawkins RF. Arteriovenous fistula after femoral vein catheterization. *JAMA.* 236:2943–2944, 1976.

54. Altin RS, Flicker S, Naidech HJ. Pseudoaneurysm and arteriovenous fistula after femoral

artery catheterization: associates with low femoral punctures. *Am J Rheum.* 152:629, 1989.

55. Yonei A, Toriumi T, Yamashita S, Kojima S. The effect of head-down positioning on percutaneous cannulation of the internal jugular or subclavian vein: a simulated study using ultrasound. *Anesthesiology.* 79:A488, 1993.

56. Sitzmann JV, Townsend TR, Siler MC, Bartlett JG. Septic and technical complications of central venous catheterization. *Ann Surg.* 202:768, 1985.

57. Damen J, Bolton D. A prospective analysis of 1400 pulmonary artery catheterizations in patients undergoing cardiac surgery. *Acta Anaesth Scand.* 30:386–392, 1986.

58. Sloan MA, Mueller JD, Adelman LS, Caplan LR. Fatal brainstem stroke following internal jugular vein catheterization. *Neurology.* 41:1092–1095, 1991.

59. Morgan R, Morrell DF. Internal jugular catheterization: a review of a potentially lethal hazard. *Anaesthesia.* 36:512–517, 1981.

60. Knoblanche GE. Respiratory obstruction due to haematoma following internal jugular vein cannulation. *Anaesth Intensive Care.* 7:286, 1979.

61. Russel JA, Joel M, Hudson RJ, Mangano DT, et al. Prospective evaluation of radial and femoral artery catheterization sites in critically ill adults. *Crit Care Med.* 11:936, 1983.

62. Gurman GM, Kriermerman S. Cannulation of big arteries in critically ill patients. *Crit Care Med.* 13:217, 1985.

63. Seneff MG. Arterial line placement and care. In: Rippe JM, Irwin RS, Alper JS, Fink MP, eds. Intensive Care Medicine. Boston: Little, Brown and Company; 1991:42.

5

Complications of Swan-Ganz Catheter

Cyril B. Tawa, M.D.
Albert E. Raizner, M.D.

DESCRIPTION OF THE PROCEDURE

The Swan-Ganz catheter is a balloon-tipped, flexible multilumen and multifunction device that is placed in the systemic venous circulation and "floated" through the right-sided heart chambers to the pulmonary circulation. It has a broad spectrum of clinical usefulness and has become one of the most frequently used devices in intensive and critical care settings.

The most common sites of access used for insertion of Swan-Ganz catheters are the internal jugular, subclavian, and femoral veins. The right internal jugular provides a nearly straight line to the right atrium and is a favorite access route. The left subclavian is used as an alternative because of the broad anatomic curve that facilitates the passage of the catheter to the right atrium. The femoral route is frequently used in the cardiac catheterization laboratory under fluoroscopic guidance.

The catheter is available in sterile, prepackaged kits that provide all the instruments needed for the procedure. The access site is prepped and draped in a sterile fashion after adequate positioning of the patient. The operator dons cap, mask, sterile gown, and gloves, and the kit is opened with the contents kept sterile. All catheter lines are flushed. The balloon is tested for leaks and all transducer ports are hooked up. Gently shaking the balloon tip should produce a smooth sinusoidal wave on the monitor.

The vein is then cannulated and an introducer sheath is advanced over the guidewire using the modified Seldinger technique. The Swan-Ganz catheter, with the protective clear contamination sleeve in place, is threaded through the introducer valve and advanced into the right atrium (20-cm mark) under continuous electrocardiographic and pressure monitoring. The balloon is inflated with 1.5 ml of air, and

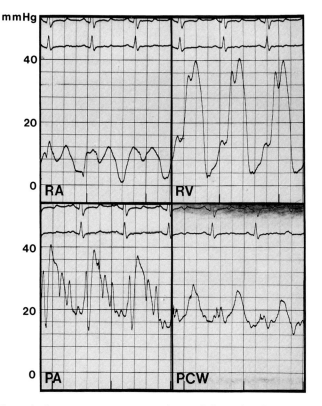

Figure 5.1. The right heart pressure tracings obtained through a Swan-Ganz catheter in a patient with a non Q wave myocardial infarction which was thought to involve the inferior left ventricular wall. The patient developed clinical signs of left and right heart failure. The pulmonary capillary wedge pressure is elevated (normal mean is <12 mmHg) with a prominent V wave suggesting mitral regurgitation secondary to papillary muscle dysfunction. There is mild pulmonary hypertension, with PA and RV systolic pressures of 40 mmHg, which is secondary to mitral regurgitation and left ventricular dysfunction. Additionally, the RV end diastolic pressure is elevated at 14 mmHg (normal <8 mmHg) and RA pressure is elevated as well (normal mean is <8 mmHg). These signs of RV dysfunction suggested concomitant RV infarction. Adjustment of inotropic agents, afterload reducing agents and volume was feasible using these hemodynamic measurements.
RA = right atrium, RV = right ventricle, PA = pulmonary artery, PCW = pulmonary capillary wedge.

the catheter is slowly advanced into the right ventricle, around the 30- to 40-cm mark, which produces a characteristic tracing on the monitor (steep upstroke with a sharp downstroke without a dicrotic notch). The catheter is advanced farther into the pulmonary artery (45- to 50-cm mark), characterized by a higher end diastolic pressure and a dicrotic notch. The catheter should then be advanced a few centimeters until a wedge tracing is obtained, recognized by damping of the pressure tracing with characteristic waveform (see figure 5.1). The balloon should then be deflated, producing a full pulmonary arterial tracing. Reinflation should reproduce a wedge tracing. The marking on the Swan-Ganz catheter at the level of the introducer sheath is recorded, and the protective contamination sleeve is pulled over the exposed catheter to the point where it enters the introducer sheath. The sheath is sutured in place and a dressing is applied over the insertion site on the patient's skin. The sterile drapes are removed and the patient is repositioned in a comfortable position. A chest roentgenogram is obtained to verify proper placement of the catheter tip in the right or left pulmonary artery, and to document the absence of a pneumothorax or tracheal shift.

HISTORY OF THE PROCEDURE

In the intensive care units of the 1960s and 1970s, preload and intravascular volume were assessed indirectly by monitoring blood pressure, heart rate, urine output, and general physical examination of the patient. Bedside central venous pressure monitoring was introduced in the 1960s but proved to be a poor indicator of left ventricular filling pressure,[1] especially in patients with cardiopulmonary disease and in elderly surgical patients. Hence, the idea of catheterization of the pulmonary artery for bedside hemodynamic measurement was developed. Dr. Swan, while watching sailboats on the beach in Santa Monica in 1967, serendipitously came up with the idea of putting a sail or a parachute on the end of a flexible catheter.[2] Simultaneously, Dr. Ganz was developing the thermodilution method for measurement of blood flow. Both investigators reported the first clinical use of the double-lumen, balloon-tipped pulmonary artery catheter in 1970.[3] The next developments were the addition of a third lumen with a port 30 cm proximal to the catheter tip for simultaneous measurement of right atrial pressure. A thermistor fitted to the catheter tip allowed temperature measurements. Injection of 10 ml of iced D5W or saline through the proximal port permitted calculation of cardiac output using the thermodilution technique. Subsequently, fiber-optic bundles were added for continuous monitoring of mixed venous oxygen saturation by reflection oximetry. The next step was the development of pacing pulmonary artery catheters for AV sequential pacing. The latest generation of pulmonary artery catheters allows determination of the right ventricular ejection fraction by using fast-response thermistors. Today, a little more than two decades after development of the original pulmonary artery catheter, it is estimated that over one million catheters are used annually in the United States. In contrast, only 6000 are used each year in the United Kingdom.[4]

INDICATIONS

Swan-Ganz catheterization is indicated for the hemodynamic monitoring of patients with significant cardiopulmonary derangement. For instance, when ventricular function is compromised in myocardial infarction, the catheter can provide crucial information on the efficacy of pharmacologic support and aid in recognition of pericardial tamponade and acute mitral regurgitation. Shock is another indication for the insertion of a pulmonary artery catheter, both as a diagnostic tool and a guide for fluid and inotropic management. A pulmonary artery catheter is generally indicated in patients with failure of two organ systems (eg, kidneys and lungs) that might have different priorities with respect to fluid administration. Right-heart catheterization is also essential to confirm the diagnosis of pulmonary hypertension and assess its reversibility. Pulmonary artery catheter insertion may also be indicated for patients undergoing surgical procedures associated with large volume requirements and fluid shifts, or before elective procedures in patients at higher risk for perioperative cardiac complications. Finally, a pulmonary artery catheter can be used to obtain blood samples from various sites of the circulation for oximetric measurements and shunt calculations.

CONTRAINDICATIONS

The only absolute contraindication to Swan-Ganz catheter insertion is the presence of a prosthetic tricuspid valve, as passage of a pulmonary artery catheter could cause valve malfunction. Relative contraindications to central vein puncture include bleeding diatheses, thrombocytopenia, and thrombolytic therapy. Severe atherosclerosis, by distorting vessel architecture, can increase the risk of inadvertent arterial puncture, causing bleeding, plaque dislodgment, and distal embolization. Caution is needed in patients with endocardial pacemaker leads, as catheter passage could dislodge a pacing electrode. The presence of left bundle branch block is another relative contraindication to pulmonary artery catheter insertion unless backup pacing is available.

COMPLICATIONS OF PULMONARY ARTERY CATHETERS

Most complications associated with pulmonary artery catheterization are minor. However, a 4% incidence of major, potentially life-threatening complications has been reported.[5]

Complications Associated with Central Vein Cannulation

Inadvertent arterial puncture has been reported in 2% to 16% of cases[5,6] and correlates with operator skill and the number of attempts. Carotid artery puncture may result in a hematoma, which should be readily recognized and managed by application of pressure over the puncture site. However, in patients with a bleeding diathesis or those receiving anticoagulation therapy in whom the artery is lacerated with a large-bore introducer sheath, a large hematoma can result, leading to rapid airway compromise requiring surgical intervention. Obviously, another cannulation attempt on the contralateral side of the neck is contraindicated owing to increased risk of respiratory and cerebral circulation compromise should a second hematoma develop. The use of ultrasound may reduce the incidence of arterial injury.[7]

Complications resulting from subclavian artery puncture are more insidious and can manifest as a hemothorax on a chest roentgenogram. Manual compression of the subclavian artery is impossible to achieve, and surgical repair of the vessel may in rare instances be needed, with concomitant needle thoracentesis or tube thoracostomy to evacuate the hemothorax and allow for lung reexpansion. Arterial puncture can be minimized by optimizing the anatomic landmarks (turning the head to the contralateral side, placing the patient in Trendelenburg's position), and by using a small-gauge needle to localize the target vessel.

Penetration of the pleura can result in a pneumothorax and has been reported in about 2% of cases.[8] It is usually a complication of an attempted subclavian puncture and is less frequent with the internal jugular approach. The incidence is increased in restless patients and in obese patients with poorly defined landmarks. Clinical manifestations include tachypnea, tachycardia, chest pain, and decreased breath sounds and respiratory excursions of the affected side. Tension pneumothorax occurs primarily in intubated patients and can rapidly progress to hemodynamic collapse. The diagnosis is made by chest roentgenography. Pneumothoraces are best prevented by optimizing the anatomic landmarks and by advancing the needle during expiration, avoiding high peak pressures if the patient is mechanically ventilated.

Treatment of a pneumothorax involves close observation and serial chest roentgenograms (in the stable, minimally symptomatic patient with a small pneumothorax) or tube thoracostomy for lung reexpansion when clinically indicated.

Puncture of the trachea or esophagus during catheter insertion is rare and can lead to subcutaneous emphysema. Close clinical observation with CT scan correlation to rule out a deep neck abscess is prudent. The use of prophylactic broad-spectrum antibiotics is controversial. Cannulation of the left internal jugular vein can damage the thoracic duct and result in a chylothorax.[9] It is diagnosed by thoracentesis and treated conservatively with local pressure, avoidance of medium- and long-chain fatty acids in the diet or hyperalimentation solution. However, a persistent chyle fistula may warrant exploration and ligation of a thoracic duct stump.

Air embolism can result from failing to backfill the introducer with blood to eliminate air before infusion or, more frequently, if the patient takes a deep inspiration when a large-bore needle or introducer is open to air. Symptoms as severe as hypotension and cardiovascular collapse can occur. Air embolism is best avoided by using Trendelenburg's position, obtaining a flashback of blood in the line before attaching intravenous fluids, and not leaving a catheter port open to air. Air embolism is treated by placing the patient in the left lateral decubitus position to trap the air in the right ventricle. Aspiration may be attempted or the air may be left to slowly dissipate through the pulmonary vasculature. Echocardiography is useful in assessing the extent of right ventricular impairment by air emboli and monitoring its recovery.

Other unusual complications of central vein puncture include Horner's syndrome secondary to injury of the preganglionic sympathetic chain, and injuries to the brachial plexus and the phrenic and recurrent laryngeal nerves.

Complications Unique to Pulmonary Artery Catheter Advancement

These include arrhythmias, right bundle branch block and complete heart block, ventricular rupture, tricuspid valve damage, and intracardiac knotting.

Arrhythmias secondary to pulmonary artery catheter advancement result from endocardial irritation by the catheter tip and are more frequent with inexperienced operators. Short runs of ventricular tachycardia are frequently noted during passage of the catheter through the right ventricular infundibulum. However, the incidence of sustained ventricular tachycardia or ventricular fibrillation necessitating emergency countershock is less than 1% occurring predominantly in patients with myocardial infarction involving the right ventricle.[10] Preliminary correction of predisposing factors to arrhythmias (such as hypokalemia, hypocalcemia, hypoxemia, and acidosis) is advisable before starting the procedure, but may not always be possible. Catheter-induced arrhythmias are treated by withdrawing the catheter to the right atrium or advancing it to the pulmonary artery. Prophylactic lidocaine administration is of no clear benefit.

Right bundle branch block is due to mechanical irritation of the bundle of His, which is located beneath the septal endocardium of the right ventricle and is suscepti-ble to trauma from the catheter tip, especially if the balloon is not fully inflated. Transient right bundle branch block is usually inconsequential, with an incidence of about 5%. Patients with a preexisting left bundle branch block can develop potentially fatal complete heart block. Therefore, a pulmonary artery catheter should be consid-ered in these patients only if pacemaker backup is available and if the data to be acquired are vital to patient management.

Cardiac tamponade resulting from perforation of the right atrium or right ventricle is rare (less than 1% of cases). It is manifested by hypotension, distended neck veins, and equalization of diastolic pressures in the heart chambers. The diagnosis is confirmed by echocardiography. Tamponade is treated by pericardiocentesis to re-move blood from the pericardial sac; emergency thoracotomy should be considered in certain cases.

Tricuspid and pulmonic valve damage can occur during catheter passage, espe-cially if the catheter is pulled back through the valves in a retrograde manner with the balloon inflated. Valvular dysfunction may also result from the mere presence of the catheters across a valve for a prolonged period of time. Clinical manifestations include new murmurs, elevated right atrial v waves and even right-sided failure. Little can be done to prevent valve damage except to withdraw the catheter gently, making sure the balloon is deflated, and to minimize long-term use of the catheter.

Intracardiac knotting has a reported incidence of less than 1% and occurs when a loop of the catheter recoils in the right ventricle or pulmonary artery. Knotting is usually associated with small-bore catheters, underinflated balloons, dilated hearts, and low flow states. This complication is best prevented by using fluoroscopy when-ever difficulty is met in advancing the catheter. J wire passage can be useful in resolving simple catheter knots. Complex knotting around intracardiac structures such as chordae tendinae or other indwelling catheters will mandate a surgical approach.

Shearing of the catheter with catheter tip embolization is a rare complication, caused by operator inexperience. Embolized fragments can usually be retrieved under fluoroscopic guidance using snaring catheters.

Complications Related to Catheter Maintenance

Infection is a prevalent complication associated with the long-term presence of a pulmonary artery catheter in the circulation. A 5.8% incidence of positive tip cultures was reported in a prospective study,[11] correlating with a higher mortality. Catheter-induced septicemia has been documented in 0.5 to 1% of patients, with an increased risk if the catheter is left in place for a prolonged period of time (0.5%/day/catheter).[12]

Routine catheter exchange over a guidewire has no effect on reducing the risk of infection. The most common causative organisms are coagulase-negative staphylococci, *Staphylococcus aureus,* and *Candida.* Treatment of catheter-related sepsis involves catheter removal, culture of the tip, antibiotic coverage according to culture isolate, and the use of a new insertion site.

Catheter-related right-sided endocardial lesions are frequent, with an incidence of 53% in a large autopsy study.[13] The pulmonic valve was most commonly affected (56%), followed by the tricuspid valve (15%), right atrium (15%), right ventricle (10%), and main pulmonary artery (5%). Most lesions consist of localized endocardial ulcerations with hemorrhage, sterile vegetations, and mural thrombi. These can serve as foci for bacterial colonization leading to infective or thrombotic vegetations.

Pulmonary infarction usually results from unexpected distal catheter migration in the pulmonary circulation, prolonged balloon inflation, or thromboembolism. The incidence of this complication has decreased from 7.2% in 1974[14] to 1.3% in a more recent series.[15] Continuous display of the pulmonary artery waveform is necessary to assure proper location of the catheter tip, and the appearance of a permanently wedged waveform mandates withdrawal of the catheter far enough to reestablish a normal pulmonary artery tracing. Daily chest roentgenograms are recommended to locate the catheter tip within the mediastinal shadow. Treatment of pulmonary infarction includes removal of the pulmonary artery catheter, oxygen supplementation, analgesics, and close clinical follow-up.

Pulmonary artery perforation or rupture are the most catastrophic complications of pulmonary artery catheterization, reported in about 0.1% to 0.2% of patients,[15,16] with an estimated mortality rate of 50%. Advancing a catheter with an underinflated balloon can result in vessel laceration, or overinflation of the balloon can cause vessel rupture. Patients of advanced age, with pulmonary hypertension, or undergoing cardiac surgery are at increased risk. Catheter-induced pulmonary artery pseudoaneurysms are rare and can cause delayed rupture within hours to weeks following catheterization.[17] Pulmonary artery rupture is prevented by minimizing balloon inflations and by inflating the balloon slowly under continuous pressure monitoring.[5]

Rupture presents with hemoptysis, hypoxia, and acute cardiopulmonary collapse, with air-space opacification noted on chest roentgenogram. Treatment involves emergent thoracotomy with vascular repair or lobectomy. Temporizing measures include turning the patient to a lateral decubitus position with the bleeding lung down, blood and volume replacement, intubation with a double-lumen tracheal tube with positive end-expiratory pressure administration, and heparin reversal.[5]

Venous thrombosis and thrombophlebitis occur in up to 20% of cases, manifested by local tenderness, pain, edema, and erythema. These are minimized by strict adherence to sterile technique during insertion, securing the catheter at the entry site to prevent movement, and changing the insertion site every 72 hours.[18] Thrombophlebitis is most common when the femoral vein is cannulated and the catheter and introducer are left in place more than 24 hours. Prompt recognition and catheter removal are the best treatment for thrombophlebitis, along with warm compress application and prophylactic gram-positive antibiotic coverage. Heparin therapy and possible vein excision may be considered if there are signs of sepsis secondary to an infected thrombus. Low cardiac output, disseminated intravascular coagulation and congestive heart failure have each been associated with a higher incidence of thrombus formation. Heparin-coated catheters markedly reduce the incidence of pericatheter thrombosis,[19] at least during the first 24 hours after insertion. However, there have been reports of heparin-induced thrombocytopenia attributed to heparin-coated pulmonary artery catheters and introducer sheaths.

Balloon rupture is a relatively innocuous complication, usually resulting from multiple inflations, or overinflation of the balloon. It tends to occur in catheters left in place for a prolonged period as lipoprotein absorption by the latex causes loss of elasticity. It is manifested by a loss of resistance when inflating the balloon and inability to obtain a wedge tracing.

CONCLUSION

Pulmonary artery catheterization can be associated with significant complications. Although most are avoidable by careful technique and close monitoring, a small risk will always be present, as is true for all invasive procedures. The decision to insert a pulmonary artery catheter should be made after carefully weighing the potential risks versus benefits pertaining to each patient. The catheter should be removed as soon as the hemodynamic information it provides ceases to be essential.

REFERENCES

1. Forrester JS, Diamond G, McHugh TJ, et al. Filling pressure in right and left sides of the heart in acute myocardial infarction: a reappraisal of central venous pressure monitoring. *N Engl J Med.* 285:190, 1971.

2. Swan HJC. The pulmonary artery catheter. *Disease a Month.* 8:478–543, 1991.

3. Swan HJC, Ganz W, Forrester J, et al. Catheterization of the heart in man with the use of flow-directed balloon-tipped catheter. *N Engl J Med.* 283:447, 1970.

4. Singer M, Bennett ED. Invasive hemodynamic monitoring in the United Kingdom: enough or too little? *Chest.* 95:623–626, 1989.

5. Ermakov S, Hoyt JW. Pulmonary artery catheterization. *Crit Care Clin.* 8:773–805, 1992.

6. Jobes DR, Schwarz AJ, Greenhow DE, Stephenson LW, Ellison N. Safer jugular vein cannulation: recognition of arterial puncture and preferential use of the external jugular route. *Anesthesiology.* 59:353–355, 1983.

7. Troianos CA, Jobes DR, Ellison N. Ultrasound-guided cannulation of the internal jugular vein: a prospective, randomized study. *Anesth Analg.* 72:823–826, 1991.

8. Steingrub JS, Celoria G, Vickers-Lahti M, Teres D, Bria W. Therapeutic impact of pulmonary artery catheterization in a medical/surgical ICU. *Chest.* 99:1451S, 1991.

9. Khalil KG, Parker FB, Jr, Mukherjee N, Webb WR. Thoracic duct injury. *JAMA.* 211:908–909, 1972.

10. Lopez-Sendon J, Lopez de Sa E, Maqueda IG, et al. Right ventricular infarction as a risk factor for ventricular fibrillation during pulmonary artery catheterization using Swan-Ganz catheters. *Am Heart J.* 119:207–209, 1990.

11. Myers ML, Austin RW, Sibbald WJ. Pulmonary artery catheter infections: a prospective study. *Ann Surg.* 201:237–241, 1985.

12. Eyer S, Brummitt C, Crossley K, Siegel R, Cerra F. Catheter-related sepsis: prospective,

randomized study of three methods of long-term catheter maintenance. *Crit Care Med.* 18:1073–1079, 1990.

13. Rowley KM, Clubb KS, Smith GJW, Cabin HS. Right-sided infective endocarditis as a consequence of flow-directed pulmonary artery catheterization. *N Engl J Med.* 311:1152–1156, 1984.

14. Foote GA, Schabel SI, Hodges M. Pulmonary complications of the flow-directed balloon-tipped catheter. *N Engl J Med.* 290:927–931, 1974.

15. Boyd KD, Thomas SJ, Gold J, Boyd AD. A prospective study of complications of pulmonary artery catheterizations in 500 consecutive patients. *Chest.* 84:245–249, 1983.

16. Shah KB, Rao TLK, Loughlin S, El-Etr AA. A review of pulmonary artery catheterization in 6245 patients. *Anesthesiol.* 61:271–275, 1984.

17. Dieden JD, Friloux LA III, Renner JW. Pulmonary artery false aneurysms secondary to Swan-Ganz pulmonary artery catheters. *AJR.* 149:901–906, 1987.

18. Masters S. Complications of pulmonary artery catheters. *Crit Care Nursing.* 9:82–91, 1989.

19. Hoar PF, Wilson RM, Mangano DT, Avery GJ, Szarnicki RJ, Hill JD. Heparin bonding reduces thrombogenicity of pulmonary artery catheters. *N Engl J Med.* 305:993–995, 1981.

— 6 —

Prevention and Treatment of Complications in Cardiac Catheterization

Stephen D. Clements, Jr., M.D.

INTRODUCTION

Cardiac catheterization is a well-established invasive procedure which is performed in large numbers in hospitals, outpatient labs and mobile cath. labs. It is an effective method for confirmation of the presence and severity of a wide variety of cardiac diseases. Although catheterization is frequently used to determine the severity of valvular, congenital and myocardial diseases characterization of the extent on coronary disease is the most common indication.

Cardiac catheterization has been performed for more than 150 years. Claude Bernard performed cardiac catheterization first, in 1844, in horses via the carotid and internal jugular approaches.[1] However, meaningful cardiac catheterization in humans required the radiographic and medical techniques of the 20th century. Forssmann, as a surgical resident, performed catheterization on himself using urethral catheters in the late 1920s.[2] Klein, in the 1930s, reported right ventricular catheterizations in humans primarily focusing on cardiac output determinations using the Fick principle.[3] Cournand and Richards studied right heart physiology in the early 1940s[4,5,6] and, later in 1947, Dexter began studies in individuals with congenital heart disease.[7] Seldinger, in 1953, introduced the percutaneous technique, which facilitated use of the retrograde aortic cannulation.[8] In 1959, Sones injected contrast into a coronary artery and opened doors that led to modern coronary arteriography.[9] Swan and Ganz, in 1970, introduced balloon-tipped catheters for right ventricular catheterization, leading to the hemodynamic monitoring of today.[10] Cardiac catheterization laid the groundwork for more advanced techniques including valvuloplasty, creation and

64

closure of septal defects, dilation of stenotic congenital lesions and the myriad of interventional coronary procedures to relieve coronary stenosis.

In all cardiac catheterizations the potential for complications exists because foreign bodies and substances are introduced into the human body. This potential for complications is enhanced since many patients are already in poor health.

INDICATIONS FOR CARDIAC CATHETERIZATION

Patients with congenital and valvular lesions can now be identified as to the anatomy and severity of the cardiac lesions by noninvasive methods such that in general, only those patients in whom surgery is contemplated are candidates for catheterization. In some cases, disorders such as an isolated atrial septal defect in a young patient may not require catheterization before surgery. Delineation of coronary anatomy may be an indication for arteriography in older patients in whom the cardiac defects are well established before surgery.

In dilated cardiomyopathy, coronary arteriography may necessitate study before listing for cardiac transplantation to insure no other mode of therapy is possible. In hypertrophic myopathy, physiologic data may be needed before correction by either pacing or surgical techniques.

In patients with suspected or known coronary disease, coronary arteriography is indicated for patients in whom noninvasive procedures fail to delineate the severity of disease and in those patients with sufficient myocardial ischemia to warrant intervention.

CONTRAINDICATIONS TO CARDIAC CATHETERIZATION

The contraindications to catheterization are generally relative. With adequate preprocedural intervention, attention to detail during the procedure (including changes in catheter insertion site) and closer observation postprocedure, most patients can undergo catheterization if needed. Table 6.1 lists the groups of patients in whom extraordinary care is needed.[11]

OCCURRENCE OF COMPLICATIONS

Despite careful techniques and attention to detail, complications still occur as a result of cardiac catheterization. Fortunately, major complications are rare: death (0.1% to 0.2%), myocardial infarction (0.06% to 0.1%), and stroke (0.07% to 0.1%).[12,13,14]

In one study reported by the Society for Cardiac Angiography and Intervention, death occurred in 0.1%, myocardial infarction in 0.06%, and stroke in 0.07% of cases. This registry of patients included 222553 patients.[13] Brachial and femoral approaches were included in this registry study with no significant difference in major complications noted in these techniques.

TABLE 6.1. High-Risk Patients Who Require Special Care Prior to Catheterization

High risk for vascular complications
Morbid obesity
Severe peripheral vascular disease
Mechanical prosthetic valve
General debility or cachexia
Low ejection fraction ($\leq 35\%$)
Anticoagulation or bleeding diathesis
Uncontrolled systemic hypertension
Patient's home a significant distance from catheterization laboratory
Diabetes mellitus that is difficult to control
Chronic corticosteroid use
History of radiographic contrast material allergy
Severe chronic obstructive lung disease
Less than 21 years of age or complex congenital heart disease, regardless of age
Recent stroke (within 1 month)
Severe ischemia during stress testing
Pulmonary hypertension
Arterial desaturation

From ACC/AHA Guidelines for Cardiac Catherization in *The Journal of American College of Cardiology* 18:(5)1149–1182, 1991. Elsevier Science Publishing Co, NY. Modified and reproduced with permission.

Other complications include arrhythmias requiring either drug treatment or a temporary pacemaker. The occurrence of these events has been reported to be from 0.3% to 0.94%.[13]

Vascular problems associated with catheterization that may require surgical intervention include femoral or brachial thrombosis, hemorrhage, pseudoaneurysm formation, or arteriovenous fistula formation. Vascular occlusion is more common in the brachial approach (0.96%) versus the femoral artery approach (0.22%). Hemorrhage from the femoral approach in a large series of procedures was in the 0.10% range versus 0.01% for brachial approach. Retroperitoneal hemorrhage, although infrequent (0.15%), is a serious complication and can result in significant morbidity and mortality.[15]

Arteriovenous fistulas and pseudoaneurysms are infrequent occurrences estimated to occur in 0.02% and 0.05% of patients, respectively.[16] False aneurysms also occur after catheterization, but arteriovenous fistulas and false aneurysms are both much more common after percutaneous transluminal angioplasty. McCann reported logistic regression analysis of vascular complications in all catheterization procedures, including angioplasty, at Duke University. He found that congestive heart failure, female sex, and angioplasty or valvuloplasty were associated with vascular injury. In addition, greater age, smaller body surface area, and less body weight also were often associated with injury.[17]

Percutaneous transluminal angioplasty or procedures that require anticoagulation for prolonged periods, particularly with use of the stent, strongly predispose the individual to serious hemorrhage and other vascular complications.

Cerebrovascular events occur in about 0.1% of individuals undergoing cardiac catheterization.[13] The mechanisms probably vary in etiology. Catheters entering the circulation via the femoral artery or femoral sheath may pick up thrombus material that may embolize to the cerebral circulation.[18,19] Catheters may dislodge atherosclerotic debris from the ascending aorta or aortic arch. Transesophageal echo has demonstrated atheromatous material in the ascending aorta that is ulcerated and pedunculated, providing a source for dislodgment by catheters or guidewires. Valvular material or intracardiac thrombi can be dislodged by catheters and wires. These events consist of embolic phenomenon to either the anterior or posterior cerebral circulation.

In one series, 5 of 12 individuals with stroke had involvement in the distribution of the posterior circulation.[20] Fortunately, many of these defects resolve in 24 hours but occasionally last longer and result in a life-threatening situation.

Embolic phenomena can occur in any vascular distribution, including renal, splenic, and mesenteric. Rarely, atherosclerotic material may be mobilized from the descending thoracic or abdominal aorta. This produces the so-called cholesterol emboli phenomenon, with obstruction of small arteries in the lower extremities resulting in varying degrees of skin necrosis.

The contrast media used in cardiac catheterization may produce adverse effects. Contrast reactions consisting of hives, hypotension, and anaphylaxis occur in about 2% of individuals.[13] In addition, the effects of contrast media on renal function can be profound, especially in the setting of renal failure (creatinine > 2.0 mg %) and diabetes.

Catheters themselves may injure the coronaries in a number of different ways. Occasionally, as the catheter engages the coronary, a small plaque may be elevated and, as injection occurs, dissection of the artery results. The dissection may propagate as it is subjected to systemic pressure and the coronary can become occluded.[21] It is possible that thrombotic material or air may be injected down a coronary artery from the catheter. Also, during power injection of the ventricles, the catheter can become entrapped, and intramyocardial injection or even myocardial perforation may occur, leading to cardiac tamponade.

There are clearly certain subsets of individuals that are at higher risk of a major complication.[13] Severity of heart disease is a strong risk factor for complication and, in particular, severe left main obstruction. Other systemic problems such as renal failure, especially when combined with diabetes, and generalized vascular disease also increase the risk of complications of cardiac catheterization.

TREATMENT AND MANAGEMENT

Complications during cardiac catheterization are relatively infrequent, and their incidence may be further reduced by use of appropriate procedures. In the event that complications do develop, prompt treatment may often minimize their severity.

The possibility of arrhythmias due to the contrast injection is always present during cardiac catheterization. If hypotension or bradycardia occurs with each contrast injection, then allowing more time for hemodynamic recovery between injections may avoid some complications of these types. The use of nonionic contrast also appears to decrease the frequency of ventricular arrhythmias requiring defibrillation.

If a history of previous reactions to contrast media is present, preparation with corticosteroids and antihistamines will usually prevent any future reactions. Prompt treatment with epinephrine and corticosteroids if hypotension or anaphylaxis occurs usually aborts the reaction. Rarely, myocardial depression in the myocardium occurs as a result of calcium antagonism and may result in left ventricular power failure; fortunately, this condition responds well to intravenous calcium administration. Newer nonionic contrast agents result in less hemodynamic compromise and less nausea but still present iodinated compounds into the circulation.

The effects of contrast media on renal function may be significant. Care must be taken to have the individual well hydrated and contrast volume should be minimized, particularly if renal failure or diabetes are present.[22]

The introduction of the catheter into the heart region may itself produce undesirable reactions. In individuals who have RBBB, care must be taken while introducing catheters into the left ventricle because transient complete heart block can occur. The same holds for LBBB and introduction of catheters into the right ventricle.[23,24] The size of the catheter employed may affect the incidence of such events. Prophylactic temporary pacing should be considered in these patients.

For diagnostic cardiac catheterization, the introduction of smaller catheters has reduced the incidence of hemorrhage. Also, individuals undergoing angioplasty with larger introducing sheaths and anticoagulants have a higher incidence of hematomas and retroperitoneal hemorrhage.

Vascular complications such as retroperitoneal hemorrhage, false aneurysm, arteriovenous fistula, and femoral thrombosis are rare in low-risk outpatients. The use of small catheters, no anticoagulants, fewer catheter changes, and the use of multipurpose catheters are all factors that minimize vascular complications.

Retroperitoneal hemorrhage is an infrequent but potentially serious complication. Individuals who, after catheterization or angioplasty, exhibit falling hematocrit, lower abdominal pain, or neurological changes in the lower extremity should be investigated early with CT scan of the abdomen, looking for retroperitoneal hemorrhage.

Arteriovenous fistulas sometimes develop after cardiac catheterization and are diagnosed by noting a continuous bruit over the puncture site. This may or may not be painful and may be present in the absence of any swelling or discoloration at the catheterization puncture site. The formation of this complication requires concomitant puncture of artery and vein. Often the vein is underlying the artery predisposing to this complication. Once arteriovenous fistulas are suspected, ultrasound visualization of the fistulous tract with color Doppler confirms the diagnosis. Some fistulas spontaneously close, some can be compressed and undergo closure, and others require surgical closure. Repeatedly, surgeons comment that the earlier the closure, the less the associated inflammatory reaction and the easier the repair.

False aneurysms are manifest by pulsatile, usually painful masses over the artery at the puncture site. Nerve compression by the mass may occur, resulting in pain radiating down the thigh. Sometimes there is a bruit over the mass from blood entering or leaving the aneurysm. Ultrasound with color Doppler also confirms the diagnosis, demonstrating a fluid-filled cavity with turbulent flow into the area and sometimes swirling blood within the aneurysm. Compression of smaller aneurysms may result in closure. Large aneurysms are often painful, difficult to compress and generally require surgical closure. (The earlier the better from the surgical standpoint). Obese or overweight patients are more likely to develop such aneurysms, since a good seal via compression of the arterial puncture site is more difficult to obtain in such individuals.

To ensure the catheter tip is properly placed, each time a catheter is positioned, a small test injection of contrast can establish the presence of rapid runoff. This rapid runoff indicates that the catheter tip is not bound, entrapped, or subintimal. Once correct placement is confirmed, one can proceed with whatever injection is needed without dissection or perforation of nearby tissues. One should also check for damping of arterial pressure before injection of contrast. Damping of pressure may indicate osteal stenosis, catheter obstruction of a small artery, or that the catheter has entered an area where it does not belong and should be withdrawn. The number of injections should be minimized in individuals with osteal right or left main stenoses. Once adequate information is obtained, the patient should be anticoagulated, the surgeon called, and a sheath left in the groin for the balloon pump if needed.

Individuals who are very ill from a recent myocardial infarction or congestive heart failure also are at greater risk for major complications from cardiac catheterization. The number of injections should be minimized in these individuals as well. If surgical intervention is needed, the patient should be anticoagulated, the surgeon called, and a sheath left in the groin should a balloon pump be needed. Occasionally, a very tightly narrowed lesion will become totally occluded after contrast injection, precipitating the need for acute intervention.

Although risks associated with cardiac catheterization can probably never be completely eliminated, consistent utilization of the preceding procedures can reduce the already low levels of complications associated with cardiac catheterization and reduce the severity of any complications that may occur. Recent experience at Emory University covering a series of 3000 selected low-risk patients receiving cardiac catheterization in the Andreas Gruentzig Outpatient Laboratory demonstrates that complications can be minimized in selected groups of patients.[25] Twenty-three and one-half percent of these individuals had normal coronary arteriograms and 10.8% had triple vessel disease. There was no mortality, five instances of ventricular fibrillation, two small cerebral emboli with subsequent total recovery, two severe allergic reactions, three pseudoaneurysms, three episodes of bleeding at home requiring reapplication of pressure, and one localized infection at the puncture site. Major complications of death, myocardial infarction, and stroke were absent or minimal in this selected group of patients, 81.8% of which were discharged home the day of the procedure. Pink reported a very similar incidence of complications in a group of 1000 outpatient cardiac catheterizations.[26]

CONCLUSION

The potential for infrequent complications associated with cardiac catheterization is always present. As cardiac catheterization is planned, potential complications should be anticipated in light of the predisposing factors. This allows alteration of the procedure to minimize complications. Being aware of the complications allows for early recognition and facilitates prompt treatment when indicated. Using the suggestions outlined earlier in this chapter, the incidence and severity of complications associated with cardiac catheterization may be further reduced.

REFERENCES

1. Cournand, A. Cardiac catheterization: development of the technique, its contributions to experimental medicine, and its initial application in man. *Acta Med Scand.* 579 (suppl):1, 1975.
2. Forssmann W. Die Sondierung des rechten Herzens. *Klin Wochenschr.* 8:2085, 1929.
3. Klein O. Zur bestimmung des zirkulatorischen minutensvohumen nach dem Fickschen. *Prinzip Munch Med.* 77:1311, 1930.
4. Cournand AF, Ranges HS. Catheterization of the right auricle in man. *Proc Soc Exp Biol Med.* 46:462, 1941.
5. Richards DW. Cardiac output by the catheterization technique in various clinical conditions. *Fed Proc.* 4:215, 1945.
6. Cournand AF, Riley RL, Breed ES, et al. Measurement of cardiac output in man using the technique of catheterization of the right auricle. *J Clin Invest.* 24:106, 1945.
7. Dexter L, Haynes FW, Burwell CS, et al. Studies of congenital heart disease, II: the pressure and oxygen content of blood in the right auricle, right ventricle, and pulmonary artery in control patients, with observations on the oxygen saturation and source of pulmonary "capillary" blood. *J Clin Invest.* 26:554, 1947.
8. Seldinger SI. Catheter replacement of the needle in percutaneous arteriography: a new technique. *Acta Radiol.* 39:368, 1953.
9. Sones FM, Shirey EK, Proudfit WL, Westcott RN. Cine coronary arteriography. *Circulation.* 20:773, 1959.
10. Swan HJC, Ganz W, Forrester J, et al. Catheterization of the heart in man with use of a flow-directed balloon-tipped catheter. *N Engl J Med.* 283:447, 1970.
11. Ad Hoc Task Force, Pepine CJ (Chairman). ACC/AAA guidelines for cardiac catheterization and cardiac catheterization laboratories. *J Am Coll Cardiol.* 18:1149–1182, 1991.
12. Kennedy JW. Complications associated with cardiac catheterization and angiography. *Cathet Cardiovasc Diagn.* 8:5, 1982.
13. Johnson LW, Lozner EC, Johnson S, et al. Coronary angiography 1984–1987: a report of the registry of the Society for Cardiac Angiography and Interventions, I: results and complications. *Cathet Cardiovasc Diagn.* 17:5, 1989.
14. Folland ED, Oprian C, Giacomini J, et al. Complications of cardiac catheterization and angiography in patients with valvular heart disease. *Cathet Cardiovasc Diagn.* 17:15, 1989.
15. Sreeram S, Lumsden AB, Miller JS, et al. Retroperitoneal hematoma following femoral arterial catheterization: a serious and often fatal complication. *Am Surg.* 59:94–98, 1993.
16. Kirsch JD, Reading CC, Charboneau JW. Ultrasound-guided compression and repair of postangiographic femoral arteriovenous fistulas. *Mayo Clin Proc.* 68:612–613, 1993.
17. McCann RL, Schwartz LB, Pieper KS. Vascular complications of cardiac catheterization. *J Vasc Surg.* 14:375–381, 1991.
18. Judkins MP, Gander MP. Prevention of complications of coronary arteriography. *Circulation.* 49:599, 1974.
19. King SB, Douglas JS. *Coronary Arteriography and Angioplasty.* New York: McGraw-Hill; 303, 1985.
20. Alio J, Esplugas E, Arboix A, Rubio F. Cerebrovascular events in cardiac catheterization. *Stroke.* 24:1264, 1993.
21. Kitamura K, Gobel FL, and Wang Y. Dissection of the left coronary artery complicating retrograde left-heart catheterization. *Chest.* 57:587–590, 1970.

22. Abraham P, Harkonen S, Kjellstrond C. Contrast nephropathy. In: SG Massry, RJ Glassock, eds. *Textbook in Nephrology*. Baltimore, MD: Williams & Wilkins; 6.206, 1983.

23. Gupta PK, Haft JI. Complete heart block complicating cardiac catheterization. *Chest.* 61:185–187, 1972.

24. Cheng TO, Bashour T, Kelser GA. Complete heart block occurring during right-heart catheterization in a patient with left bundle branch block and prolonged P-R interval studied by bundle of his recording and atrial pacing. *Med Ann DC.* 41:742–743, 1972.

25. Clements SD, Gatlin S. Outpatient cardiac catheterization: a report of 3000 cases. *Clin Cardiol.* 14:477–480, 1991.

26. Pink S, Fiutowski L, Gianelly RE. Outpatient cardiac catheterization: analysis of patients requiring admission. *Clin Cardiol.* 12:375–378, 1969.

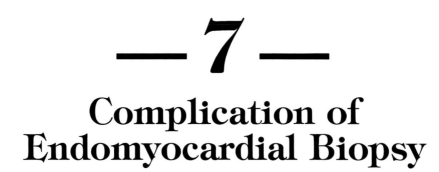

— 7 —

Complication of Endomyocardial Biopsy

Edward K. Kasper, M.D.
Kenneth L. Baughman, M.D.

TECHNIQUE OF ENDOMYOCARDIAL BIOPSY

Right ventricular endomyocardial biopsy can be performed percutaneously from the right internal jugular, right subclavian, and right or left femoral veins. The most frequently used approach is from the right internal jugular vein. Certain equipment and techniques are common to all of these approaches.

The patient should avoid eating for 8 hours before the procedure. No premedications are given before routine endomyocardial biopsy. Blood pressure, heart rate, rhythm, and peripheral oxygen saturation are noninvasively monitored throughout the procedure. The skin of the right neck is prepped using povidone-iodine and alcohol, and the area is isolated using sterile towels. An ether shield is useful to allow isolation of the field without covering the face of the patient.

The right internal jugular vein usually lies lateral to and above the carotid artery beneath the lateral edge of the medial head of the sternocleidomastoid muscle. It is usually located within 2 cm of the skin surface regardless of the size of the neck. It is important to define the area of the internal jugular vein before attempting any cannulation, as landmarks may subsequently become altered.

Once identified, the area is anesthetized with lidocaine along the anticipated venous pathway. We attempt internal jugular vein cannulation in the middle third of the neck, thus avoiding the apical pleural reflections and allowing compression of the carotid artery should puncture occur. The probing needle is initially directed toward the right nipple at a 45-degree angle to the plane of the neck. If the vein is not found, the needle is redirected more laterally and then medially only if the vein is still not found. Once the vein is found, the probing needle is withdrawn and a 2-mm slit is made at the insertion site with a No. 11 surgical blade.

The internal jugular vein is then cannulated using an 18-gauge Amplatz needle attached to a 10-ml syringe. A 9 French sheath is then inserted over a 0.38-in guide-wire positioned in the internal jugular vein through the Amplatz needle. The sheath is aspirated of blood and then flushed with heparinized solution.

The physicians at Johns Hopkins have continued to use fluoroscopy to direct the course of the biopsy forceps for routine endomyocardial biopsies. Others use echocardiographic guidance exclusively.[1] If the tip of the forceps can be visualized, either technique should reduce the risk of perforation. The 50-cm Caves-Schultz bioptome or a similarly shaped disposable bioptome is inserted with the tip pointed toward the lateral border of the right atrium. In the mid-right atrium, the tip of the bioptome is rotated anteriorly 180 degrees and advanced across the tricuspid valve. This approach avoids the posteromedially located coronary sinus, and can be used from either the right internal jugular or subclavian veins. If resistance is met, the bioptome should be withdrawn to the right atrium and a different angle of entry should be used. The bioptome is stiff and must be guided (not forced or prolapsed) through the cardiac chambers.

The bioptome is advanced within the right ventricle until the endocardium is encountered. This is confirmed by the appearance of premature ventricular depolarizations. The bioptome is directed posteromedially toward the right ventricular septum. The anteriorly positioned right ventricular freewall is only 1 to 2 mm thick and biopsy of this wall presents a high risk of perforation. The septum is located at a 45-degree angle to the plane of the patient's chest. The bioptome handle should be directed perpendicular to this plane. Echocardiography is particularly useful in making certain the bioptome is directed toward the septum and not the freewall. The bioptome is then withdrawn 1 to 2 cm and the jaws are opened. The bioptome is then slowly advanced to engage the septum, the jaws are closed, and the encapsulated specimen is then removed by gently pulling on the shaft of the bioptome. The bioptome may require a tug on removal, but a biopsy that requires more force may imply extensive scar tissue, a nearly transmural biopsy, or entrapment within the tricuspid apparatus. If this occurs, the specimen should be released and the bioptome redirected toward a different site. Sharp or visceral chest pain may imply a perforation, but the patient commonly experiences a tugging sensation during specimen removal. Repeated biopsies may mandate variation of the bioptome position within the right ventricle. Usually, three to five specimens are taken.

The approach from the femoral vein requires different equipment and technique. A 98-cm femoral venous bioptome sheath with a 135-degree dogleg angle is used to position the bioptome in the right ventricle. This angulation prevents insertion of the long sheath without a central wire guide. The wire guide and the long sheath are inserted through a 9 French sheath introduced into the left or right femoral vein using the Seldinger technique under sterile conditions following 1% local lidocaine anesthesia. Once the tip of the long sheath is in the high right atrium, the central guidewire is slowly withdrawn to allow the natural bend in the long sheath to direct the tip into the right ventricle. The long venous sheath comes in only one size. The short dogleg portion of the catheter may be too long for the transverse length of the right ventricle. If inserted, the end of the sheath may rest against the right ventricular freewall endocardium.

Insertion of the bioptome through the sheath may perforate the freewall. Therefore, the dogleg arm of the sheath may need to be shortened before insertion. The amount that the dogleg short arm of the sheath needs to be shortened can be judged by positioning the sheath on the outside of the chest over the silhouette of the heart using fluoroscopy. The long sheath is continuously flushed with heparinized solution to prevent clot formation. A 104-cm bioptome is then inserted through the long sheath, and right ventricular placement is confirmed by the appearance of premature ventricular depolarizations. As the stiff bioptome approaches the bend in the long sheath, the angle may straighten and move forward, resulting in loss of proper position within the right ventricle. When the bioptome tip is properly placed, it is advanced to contact the endomyocardial wall gently. The bioptome is then withdrawn 1 to 2 cm, the jaws opened, and the bioptome is again advanced until contact with the wall is again made. The bioptome is closed firmly and the specimen removed. The same amount of force is necessary to pull the specimen from the right ventricular septum using this approach as from the internal jugular vein approach. This is a matter of experience.

Following the procedure, the venous sheath is removed and gentle pressure is applied to obtain hemostasis. A bandage is applied and the patient is free to return home. If the procedure was complicated, or if a femoral approach was used, then a period of observation is necessary. Postprocedure chest radiography is not routinely performed. The patient can remove the bandage the following day. It is the responsibility of the operator to make sure the appropriate specimens are sent to pathology. The sectioned specimen should be reviewed by the operator with a pathologist to ensure adequacy of the specimen and to review any pathologic findings.

HISTORY OF MYOCARDIAL BIOPSY

The era of the modern percutaneous transvenous endomyocardial biopsy was introduced by Sakakibara and Konno in 1962.[2] Before this, there had been several descriptions of transthoracic needle biopsy of the left ventricle. The Konno bioptome was a large-diameter, stiff forceps that required brachial artery cutdown for insertion. In 1974, P.J. Richardson of King's College Hospital, London introduced the King's bioptome,[3] which was both smaller in diameter and more flexible. This bioptome could be inserted through either the internal jugular, subclavian, or femoral veins. In 1975, Caves introduced a bioptome developed at Stanford[4] (the Caves-Schultz bioptome), which remains the most frequently used bioptome today. The shaft is relatively flexible and measures 50 cm in length. Opening and closing the forceps handle controls both the jaws and the degree of curvature of the shaft. The jaws consist of one movable and one fixed hollow cup of 1.5 mm diameter. The edges of the cups are sharp in order to remove specimens by cutting rather than avulsion. Disposable bioptomes have been developed more recently. Currently, endomyocardial biopsy has progressed from a rather crude, rarely performed transthoracic procedure with considerable risk to a reliable and safe outpatient procedure. A large transplant center will perform several hundred myocardial biopsies each year.

INDICATIONS FOR MYOCARDIAL BIOPSY

The indications for endomyocardial biopsy remain controversial.[5] There are several well-recognized indications. These include monitoring for rejection in cardiac transplant recipients, grading the cardiotoxic effects of doxorubicin on the myocardium and differentiating between restrictive and constrictive heart disease. Other less well accepted indications include the detection of myocarditis and the diagnosis of specific causes of heart muscle disease such as amyloidosis. The argument against endomyocardial biopsy is that it infrequently finds a treatable cause of specific heart muscle disease.[5] Billingham, however, feels that endomyocardial biopsy, when intelligently examined, is a useful tool for the study of many cardiac disease states.[6] In truth, most biopsies of patients with a dilated cardiomyopathy will show changes consistent with an idiopathic process. These changes likely represent the limited number of ways the myocardium can respond to a variety of insults. Whether or not this is important knowledge to the treating clinician in managing a patient with dilated cardiomyopathy is uncertain. The authors feel strongly that this knowledge is both useful to the clinician and important to the patient who seeks an explanation for why this disorder has occurred. Biopsy results are most important in those patients who are young, have a recent onset of dilated cardiomyopathy (less than 6 months), have a suspected specific heart muscle disease, or who are cardiac transplant candidates.

The most exciting use for specimens obtained at endomyocardial biopsy is in the novel techniques used for studying pathophysiology at the subcellular and molecular level. Endomyocardial biopsy has been used to obtain tissue to study alterations of gene expression in the failing human heart[7] and to detect enteroviral genome in patients with dilated cardiomyopathy.[8] These are but two of the many recent studies that link the basic scientist to the clinician through endomyocardial biopsy.

CONTRAINDICATIONS TO MYOCARDIAL BIOPSY

There are few absolute contraindications to endomyocardial biopsy. This procedure should be avoided in patients with an uncorrected bleeding disorder and in those who cannot cooperate with the procedure. The patient should be stabilized before endomyocardial biopsy but there are occasions when emergency biopsies are required in unstable patients. This procedure should be avoided in patients with altered mentation who are unable to recognize the visceral pain of cardiac perforation.

COMPLICATIONS OF MYOCARDIAL BIOPSY

Virtually all complications of endomyocardial biopsy occur during the procedure. Endomyocardial biopsy is safely performed as an outpatient procedure with complications related to either the introduction of the venous sheath or to the biopsy itself. There is a difference in the incidence of complications related to the type of patient undergoing the procedure. Cardiac transplant recipients have fewer complications overall than do patients with dilated cardiomyopathy. Table 7.1 shows the combined

TABLE 7.1.   Complications of Endomyocardial Biopsy

Complication	DCM n = 546 # (%)	TX n = 2,454 # (%)
During Introduction	15(2.7)	56(2.3)
Arterial Puncture	12(2.2)	44(1.8)
Prolonged Bleeding	1(0.2)	10(0.4)
Vasovagal	2(0.4)	2(0.08)
Pneumothorax	0	0
Neurologic Event	0	0
Infection	0	0
During Biopsy	18(3.3)	18(0.7)
Arrhythmias		
Supraventricular	5(0.9)	6(0.2)
Ventricular	1(0.2)	0
Conduction Defect		
Bradycardia	1(0.2)	1(0.04)
RBBB	1(0.2)	1(0.04)
CHB	1(0.2)	1(0.04)
CHB (LBBB)	2(0.4)	0
Unspecified	0	1(0.04)
Perforation (Possible)		
Pain with Biopsy	3(0.5)	2(0.08)
Hypotension	1(0.2)	0
Perforation (Definite)	3(0.5)	0
Pericardial Fluid	1(0.2)	0
Death	2(0.4)	0
Allergic Reaction	0	5(0.2)
Pacemaker Dislodgment	0	1(0.04)

CHB, Complete heart block; DCM, Dilated cardiomyopathy; LBBB, Left bundle branch block; RBBB, Right bundle branch block
TX, Patients who have undergone cardiac transplant

results from two published reports from Johns Hopkins on the complications of endo-myocardial biopsy in adults with cardiomyopathy[9] and cardiac transplantation.[10]

Right Ventricular Perforation

The most life-threatening complication of endomyocardial biopsy is right ventricular perforation leading to pericardial tamponade. The risk of this complication can be decreased by directing the bioptome toward the interventricular septum. Confirmation of a posterior direction of the bioptome tip in the left anterior oblique projection or the use of echocardiography may be useful in making sure the biopsy comes from the interventricular septum. The risk of bleeding into the pericardium after a perforation is increased by right ventricular hypertension or any bleeding diathesis.

At Johns Hopkins, well over 6000 biopsies have been performed on cardiac transplant recipients without a documented right ventricular perforation. There have been three definite perforations in adult patients with dilated cardiomyopathy; two died and one required emergency cardiac surgery to repair the puncture. Both of the deaths occurred in patients with altered mentation who were unable to describe the sharp pain characteristic of cardiac perforation, and presented as vascular collapse without warning. The true incidence of perforation is probably higher. Any patient complaining of a sharp pain while the bioptome is within the heart should be considered to have had pericardial irritation as a result of cardiac perforation. This pain is distinct from the tugging sensation that patients may complain of during withdrawal of the specimen. It is important to monitor the blood pressure frequently in order to diagnose pericardial tamponade and vascular collapse immediately.

Patients with possible perforation should be monitored closely, and no further biopsies should be performed until the significance of their complaint is determined. Emergent echocardiography should be used to exclude a pericardial effusion. Cardiovascular collapse or electromechanical dissociation occurring during the procedure should be considered to be due to cardiac perforation with resultant tamponade. Emergency pericardiocentesis should be performed immediately from a subxiphoid approach. Pericardial exploration and suture of the right ventricular perforation should performed quickly as the pericardium may be difficult to drain adequately because of clotted blood within the pericardial sac.

Arrhythmias

Premature ventricular depolarizations should be expected to occur upon contact of the bioptome with the endocardium. Short bursts of couplets or triplets are also common and are usually responsive to removal of the bioptome back into the right atrium. Sustained ventricular tachycardia may occur and can be treated with either antiarrhythmic therapy or electric cardioversion. Patients who have a history of ventricular ectopy with a previous biopsy or who have known ventricular tachycardia may be prophylactically treated with an antiarrhythmic. Appropriate medications and cardioversion equipment should be immediately available.

Supraventricular tachycardia can be induced by passage of the bioptome through the right atrium. Adenosine, verapamil, or overdrive pacing are usually successful in converting the patient back to normal sinus rhythm. Finally, as with any procedure involving right ventricular manipulation, pressure against the interventricular septum in the region of the tricuspid valve may result in right bundle branch block. Patients with a preexisting left bundle branch block may develop complete heart block. Removal of the bioptome from the right ventricle may resolve the conduction delay, but temporary transvenous pacing must be immediately available if needed. The electrocardiogram should be continuously monitored. Biopsy of the high interventricular septum should be avoided as this may damage antegrade conduction more permanently.

Pacemaker Lead Dislodgment

Pacemaker dislodgment is rare and may happen during the rapid recoil of the endocardium after the biopsy specimen is removed. It is not usually due to engagement of the lead itself. Biopsies should be taken from an area of the right ventricle that is remote from the pacemaker lead. This will minimize both the risk of lead dislodgment and lead perforation, which can occur as the endocardium is pulled up during specimen removal. Screw-in leads may decrease the risk of this complication, and should be considered in cardiac transplant recipients in need of a pacemaker, as they will also undergo many subsequent cardiac biopsies.

Pneumothorax

Cannulation of the right internal jugular or right subclavian veins can be complicated by pneumothorax of the right lung. This can be minimized by careful cannulation technique using a midneck approach to the internal jugular vein. The internal jugular vein is rarely more than 2 cm from the skin surface; deeper probing, especially with the Amplatz needle, should be avoided.

Carotid Artery Puncture

This is the most frequent complication of internal jugular vein cannulation. The carotid artery is immediately adjacent to the internal jugular vein. This complication can be minimized by the use of a probing needle to find the vein before the larger Amplatz needle is used. An ultrasound device may also be used to find the internal jugular vein and define its relationship to the carotid artery before any cannulation attempt.[11] A smaller 4 French needle with a special guidewire instead of the larger Amplatz needle can also be used. Should arterial puncture occur, the needle should be withdrawn and gentle pressure applied to obtain hemostasis. Cannulation of the carotid or subclavian arteries with the 9 French sheath is of greater concern. Arterial access should be detected by the greater oxygenation of arterial blood before insertion of the sheath. If there are any questions, passage of the guidewire below the diaphragm into the inferior vena cava should be demonstrated before there are any attempts to pass the sheath. If a carotid or subclavian artery is cannulated with the 9 French sheath, immediate consultation with a vascular surgeon is necessary before pulling the sheath.

Miscellaneous

Nerve paresis due to infiltration with lidocaine may result in a Horner's syndrome or vocal cord paralysis. This complication is usually temporary. Venous hematoma usually results in no significant morbidity but may hinder future biopsy attempts. Adequate attention to technique is important. Finally, five patients at Johns Hopkins have had allergic reactions to the reusable Caves-Schultz bioptome or the solution used to sterilize the instrument between procedures.

SUMMARY

The vast majority of complications of transvenous endomyocardial biopsy are minor and have no sequelae. Greater than two thirds are related to vascular access. Right ventricular perforation is rare but can be fatal. Endomyocardial biopsy is a safe and reliable means of obtaining myocardial tissue.

REFERENCES

1. Pierard L, ElAllaf D, D'Orio V, et al. Two-dimensional echocardiographic guiding of endomyocardial biopsy. *Chest.* 85:759, 1984.
2. Sakakibara S, Konno S. Endomyocardial biopsy. *Jpn Heart J.* 3:537, 1962.
3. Richardson PJ. King's endomyocardial bioptome. *Lancet.* 1:660, 1974.
4. Caves PK, Stinson EB, Graham AF. Percutaneous transvenous endomyocardial biopsy. *JAMA.* 225:288, 1973.
5. Mason JW, O'Connell JB. Clinical merit of endomyocardial biopsy. *Circulation.* 79:971, 1989.
6. Billingham ME. Acute myocarditis: is sampling error a contraindication for diagnostic biopsies? *JACC.* 14:921, 1989.
7. Feldman AM, Ray PE, Silan CM, et al. Selective gene expression in failing human heart: quantification of steady-state levels of messenger RNA in endomyocardial biopsies using the polymerase chain reaction. *Circulation.* 83:1866, 1991.
8. Jin O, Sole MJ, Butany JW, et al. Detection of enterovirus RNA in myocardial biopsies from patients with myocarditis and cardiomyopathy using gene amplification by polymerase chain reaction. *Circulation.* 82:8, 1990.
9. Deckers JW, Hare JM, Baughman KL. Complications of transvenous ventricular endomyocardial biopsy in adult patients with cardiomyopathy: a seven-tier survey of 546 consecutive diagnostic procedures in a tertiary referral center. *JACC.* 19:43, 1992.
10. Baraldi-Junkins C, Levin HR, Kasper EK, et al. Complications of endomyocardial biopsy in heart transplant patients. *J Heart Lung Transplant.* 12:63, 1993.
11. Denys BG, Uretsky BF, Reddy PS. Ultrasound-assisted cannulation of the internal jugular vein: a prospective comparison to the external landmark–guided technique. *Circulation.* 87:1557, 1993.

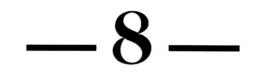

— 8 —

Complications of the Intraaortic Balloon Pump

Andrew L. Smith, M.D.

DESCRIPTION OF PROCEDURE

The intraaortic balloon pump provides mechanical circulatory assist for a variety of life-threatening cardiovascular conditions. The balloon catheter is positioned in the descending thoracic aorta and rapidly inflates in diastole and deflates in systole, resulting in diastolic pressure augmentation and reduction of peak systolic left ventricular pressure. The intraaortic balloon pump decreases myocardial work, decreases left ventricular end diastolic pressure, increases cardiac output, and improves coronary artery perfusion pressure.[1,2]

In recent years, the intraaortic balloon pump has most commonly been inserted percutaneously through the common femoral artery. This procedure can be carried out in the catheterization laboratory, intensive care unit, or operating room. Fluoroscopic guidance is helpful but not mandatory. In the setting of hemodynamic compromise, pulmonary artery catheterization and hemodynamic monitoring are generally used to assist in the medical management during the period of mechanical support.

Using sterile technique and following local anesthesia, a J-tipped guidewire is passed through an insertion needle retrograde into the thoracic descending aorta. Following dilatation of the subcutaneous tissue and artery with a dilator, a 10 French arterial sheath is inserted over the guidewire. An 8.5 or 9.5 French balloon catheter is then inserted over the guidewire through the sheath and advanced up the descending thoracic aorta such that the tip is distal to the origin of the left subclavian artery. The central guidewire is withdrawn and connected to a pressure transducer via plastic extension tubing. The balloon is connected to a pump console, which drives the gas-mediated counter pulsation.[3] In recent years, sheathless systems have been devised and are presently under investigation.

A surgical cutdown technique is employed in selected instances such as when the patient is on cardiopulmonary bypass or in patients with significant peripheral vascular disease in whom percutaneous insertion is more difficult. In rare instances, the balloon may be inserted through a side arm Dacron graft sewn to the femoral artery. Approaches involving direct insertion into the ascending or descending aorta, axillary artery, subclavian artery, or iliac arteries are occasionally utilized.

Following balloon insertion, patients are anticoagulated with heparin. Heparin is generally discontinued one to several hours before intraaortic balloon catheter removal. Anticoagulation is commonly not given to patients immediately following bypass surgery. Balloons inserted percutaneously are removed at the bedside and the femoral artery is compressed manually. Release of pressure both on the distal artery and proximal artery for several seconds before the onset of compression allows for back bleeding, which helps prevent embolization of thrombi to the distal extremity. Balloon pumps inserted surgically are removed in the operating room under direct visualization.

HISTORY OF PROCEDURE

The intraaortic balloon pump was developed by Moulopoulos et al in 1962.[4] The first clinical use of the pump was in the late 1960s as an assist device for patients with cardiogenic shock. Following this, the balloon pump gained widespread acceptance in the treatment of refractory left ventricular failure, unstable angina, and complicated acute myocardial infarctions, and in patients difficult to wean from cardiopulmonary bypass.[5,6] The use of these catheters increased in 1980 with the availabiilty of the percutaneous system. The intraaortic balloon pump continues to undergo modification, the most recent development involving the institution of a sheathless balloon. Unfortunately, the relatively large size of the balloon pump catheters continues to be a limiting factor associated with a high vascular complication rate.

The short-term use of the intraaortic balloon pump for unstable angina has diminished in recent years owing to the use of early coronary revascularization by surgery or balloon angioplasty. In contrast, prolonged uses of the pump have been employed as a bridge to cardiac transplantation in a growing number of patients. These patients may alternatively be managed with implantable left ventricular assist devices.[7]

INDICATIONS FOR THE INTRAAORTIC BALLOON PUMP

The intraaortic balloon pump has the hemodynamic effects of lowering peak systolic pressure, reducing afterload, raising diastolic pressure, reducing left ventricular end diastolic pressure, decreasing myocardial oxygen consumption, improving cardiac output, and improving coronary artery blood flow.[1,2] The balloon pump is utilized for life-threatening cardiovascular conditions in which pharmacologic or interventional therapies have been inadequate. Table 8.1 summarizes the various indications for intraaortic balloon pump use.

TABLE 8.1. Indications for Placement of an Intraaortic Balloon Pump

---

Acute myocardial ischemia
  Unstable angina
  Refractory ventricular tachyarrhythmias of ischemic etiology
  Procedural support for angiography or angioplasty
  Myocardial infarction (to limit size of infarct)
Cardiogenic shock
  Peri-infarction
  Cardiomyopathy
    Bridge to cardiac transplantation
Mechanical complications of acute myocardial infarction
  Ventricular septal defect
  Acute mitral regurgitation
  Volume-inclusive left ventricular aneurysm
Perioperative support
  Weaning from cardiopulmonary bypass
  Perioperative low cardiac output states
  Noncardiac surgeries in high-risk cardiac patients
  Postangioplasty coronary dissection or abrupt closure

From: Benn A, Feldman T. The technique of inserting an intraaortic balloon pump. *J Crit Illness.* 7:437, 1992. Reproduced with permission of publisher and author.

CONTRAINDICATIONS

Contraindications to the use of the intraaortic balloon pump are listed in Table 8.2. Because the intraaortic balloon pump is a costly and temporary measure associated with discomfort and morbidity, it is not indicated for cardiovascular conditions in which there is no definitive therapy. Diastolic counterpulsation increases aortic regurgitation and results in a deterioration in hemodynamics in patients with significant aortic regurgitation. Aortic counterpulsation is also contraindicated in the setting of aortic aneurysm or dissection. Severe iliofemoral disease is a relative contraindication and is associated with failure of successful intraaortic balloon placement and a higher incidence of vascular complications.

TABLE 8.2. Contraindications to IABP Placement

Lack of definitive therapy for underlying pathology
Significant aortic insufficiency
Thoracic or abdominal aortic aneurysm
Severe iliofemoral vascular disease
Clotting disorder

From: Benn A, Feldman T. The technique of inserting an intraaortic balloon pump. *J Crit Illness.* 7:438, 1992. Reproduced with permission of author and publisher.

TABLE 8.3. Complications of the IABP

Major	
Limb ischemia requiring surgery	10%
Bleeding/pseudoaneurysm requiring arterial repair	<4%
Aortic or iliofemoral dissection	<2%
Limb loss	<2%
Septicemia	<1%
Organ embolization (kidney, bowel, spinal cord)	<1%
Femoral nerve palsy/neuritis	<1%
Lymphocele	<1%
Balloon rupture with gas embolization	<1%
Death	<1%
Minor	
Limb ischemia resolving with balloon removal	5% to 30%
Hematoma requiring transfusion	<5%
Superficial wound infection	
Surgical	<5%
Percutaneous insertion	<1%
Hemolytic anemia	<1%
Thrombocytopenia	<1%

COMPLICATIONS

Despite significant technical improvements, the complication rate of intraaortic balloon pump use remains considerable. Reports of intraaortic balloon pump use in recent years suggest that the complication rate is 15% to 40%. Limb ischemia accounts for 80% of these complications. Ischemia may result from reduction of the functional blood vessel luminal size by the balloon pump or from thromboembolic complications. Table 8.3 lists the major and minor complications and their associated rates based on recent literature.

The actual incidence of these complications is likely underreported. Autopsy studies indicate that a number of balloon pump complications are not clinically recognized.[13] It should also be pointed out that the use of vasoconstrictor agents often necessary for hemodynamic support in critically ill patients may contribute to ischemic complications. In 5% to 10% of patients there may be a failure to insert the balloon pump for technical reasons.

Management of complications relies on prompt recognition. Pulses should be monitored closely after balloon insertion. Loss of the pulse by Doppler or evidence of tissue ischemia necessitates removal of the balloon pump. If balloon pump use is mandatory, reinsertion on the contralateral side can be attempted. Another approach is to perform revascularization with femorofemoral bypass in order to retain the use of the balloon pump.[8] In the setting where the balloon pump is removed, if removal does not restore perfusion, thrombectomy is required.

Vascular dissection or perforation is generally the result of difficult balloon insertion and can potentially result in rapid blood loss requiring transfusion and surgical intervention. Balloon rupture, an uncommon occurrence, may be recognized by the appearance of blood in the helium tubing. This complication is best avoided by advancing the wire only when there is no resistance. This problem necessitates prompt removal of the balloon catheter to avoid entrapment.

Superficial infection, almost exclusively seen after surgical placement, respond well to dressing changes and antibiotic therapy.

Risk factors for vascular complications include history of peripheral vascular disease, female sex, obesity, diabetes mellitus, and percutaneous versus surgical catheter insertion.[8–12] Catheter placement in obese patients may be more difficult and this likely accounts for the higher complication rate. Females generally have smaller arteries, making catheter placement more difficult and occlusive complications higher. Diabetics generally have a higher incidence of wound complications. Most studies support a lower incidence of complications in balloons inserted by surgical cutdown versus by the percutaneous approach. The surgical approach, however, may result in a time delay to balloon insertion and may not be judicious in the management of the acutely ill patient. In selected patients, such as those with peripheral vascular disease or obesity, surgical insertion should be considered.

SUMMARY

The intraaortic balloon pump may be life-sustaining in a number of cardiovascular conditions, but is associated with a high complication rate. The majority of complications are vascular and are more likely to occur in patients with preexisting peripheral vascular disease. Awareness of the potential complications of this therapy is necessary for appropriate measures to be instituted promptly. The recent trend in technology has been toward smaller balloon catheters and the development of sheathless systems.[14] It is anticipated that complications will diminish as newer technologies are developed.

REFERENCES

1. Weber KT, Janiki JS. Intra-aortic balloon counterpulsation: A review of physiologic principles, clinical results, and device safety. *Ann Thorac Surg.* 17:602–636, 1974.
2. Fuchs RM, Brin KP, Brinker JA, et al. Augmentation of regional coronary blood flow by intra-aortic balloon counterpulsation in patients with unstable angina. *Circulation.* 68:117–123, 1983.
3. Benn A, Feldman T. The technique of inserting an intra-aortic balloon pump. *J Crit Ill.* 7:435–444, 1992.
4. Moulopoulos SD, Topaz S, Kolff WJ. Diastolic balloon pumping (with carbon dioxide) in the aorta - A mechanical assistance to the failing circulation. *Am Heart J.* 63:669–675, 1962.
5. Willerson JT, Curry GC, Watson JT, et al. Intra-aortic balloon counterpulsation in patients in cardiogenic shock, medically refractory left ventricular failure and/or recurrent ventricular tachycardia. *Am J Med.* 58:183–191, 1975.

6. Pennington DG, Swartz M, Codd JE, et al. Intra-aortic balloon pumping in cardiac surgical patients: a nine-year experience. *Ann Thorac Surg.* 36:125–131, 1983.

7. Miller CA, Pae WE, Pierce WS. Combined registry for clinical use of mechanical ventricular assist pumps and total artificial heart in conjunction with heart transplantation. *J Heart Transplant.* 9:453–458, 1990.

8. Miller JS, Dodson TF, Salam AA, et al. Vascular complications following intra-aortic balloon pump insertion. *Am Surg.* 58:232–238, 1992.

9. Makhoul RG, Cole CW, McCann RL. Vascular complications of the intra-aortic balloon pump: An analysis of 436 patients. *Am Surg.* 59:564–568, 1993.

10. Eltchaninoff H, Dimas AP, Whitlow PL. Complications associated with percutaneous placement and the use of intra-aortic balloon counterpulsation. *Am J Cardiol.* 71:328–332, 1993.

11. Alderman JD, Gabliani GI, McCabe CH, et al. Incidence and management of limb ischemia with percutaneous wire-guided intraaortic balloon catheters. *J Am Coll Cardiol.* 9:524–530, 1987.

12. Goldberg MJ, Rubenfire M, Kantrowitz A, et al. Intra-aortic balloon pump insertion: a randomized study comparing percutaneous and surgical techniques. *J Am Coll Cardiol.* 9:515–523, 1987.

13. Isner JM, Cohen SR, Virmani R. Complications of the intra-aortic balloon counterpulsation device: clinical and morphologic observations in 45 necropsy patients. *Am J Cardiol.* 45:260–269, 1980.

14. Tatar H, Cicek S, Demirkilic U, et al. Vascular complications of intra-aortic balloon pumping: unsheathed versus sheathed insertion. *Ann Thorac Surg.* 55:1518–1521, 1993.

— 9 —

Transesophageal Echocardiography: Indications and Complications

Brent D. Videau, M.D.
Vipul Shah, M.D.
David Caras, M.D.
Randolph P. Martin, M.D.

DESCRIPTION OF THE PROCEDURE

The echocardiographic laboratory of the 1990s has stepped into the forefront of cardiology by performing several important functions. These include evaluation of the structure and function of the heart, assessment of hemodynamic measurements, estimation of the severity of regurgitant lesions, and determination of the significance of coronary artery stenosis and valvular disease using different forms of stress.[1] One diagnostic technique that has propelled echocardiology from a noninvasive procedure to a semi-invasive procedure is transesophageal echocardiography (TEE).

Transesophageal echocardiography is a semi-invasive procedure that requires intubation of the esophagus with a semirigid probe. The unique vantage point from the esophagus provides views of specific cardiac structures that are not adequately provided by transthoracic echocardiography (TTE).[2] Anatomical details of various conditions such as endocarditis and prosthetic valvular dysfunction are better seen by TEE. However, complications may occur, the majority of which are minor. Death is extremely rare and occurred in only .0098% of patients in the largest study. TEE is a safe and effective procedure as long as the physician learns to recognize and treat these potential complications.

HISTORY OF THE PROCEDURE

The evolution from the first application of M-mode transesophageal echocardiography to the current status of two-dimensional color Doppler TEE has occurred over a relatively short period of time. The early echoprobes were simply modified esophageal endoscopes. Frazin developed M-mode TEE with the hope that it could overcome the difficulty in obtaining echocardiograms in patients with emphysema or obesity.[3] This primitive M-mode probe was first applied to a cardiac surgical patient in 1978.[4]

Further modifications to the echoscope were made and by 1982, Schluter et al incorporated a phased array system into the tip of a flexible gastroscope.[5] This probe design became the standard for image acquisition. In this same year, Souquet[6] and Hanrath[7] suggested a rotating phased-array transducer to provide greater imaging flexibility. This transducer was later redesigned by Souquet in 1985.

TEE became increasingly popular with further improvements in probe design and image resolution, especially when color flow images were introduced and reported by Kyo et al in 1987.[8]

In 1989 Omoto et al developed a biplane TEE probe that further facilitated the ability to study intracardiac and intravascular events.[9] The 1990s brought the emergence of the multiplane transesophageal probe and further improvements in the size and flexibility of the probe.

INDICATIONS FOR TEE

Transesophageal echocardiography is now established as an important diagnostic technique for a variety of cardiovascular diseases and is being applied in an increasingly large number of clinical settings[10] (Table 9.1). This technique allows anatomical interrogation of cardiac regions that are difficult to detect by precordial ultrasound. Thus TEE is indicated for conditions in which conventional transthoracic echocardiography is inadequate, such as those with poor acoustic windows due to obesity, emphysema, and thoracic skeletal abnormalities. Other conditions in which TEE is useful include evaluation of prosthetic valvular dysfunction[11] or endocarditis. TEE is superior in evaluating the heart as a source of emboli as well as identifying those patients at risk for emboli following electrical cardioversion.[12] TEE is playing an increasingly important role in the evaluation of aortic diseases such as aortic dissection,[13] transection,[14] and atherosclerotic disease.

In addition to the preceding, TEE has found numerous uses outside the imaging laboratory. TEE is used in the operating room to assess the results of cardiac surgery and monitor cardiac systolic and diastolic function during surgery. Its use has extended to the intensive care unit[15] where transthoracic imaging may be suboptimal to the electrophysiology lab, where it assists in guidance of catheter ablation.[16]

TABLE 9.1.   Indications for Use of Transesophageal Echocardiography

---

In outpatients
   Endocarditis
   Atrial mass (thrombus)
   Prosthetic valve dysfunction
   Cardiac source of embolus
   Aortic pathology
   Native valvular regurgitation
   Congenital heart disease
   Inadequate transthoracic echocardiography images
In critically ill patients
   Inadequate transthoracic echocardiography images
   Hypotension
   Low cardiac output
   Tamponade
   Acute valve dysfunction
   Active endocarditis
   Acute aortic pathology
In patients undergoing surgery
   Left ventricular function monitoring (during valve repair or replacement)
   Intracardiac air embolus
   Complex congenital heart disease
   Aortic pathology
In the catheterization laboratory
   Assist in balloon valvuloplasty
   Guide catheter ablation

Modified from: Martin RP et al. Heart disease and stroke, 2:121–130, 1993. Reproduced with permission from American Heart Association.

CONTRAINDICATIONS TO TEE

Despite the increasing popularity of TEE, there are contraindications to the performance of a transesophageal echocardiogram. The major limitation is esophageal disease. Before using TEE a brief history of symptomatology related to the gastrointestinal tract needs to be obtained. This should include any history of dysphagia, odynophagia, hematemesis, esophageal varices, or radiation to the chest. The presence of any one of these may preclude a TEE without further consultation with a gastroenterologist and perhaps a barium esophagram. Another contraindication of TEE is severe cervical neck disease as seen in some patients with rheumatoid arthritis. It is routine to ask the patient to keep his or her head flexed during the examination. However, in the presence of rheumatic involvement of the atlantoaxial joint this may not be possible and even may be harmful to the patient. Table 9.2 lists the absolute and relative contraindications to a TEE.

COMPLICATIONS WITH TEE

Complications with transesophageal echocardiography are exceedingly rare. Two large trials reported a major complication rate of 0.18% and 0.5%.[1,17] There are

TABLE 9.2. Absolute and Relative Contraindications to a TEE

Absolute	Relative
esophageal disease	hiatal hernia
esophageal diverticulum	active gastric ulcer
tumors/tears/perforations	loose teeth
recent esophageal or gastric surgery	radiation to mediastinum
esophageal varices	atlantoaxial dislocation

numerous smaller studies all with complication rates below 1%.[18] Complications can be either major or minor and for the purposes of classification can be divided into probe related (mechanical), procedure related, or related to medication.

Probe-Related Complications

Probe-related complications conceivably may include mechanical, biological, and thermal injury due to direct ultrasound energy transmission. To date there has been no study that has shown trauma to the esophagus due to prolonged esophageal intubation with the transesophageal probe.[19] In one study, continuous imaging and manipulation of the esophageal probe was performed for up to 8.5 hours in fully heparinized animals with no evidence of pathologic damage to the esophageal mucosa on detailed macroscopic and histologic examination.[20] In addition, no thermal injury was noted despite the prolonged intubation. No reports of thermal injury have appeared in the literature.

Perforation associated with flexible esophagoscopy ranges from 0.02% to 0.03%,[29] with perforation occurring most commonly in the region of the cricopharyngeal muscle. Fortunately, there have been very few reported incidences of perforation secondary to TEE, presumably because of adequate screening for esophageal disease.[21]

Despite this data it seems prudent to restrict the duration of imaging and Doppler studies with TEE to the minimum time required to resolve the clinical question posed. Systemic heparinization was not found to increase risk in these animals, although it has been reported to worsen such complications as Mallory-Weiss syndrome.[21]

Mechanical problems with the steering mechanism of the transducer are rapidly becoming obsolete as technologic advances continue to improve probe design. Previous reports mainly pertained to problems from the buckling of the tip of the probe during insertion. In one study this technical problem was reported in four patients and attributed to flaccidity of the steering cables.[22] In all cases in which problems were reported, the knob controlling the flexion was fixed in the extreme anteflexion (clockwise) position. To prevent this complication, the operator should be familiar with the normal flexion of the TEE probe, and any excessive flaccidity warrants further investigation. Probe flexion should be checked before each procedure. Figure 9.1 demonstrates accepted procedure for removal of a flexed TEE probe.

There has been some question of the safety of the biological effects of the ultrasound energy to the personnel in the surgical operating room; however, current evidence suggests that TEE presents no appreciable risk to the surgeon or other

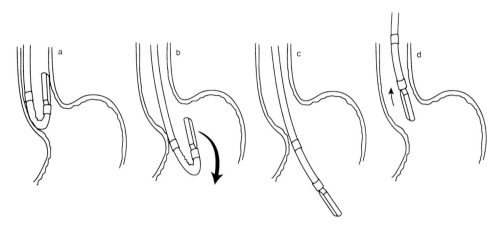

Figure 9.1.   Figure 1 is a schematic diagram illustrating the following: A) Probe flexed upon itself in the lower esophagus; B) advancing the probe into the stomach; C) extending the probe to straighten it out; and D) smooth withdrawal.

medical or nursing staff.[17] Scanning should be performed only as needed, thus minimizing the output. Ultrasound energy attenuates rapidly as it travels through esophageal, pericardial, or myocardial tissue, decreasing by 91% after 7 cm. Thus, only infinitesimal amounts of ultrasound energy reach the eyes of the medical staff.[23]

Probe-related compression of structures in the vicinity of the esophagus is rare, but has been reported. One such case involved bronchial airway obstruction in a 5½-year-old male using a 9-cm conventional echo probe.[24] These complications emphasize that in performing a TEE one must be cognizant of adjacent structures that could be compressed, especially if large probes are used in small patients.

Procedure-Related Complications

Complications related to the TEE procedure can be subdivided into three categories: cardiac, pulmonary, and bleeding.

Cardiac Complications

Cardiac complications include hemodynamically significant ventricular tachycardia, supraventricular tachycardia (SVT), bradyarrhythmias (including AV block), hypotension, hypertension, and precipitation of angina. Almost all studies have shown a very low incidence of induction of sustained ventricular or supraventricular arrhythmias.[1,17,18] In the majority of cases the arrhythmia terminates when the offending agent, the probe, is removed. Occasionally, especially with SVT, pharmacologic therapy is necessary for termination. Bradyarrhythmias have also been reported and are responsive to atropine. Using glycopyrrolate may serve as a deterrent to bradyarrhythmias because of its atropinelike properties.[1] The majority of bradyarrhythmias are due to a vasovagal response. Hemodynamic changes in heart rate (HR) and blood pressure (BP) are mild and occur mostly in elderly patients.[27] Engberding et al studied changes in BP and HR in 44 consecutive patients undergoing TEE without sedation and measured only a mild increase in BP and HR after insertion of the TEE probe.[25] Geibel et al performed blood pressure measurements in 54 unsedated patients during TEE and found that 77% showed an increase of systolic blood pressure from a mean of 125 ± 16 to 141 ± 16[26] mm Hg.

Rarely do these complications require the TEE procedure to be aborted. The patient should be monitored continuously, with standard limb leads and BP measurements recorded every three minutes. Being elderly[27] (age >70 years) and being on a ventilator are independent predictors for the development of hypotension and warrant judicious use of sedation.[28]

Pulmonary Complications

Pulmonary complications such as bronchospasm, laryngospasm, and hypoxia have also been reported in the literature.[1,17,18] Laryngospasm can occur during instillation of local anesthetic to the pharynx or when the echoscope touches the uvula. Typically the patient presents with loss of speech, stridor or wheezing, and the sensation of not being able to breathe. Laryngospasm is rarely life threatening and usually resolves in 15 to 20 minutes. Avoidance is accomplished by gently anesthetizing the posterior pharynx and avoiding voluminous spraying. In the Mayo experience, laryngospasm occurred in 0.2% of procedures.[1] Hypoxia can be avoided by monitoring oxygen saturation in all patients and by providing supplementation by nasal cannula when indicated.

There are numerous minor complications that in some circumstances could lead to abortion of the procedure. Nausea, vomiting, and intolerance of the echoscope are a few examples. When these problems arise, one should pursue a goal-directed exam so as to obtain the information needed rather than an elaborate exam. In the two largest trials, less than 0.01% of procedures were aborted secondary to procedure intolerance.[1,17]

Another pulmonary complication that was observed in four patients at the University of Ottawa Heart Institute was tracheal intubation.[18] The patients developed stridor and an incessant cough. Other clues include inability to advance the probe beyond 30 cm from the teeth and poor image quality except of the aorta, which can easily be visualized because of its proximity to the trachea. This complication requires immediate extubation and suction.

Bleeding Complications

Bleeding from diagnostic endoscopy, even with biopsy, is rare, with a reported incidence of 0.03%.[20,29] Blood-tinged sputum can occur and is frequently due to minor mucosal injury incurred during initial passage of the probe.[1]

Systemic heparinization or Coumadinization has not been found to be a contraindication to TEE as long as there is not active esophageal or gastric bleeding and measures of clotting time are within a therapeutic range. In our experience, thrombocytopenia with platelet counts of 30000 and above has not been associated with an increased rate of bleeding.

DEATH FROM TEE

Death from transesophageal echocardiography is exceedingly rare. There have been only a handful of cases reported. One death was reported in the Mayo series.[1] A 64-year-old obese woman with Type II diabetes died after she had an acute fatal episode of respiratory distress 5 to 10 minutes after completion of the TEE. The patient was unable to be resuscitated from ventricular fibrillation. Autopsy confirmed myocarditis as the likely mechanism.

The European multicenter study also reported one death (.0098%) in a patient who had a malignant lung tumor that had infiltrated into the esophagus.[17] During introduction of the probe, there was laceration of the tumor, leading to massive hematemesis and death. Another reported death occurred in a 28-year-old male who underwent a TEE to look for a source of embolus.[29] During manipulation of the probe in the gastric fundus he had the sudden onset of a tonic-clonic seizure and was in pulseless electrical activity. He could not be revived, and autopsy revealed a ruptured apical pseudoaneurysm that was seen on TEE but missed by transthoracic echo. The authors speculate that the pseudoaneurysm ruptured during the TEE possibly because of probe manipulation within the fundus of the stomach.

BACTERIAL ENDOCARDITIS

A brief mention of bacterial endocarditis as a complication of TEE is warranted. The literature suggests that the risk of bacteremia from TEE is minimal. There has been one case report that suggests a temporal relationship between TEE and the development of bacterial endocarditis.[30] Another series of four patients suggests that the risk is high. However, all organisms isolated in this study were mouth flora.[31] Thus, the evidence of bacterial endocarditis as a complication of TEE is scant and controversial. The final recommendations from the American Heart Association on the use of antibiotic prophylaxis are pending. Currently, prophylaxis is recommended for those who are at highest risk, namely, patients with prosthetic heart valves, devices, poor dentition, or those with a history of recurrent endocarditis.[32]

COMPLICATIONS SECONDARY TO MEDICATION

Complications during TEE may be related to topical anesthetics or other medications used during the procedure. Because of the high vascularity of the tracheobronchial tree, plasma concentrations similar to those seen with intravenous lidocaine have been noted 12 to 15 minutes after administering a laryngotracheal spray. Patients may experience toxic effects if given over 3 mg/kg of lidocaine over a short period of time. Each spray of 10% xylocaine oral spray is equivalent to 10 mg, so approximately 20 sprays to a 70-kg patient may lead to toxicity.

Another rare complication of topical anesthetics is toxic methemoglobinemia.[33] There has been a case report during TEE involving a 64-year-old man with aortic stenosis. This is seen most frequently in adults with congenital deficiency of the methemoglobin reductase enzyme and results in cyanosis and a drop in oxygen saturation. The symptoms can include headache, weakness, dyspnea, and cyanosis. The drop in oxygen saturation may not be detected by pulse oximetry because the spectroscopic method cannot distinguish between methemoglobin and reduced hemoglobulin. The treatment is a reducing agent such as methylene blue at a dose of 1 to 2 mg/kg intravenous over 5 to 15 minutes.

REFERENCES

1. Khandheria BK. The transesophageal echocardiographic examination: is it safe? *Echocardiography: J CV Ultrasound Allied Tech.* 11:55–63, 1994.
2. Nanda NC, Pinheiro L, Sanyal RS, Storey O. Transesophageal biplane echocardiographic imaging: technique, planes, and clinical usefulness. *Echocardiography: J CV Ultrasound Allied Tech.* 7:771–788, 1990.
3. Frazin L, Talano JV, Stephanides L. Esophageal echocardiography. *Circulation.* 54:102, 1976.
4. Oka Y, Matsumoto M, et al. Clinical application of transesophageal echocardiography. Post Graduate Assembly, New York Society of Anesthesiologists, 1979.
5. Schlüter M, Langenstein BA, Polster J. Transesophageal cross-sectional echocardiography with a phased-array transducer system: technique and initial clinical results. *Br Heart J.* 48:67, 1982.
6. Souquet J. Phased-array transducer technology for transesophageal imaging of the heart: current status and future aspects. In: Hanrath P et al, eds. Cadiovascular Diagnosis by Ultrasound. The Hague: Martinus Nijhoff; 251, 1982.
7. Hanrath P et al. Transesophageal horizontal and sagittal imaging of the heart with a phased-array system: initial clinical results. In: Hanrath P et al, eds. Cardiovascular Diagnosis by Ultrasound. The Hague: Martinus Nijhoff; 280, 1982.
8. Kyo S, Takamoto S, Matsumura M, et al. Immediate and early postoperative evaluation of results of cardiac surgery by transesophageal two-dimensional doppler echocardiography. *Circulation.* 76:V113, 1987.
9. Omoto R, Kyo S, Matsumura M. Bi-plane color transesophageal doppler echocardiography (color TEE): its advantages and limitations. *Int J Cardiac Imaging.* 4:57, 1989.
10. Martin RP, Shah V. When to refer a patient for transesophageal echocardiography. *Heart Disease Stroke.* 2:121–130, 1993.
11. Alam M, Serwin JB, Rosman HS. Transesophageal echocardiographic features of normal and dysfunctioning bioprosthetic valves. *Am Heart J.* 121:1149, 1991.
12. Manning WJ, Siverman DI, Gordon SPF. Cardioversion from atrial fibrillation without anticoagulation with use of transesophageal echocardiography to exclude the presence of atrial thrombi. *N Eng J Med.* 328:750–755, 1993.
13. Nienaber CA, Spielmann RP, Kodolitsch YV. Diagnosis of thoracic aortic dissection. *Circulation.* 85:434–447, 1992.
14. Shapiro MJ, Yanofsky SD, Trapp J. Cardiovascular evaluation in blunt thoracic trauma using transesophageal echocardiography (TEE). *J Trauma.* 31:835–839, 1991.
15. Ofili EO, Labovitz AJ. Transesophageal echocardiography: expanded indications for ICU use. *J Crit Illness.* 7:85–96, 1992.

16. Saxon LA, Stevenson WG, Fonarow GC, et al. Transesophageal echocardiography during radiofrequency catheter ablation of ventricular tachycardia. *Am J Cardiol.* 72:658–661, 1993.

17. Daniel WG, Erbel R, Kasper W. Safety of transesophageal echocardiography: a multicenter survey of 10419 examinations. *Circulation.* 83:817–821, 1991.

18. Chan KL, Cohen GI, Sochowski RA. Complications of transesophageal echocardiography in ambulatory adult patients: analysis of 1500 consecutive examinations. *JASE* 4:577–582, 1991.

19. Urbanowicz JH, Kernoff RS, Oppenheim G. Transesophageal echocardiography and its potential for esophageal damage. *Anesthesiology.* 72:40–43, 1990.

20. O'Shea JP, Southern JP, D'Ambra MN. Effects of prolonged transesophageal echocardiographic imaging and probe manipulation on the esophagus: an echocardiographic pathologic study. *JACC.* 17:1426–1429, 1991.

21. Dewhirst WE, Stragand JJ, Fleming BM. Mallory-Weiss tear complicating intraoperative transesophageal echocardiography in a patient undergoing aortic valve replacement. *Anesthesiology.* 73:777–778, 1990.

22. Kronzon I, Gziner DG, Katz ES. Buckling of the tip of the transesophageal echocardiography probe: a potentially dangerous technical malfunction. *JASE.* 5:285–287, 1992.

23. Villforth JC. *Diagnostic Ultrasound Guidance Update.* US Department of Health and Human Services, 14–37, 1987.

24. Gilbert TB, Panico FG, McGill WA et al. Bronchial obstruction by transesophageal echocardiography probe in a pediatric cardiac patient. *Anesth Analg.* 74:156–158, 1992.

25. Engberding R, Hasfeld I, Chiladakis I. Transöphagaeale echokardiographie: erhöhtes untersuchungsrisiko durch blutdruckanstieg und herzhythmustörungen? *Herz Kreisi.* 20:233–236, 1988.

26. Geibel A, Kasper W, Behroz A. Risk of transesophogeal echocardiography in awake patients with cardiac diseases. *A J Cardiol.* 62:337–339, 1988.

27. Ofili Eo, Rich MW. Safety and usefulness of transesophageal echocardiography in persons aged ≥70 years. *Am J Cardiol.* 66:1279–1280, 1990.

28. Stoddard MF, Longaker RA. The safety of transesophageal echocardiography in the elderly. *Am Heart J.* 125:1358–1362, 1993.

29. Sastry BKS, Krishna RN, Ventkateshwer RG. An unusual complication during a transesophageal echocardiographic procedure in a patient with left ventricular pseudoaneurysm. *Echocardiography: J CV Ultrasound Allied Tech.* 11:51–54, 1994.

30. Foster E, Kusumoto FM, Sobol SM. Streptococcal endocarditis temporally related to transesophageal echocardiography. *JASE.* 3:424–427, 1990.

31. Gorge G, Erbel R, Henrichs KJ. Positive blood cultures during transesophageal echocardiography. *JASE.* 3:177–180, 1990.

32. Khandheria BK. Prophylaxis or no prophylaxis before transesophageal echocardiography. *JASE.* 5:285–287, 1992.

33. Marcourtz PA, Williamson BD, Armstrong WF. Toxic methemoglobinemia caused by topical anesthetic given before transesophageal echocardiography. *JASE.* 4:615–618, 1991.

— 10 —

Complications of Pericardiocentesis

Jerre F. Lutz, M.D.

HISTORY OF THE PROCEDURE

In 1649, Riolan first suggested trephining the sternum as a rudimentary form of pericardiotomy in the treatment of tamponade.[1] In 1819, Romero introduced open pericardiotomy through the fifth left intercostal space. There was unfortunately a high incidence of secondary infection in the preantibiotic era.[2] In 1840, Schuh and Kara-haeff used pericardiocentesis through the closed chest for relief of hemorrhagic effusion.[2,3] In their first case, they attempted to remove fluid from the third left intercostal space but met with more success when the fourth interspace was used. Their first patient, a 24-year-old female, died five months postprocedure as a result of malignant effusion. In 1911, Marfan introduced the subxiphoid approach for pericardiocentesis.[4] Bishop et al[5] described electrocardiographic monitoring of the procedure in the 1960s, whereas ultrasound-guided pericardiocentesis is now the standard.[6]

In the last decade there has been increasing favor to return to the open approach of pericardiotomy in elective cases as a result of the high frequency of recurrent effusion (often with tamponade) and a low yield as to the etiology from fluid attained with the closed procedure.

TECHNIQUE OF PERICARDIOCENTESIS

The patient in whom an elective pericardiocentesis is to be performed is placed in a sitting or semiupright position to move the pericardial fluid anteriorly and inferolaterally. Pillows may be placed posteriorly to aid extension of the spine. Resuscitation equipment should be readily available. The patient should be premedicated with

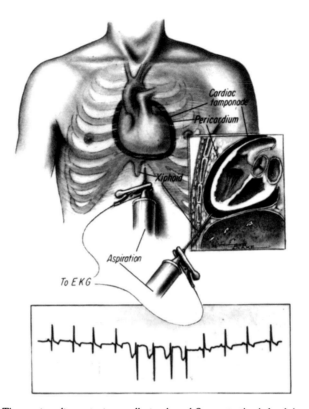

Figure 10.1. The pericardiocentesis needle is placed 2 cms to the left of the xiphoid process and directed toward the mid scapular region. An electrocardiogram is attained by attaching alligator clamps to the electrode needle and to the V, lead of an electrocardiogram recording device. A negative deflection of the QRS with ST elevation represents contact with the epicardium. The needle is withdrawn slowly and the ecg results to baseline once the needle loses contact with the myocardium. Reproduced with permission from: Ebert PA. In: Sabiston DC, Spencer FC (eds) The Pericardium in Gibbon's Surgery of the Chest. 4th edition, 1983. WB Saunders, Philadelphia, 1983, p. 996.

atropine to prevent vagal reflexes. Experienced personnel in the cardiac cath lab, echo lab, or ICU should assist the physician with ECG monitoring of the procedure.

Electrocardiographic and ultrasound monitoring may both be used. Echocardiography can identify the place on the body wall closest to the fluid that permits an entry tract that prevents puncture of an underlying vital structure.[6,7] Before ultrasound guidance, the subxiphoid approach was the most commonly used entrance site. The needle advanced through the diaphragm into the pericardial space while vital structures such as the pleural spaces, mammary arteries, and coronary arteries were avoided (Figure 10.1). This method uses a puncture site 2 cm below the xiphoid to the left of midline. Following sterile technique, a skin bleb is made using 1% lidocaine. A 20-gauge, 3-in needle is advanced at an angle of 45 degrees to the horizon toward the left shoulder. The needle should be aspirated and lidocaine administered throughout the path. Once pericardial fluid is attained, the needle should be clamped at the skin level to mark the depth and prevent further advancement. A large-bore needle, such as a 6-in No. 16 spinal needle, can be advanced at the same angle to a similar depth. If the pericardiocentesis is purely diagnostic, a three-way adapter may be attached to facilitate fluid withdrawal without introduction of air. A hemostat attached to the needle permits advancement to a similar depth as the smaller-bore needle. An alligator clamp attached to the spinal needle and to the V lead of the electrocardiographic monitor permits monitoring of the needle tip. ST elevation and ventricular ectopy indicate epicardial injury of the right ventricular wall.[5] Similarly, PR depression or elevation with atrial premature beats indicate atrial tissue has been inadvertently entered (Figure 10.2). The cardiac chambers can be entered without ST change or ectopy on occasion. Intrapericardial position can be confirmed at the bedside by removing blood from the suspected pericardium. The constant churning effect of cardiac systole defibrinates blood products in the pericardial space and prevents clotting, whereas intracardiac blood clots.

Intrapericardial fluid, even if bloody, has a lower hematocrit than blood attained from the right ventricle.[8] Saline injection through the needle can identify the needle

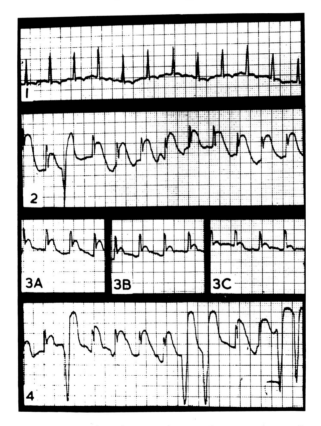

Figure 10.2A.   Serial tracings of an electrocardiogram during aspiration of an effusion. Panel 1 shows the control tracing with T wave inversion secondary to pericarditis. Panel 2 shows one PVC and an acute injury current with the electrode needle touching the epicardium. Panel 3A shows acute injury with the needle touching the epicardium while panel 3B shows the injury to be less well marked as the needle is withdrawn. Panel 4 reveals 5 PVC's and an acute injury pattern as the needle is advanced in another portion of the epicardium. The changes noted in panels 2, 3 and 4 indicate epicardial damage or irritation. Gotsman MS & Schrire V. A Pericardiocentesis Needle. Reproduced with permission from British Heart J. 28:566–9, 1966.

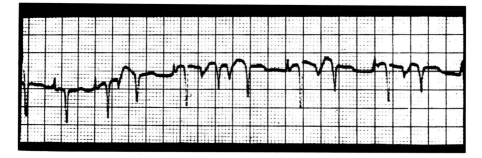

Figure 10.2B. Atrial premature beats with a current of injury showing the effect of needle injury to right atrial muscle. Gotsman MS & Schrire V. A Pericardiocentesis Electrode Needle. Reproduced with permission from *Br Heart J* 28:566–9, 1966.

tip site as intrapericardial or intracardiac using echocardiographic guidance. The needle may also be attached to a pressure transducer and monitored continuously during the procedure.

Fluid may be submitted for cell counts, protein, glucose (with concomitant serum glucose), LDH, and cytology as well as cultures for bacteria, tuberculosis, and fungi. Gram stains for bacteria and a Ziehl-Neelsen stain for tuberculous bacilli may also be performed. Air may be injected into the pericardial space to evaluate pericardial thickness by radiographic techniques. The intrapericardial position must be confirmed before air injection because air injected into the right ventricle may lead to a potentially fatal air embolus.[9] If the pericardiocentesis is to be therapeutic, a 0.035-cm guidewire may be inserted through the large-bore needle, followed by a dilator and an 8 French pigtail or multiholed intracath (Figure 10.3). This permits safe removal of substantial amounts of fluid without needle abutment against the beating heart, thus lessening the likelihood of cardiac laceration. Approximately 70% of pericardiocenteses are performed for therapeutic reasons, whereas only 21% are pure diagnostic techniques.[6] The catheter may be capped with a three-way stopcock that allows serial aspirations from the pericardium with deposition into a closed system. Echocardiography now indicates an optimal position on the chest wall other than the subxiphoid route 64% of the time.[6] The apical portal is located 2 cm inside the maximum cardiac impulse at the fourth interspace.[10]

The apical approach is similar in technique except there is a higher likelihood of cardiac perforation, making attention to depth all the more important. Echocardiography may also indicate a parasternal entrance site as optimal. The catheter may be removed immediately after the procedure or left as an indwelling drain for several days. Continued sterile technique is of utmost importance to prevent secondary infection.

Pericardiocentesis followed by dilatation of the pericardium with a percutaneous balloon is presently being evaluated. There is an 85% immediate success rate, but the long-term success rate is not known. Indications for this procedure rather than conventional pericardiocentesis or surgical pericardiotomy are presently being evaluated.[11]

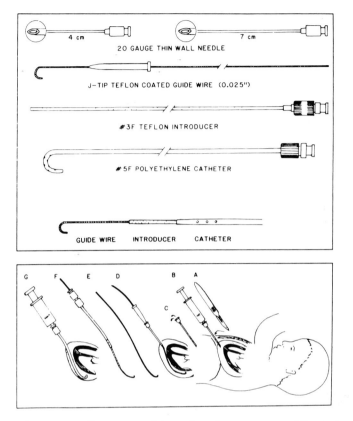

Figure 10.3. Diagramatic illustrations of the technical components of the pericardiocentesis set as well as the sequence of the procedure. Reproduced with permission from Park SC, Pahl E, Ettedgui JA, et al. Experience with a Newly Developed Pericardiocentesis Set. *AJC* 66:1528–1531, 1990.

INDICATIONS FOR PERICARDIOCENTESIS

Pericardiocentesis may be performed solely to recover fluid for diagnostic purposes, relieve tamponade, study the physiologic effect of fluid removal on elevated venous pressure in patients in whom more than one cause is present (such as a cancer patient with pericardial effusion and superior vena caval obstruction), and decompress the pericardium before pericardiectomy (to lessen the risk of anesthesia).

Not all pericardial fluid has to be tapped. Some patients with small or moderate effusions secondary to treatable conditions may be observed so long as no hemodynamic compromise exists. If the etiology of a small effusion is unclear, diagnostic pericardiocentesis may be indicated. Because the yield of an etiology is not always attained with a successful procedure, close observation or a more invasive procedure such as a pericardial window are alternatives. In the setting of a large effusion, pericardial tamponade, hypotension, and a pretamponade state in which observation is hazardous are all indications for pericardiocentesis.[6]

CONTRAINDICATIONS TO PERICARDIOCENTESIS

Elective pericardiocentesis should be delayed until correction of low platelets or abnormal coagulation factors has occurred. Inadvertent sticks of the right ventricle are poorly tolerated in these settings.

Open thoracotomy is preferable in severe suppurative pericarditis and recurrent malignant effusions, or for dialysis patients with tamponade.[12]

One should avoid pericardiocentesis if the effusion is loculated posteriorly or if there is less than 1 cm of anterior effusion.[13]

COMPLICATIONS OF THE PROCEDURE

Because pericardiocentesis is often performed in life-threatening circumstances, the exact incidence of complications is difficult to ascertain. However, data are available in specific subgroups of patients. Most of the data were obtained in nonemergent procedures.

Fluid is readily attained in 90% of large effusions but only 50% of small or posterior effusions.[14] Fluid diagnostic of a specific etiology is attained in only 24% of cases.[14] Cytologic examinations appear to be quite reliable (80% to 90%) if the primary is carcinomatous (especially lung or breast cancer)[13,14,15] but much less reliable if the primary is a lymphoma or mesothelioma.[14] False positives are similarly unusual.[13,15] Elevated CEA (Carcinoembryonic Antigen) levels in the pericardial fluid may also identify those patients who have neoplastic effusions but negative cytology.[13]

Most complications of pericardiocentesis are traumatic. Laceration of vascular structures including the right atrium, right ventricle, and coronary arteries have been reported. Laceration of avascular structures including the stomach, lung, and colon have also occurred. Additional complications include pneumothorax, cardiac tamponade, and arrhythmias.[14,16,17] Premature atrial and ventricular beats are almost expected, whereas serious arrhythmias such as ventricular fibrillation or sustained ventricular tachycardia are uncommon. Indwelling catheters predispose to secondary infection.[14] Pulmonary edema may follow large-volume pericardiocentesis. This phenomenon has been attributed to the same preload-afterload mismatch that precipitates pulmonary edema following large-volume paracentesis or thoracentesis.[18]

In 165 procedures performed in 123 patients over a 6-year period, the Stanford group reported five deaths: two soon after the procedure in critically ill patients, two in whom surgical delay was felt to be a contributing factor, and one with a secondarily infected sheath who developed purulent pericarditis. There were also five cases of tamponade, eight cases of clear fluid becoming bloody secondary to trauma, and one episode of ventricular tachycardia. "Several" patients had vagal episodes during the procedure.[14]

Callahan et al.[6] reported the Mayo experience with two-dimensional, echocardiographically guided pericardiocentesis in 132 consecutive procedures in 117 patients over a 4-year period. There were no deaths, one pneumothorax, one pneumopericardium, and three minor complications, including one vagal episode and two patients in whom the right ventricle was entered but not dilated.

Duvernoy et al.[19] reported the complications of 352 cases of fluoroscopically guided periocardiocentesis. Included were three cardiac perforations, two cardiac arrhythmias, four cases of arterial bleeding, two pneumothoraces, and one major vagal reaction.

Rostand and Rutsky[20] summarized the results of pericardiocentesis in several series of patients with uremic pericarditis. Tamponade was precipitated in 3%, myocardial laceration in 3%, cardiac arrest in 2%, and death in 3% of cases. The pericardial fluid was felt to be inadequately drained in 28% of cases. Because of the altered anatomy, altered platelet function, and high incidence of concomitant hypertension, these results probably define a high-risk subset.

These results suggest that pericardiocentesis is a relatively high-risk procedure. To decrease the frequency of complications, one must rely on meticulous attention to technique, refer high-risk patients for thoracotomy, and follow sterile wound precautions in those patients with a residual surgical drain postprocedure.

REFERENCES

1. Riolan J. *Encheiridium Anatomicum et Pathologicum Lugduni Batavorum.* Ex officina Adriani Wyngaerden, Leyden. Vol. 2(2):206, 1649.

2. Romero cited by Baizeau: Mémoire sur le ponction du péricarde, envisagée au point du vue chirugical. *Gaz hebd de méd Par.* (2^{me}série) 5:515–562, 1868.

3. Kilpatrick ZM, Chapman CB. On pericardiocentesis. *Amer J Cardiol.* 15:722–726, 1965.

4. Marfan AB. Ponction du péricarde par l'epigastre. *Ann de méd et chir.* 15:529, 1911.

5. Bishop LH, Jr, Estes EH, Jr, McIntosh HD. Electrocardiogram as a safeguard in pericardiocentesis. *JAMA.* 162:264, 1956.

6. Callahan JA, Seward JB, Nishimura RA, et al. Two-dimensional echocardiographically guided pericardiocentesis: experience in 117 consecutive patients. *Amer J Cardiol.* 55: 476–479, 1985.

7. Callahan JA, Seward JB, Tajik AJ. Cardiac tamponade: pericardiocentesis directed by two-dimensional echocardiography. *Mayo Clin Proc.* 60:344–347, 1985.

8. Miller JI. *Pericardiectomy.* In: Update III to 4th ed. *The Heart.* Hurst JW, ed. New York, NY: McGraw-Hill; 1982:147–158.

9. Chandraratna PAN, First J, Langevin E, O'Dell R. Echocardiographic contrast studios during pericardiocentesis. *Ann Int Med.* 87:199–200, 1977.

10. Fowler N; Hurst JW, Logue RB, (eds.) *Pericardial Disease in The Heart, Arteries, and Veins.* 1st ed. New York, NY: McGraw-Hill; 1966:846–858.

11. Lemmon MS, Rodriguez S, Ziskind AA. Percutaneous balloon pericardiotomy: an advance in treating pericardial effusion and tamponade primary. *Cardiology.* 20(7):38–42, 1994.

12. Kapoor AS, Kapoor AS, ed. *Technique of Pericardiocentesis and Intrapericardial Drainage in Interventional Cardiology.* New York, NY: Springer-Verlag; 1989:146–153.

13. Hancock EW. Neoplastic pericardial disease. *Cardiol. Clin.* 8(4):673–696, 1990.

14. Krikorian JG, Hancock EW. Pericardiocentesis. *Amer J Med.* 65:808–813, 1978.

15. Wiener HG, Kristensen IB, Haubek A, Kritensen B, Baandrup U. Diagnostic value of pericardial cytology. *Acta Cytologica.* 35:149–153, 1991.

16. Baue AE, Blakemore WS. The pericardium. *Ann Thoracic Surg.* 14:81–106, 1972.

17. Wong B, Murphy J, Chang CJ, Hassenein K, Dunn M. The risk of pericardiocentesis. *Amer J Cardiol.* 44:1110–1114, 1979.

18. Vandyke WH, Cure J, Chakko CS, Gheorghiade M. Pulmonary edema after pericardiocentesis for cardiac tamponade. *N Eng J Med.* 309:595–596, 1983.

19. Duvernoy O, Borowiec J, Helmius G, Erikson U. Complications of percutaneous pericardiocentesis under fluoroscopic guidance. *Acta Radiol.* 33:309–313, 1992.

20. Rostand SG, Rutsky EA. Pericarditis in end-stage renal disease. *Cardiol Clin.* 8(4):701–716, 1990.

— 11 —

Complications of External Cardioversion-Defibrillation

M. Erick Burton, M.D.

DESCRIPTION OF PROCEDURE

The principal aim of cardioversion-defibrillation is to deliver an electrical current between two electrodes resulting in depolarization of a critical mass of cardiac tissue,[1] momentarily terminating the arrhythmia and allowing the sinus node to regain function as the dominant pacemaker. The delivery of an electrical impulse synchronized to the electrocardiogram is termed cardioversion; delivery of an unsynchronized impulse is properly termed defibrillation.[2] The cardioverter-defibrillator uses an inductor to store energy onto an internal capacitor that is then delivered between the two electrodes when the circuit is closed. Most commercially available external devices use a dampened sinusoidal waveform in contrast to implantable cardioverters-defibrillators, which use a truncated exponential waveform. The energy is measured in watt-seconds or joules (J). The amount of energy delivered depends on the impedance (resistance) between the electrodes and is less than the amount of energy stored on the capacitors.[3] The higher the impedance, the lower the delivered energy. Older models allow the operator to choose the amount of energy stored on the capacitor (up to 400 J); newer devices show the amount of energy delivered through 50-ohm circuit.[4] It is the delivered energy or, more appropriately, the delivered current density (current per unit area) that traverses the myocytes of the chambers to be cardioverted-defibrillated that determines success.[5]

External cardioversion-defibrillation occurs in two settings, emergent or urgent termination of hemodynamically compromising tachyarrhythmias and elective conversion of less threatening arrhythmias. Patients scheduled for elective cardioversion should be in a fasting or postabsorptive state. Serum electrolyte levels, particularly serum potassium, should be normal. Knowledge of renal function is helpful in guiding the dosage of adjunctive medications. Patients without clinical evidence of digitalis

103

toxicity may continue to take this agent until the day of the procedure.[6] If there is clinical evidence of digitalis toxicity, the serum digoxin level should be checked and the procedure delayed. Secure intravenous access should be obtained and appropriate cardiac monitoring initiated. Noninvasive continuous monitoring of blood hemoglobin oxygen saturation provides useful information on the patient's respiratory status throughout the procedure.

Transthoracic electrode position and size are important determinants of successful cardioversion. Anteroposterior positioning provides a current vector that traverses the largest amount of atrial tissue, although anterolateral positioning is acceptable. An electrode size between 8 cm^2 to 12 cm^2 is desirable. If the electrodes are too small, current is concentrated and myocardial damage is a concern; if the electrodes are too large, the current density is not great enough for successful termination of the arrhythmia.[7]

In an elective cardioversion, the patient should be anesthetized or sedated by a qualified physician in an area suitable for the intravenous administration of a general anesthetic and for performance of cardiopulmonary resuscitation if necessary. Recent studies illustrate the feasibility of performing cardioversion in an outpatient office setting[8] and in the more traditional hospital setting. A number of different protocols for sedation are efficacious.[9] All successful protocols induce a state of analgesia and amnesia, the importance of which cannot be overemphasized. Once an adequate level of sedation is present, delivery of energy synchronized to the QRS complex on the electrocardiogram can be performed. Synchronization of electrical discharge on the QRS is necessary to prevent inadvertent ventricular fibrillation by discharging in the "vulnerable" period of ventricular repolarization.

The initial shock for atrial fibrillation should be 200 J because 85% of those who are ultimately able to be electrically cardioverted to normal rhythm will do so at 200 J but only 50% of patients will cardiovert with 100 J.[7] If unsuccessful, the next shock should be 360 J. If this second shock is unsuccessful another 360-J shock is reasonable because data suggest repetitive shocks lower chest impedance and thus increase current flow.[10] If atrial fibrillation persists after the preceding protocol, it is unlikely continued shocks will be successful without a change in electrode position or infusion of an antiarrhythmic agent before repeat attempts. Atrial flutter, ventricular tachycardia, and most forms of reentrant supraventricular tachycardia require less energy to terminate than atrial fibrillation. Thus it is reasonable to start at 50 J to 100 J for these arrhythmias. After the procedure, a 12-lead ECG should be obtained to evaluate the stability of the rhythm, and the patient should be monitored for at least one hour.

In emergent situations, time is of the essence. Restoration of a hemodynamically stable cardiac rhythm is paramount, as studies have demonstrated that defibrillation thresholds increase with prolonged tachyarrhythmias.[11] Emergent defibrillation of ventricular fibrillation should be performed in an unsynchronized mode because the low-amplitude fibrillatory waves can inhibit the discharge of the defibrillator in the synchronized mode.

HISTORY OF PROCEDURE

The association of electrical energy and cardiac rhythm dates back 200 years to the pioneering experiments of Galvani and Volta.[12] The ability to induce ventricular fibrillation in dogs was described by Hoffa and Ludwig in 1850.[13] Ventricular defibrillation using electrical current was first described in 1899 by Prevost and Battelli.[14] In 1947, Beck applied 120 volts from a 60-Hz power line to transventricular electrodes and electrically defibrillated the first human heart.[15] Zoll's successful reversion of ventricular fibrillation with AC current in 1956 was the first description of closed-chest external electrical defibrillation.[16] Synchronized elective DC cardioversion of atrial fibrillation was reported six years later by Lown.[2] A number of modalities now exist for the safe, effective delivery of electrical energy to convert cardiac arrhythmias including transesophageal[17] and intracardiac[18] as well as the traditional transcutaneous approach.

INDICATIONS

Both supraventricular and ventricular arrhythmias refractory to medical therapy can be effectively treated with electrical cardioversion. Patients with supraventricular arrhythmias are usually electively cardioverted unless there is concomitant hemodynamic embarassment. Patients with ventricular arrhythmias who require cardioversion are usually converted more urgently.

An estimation of the likelihood of acute success and long-term maintenance of sinus rhythm is important before elective cardioversion of supraventricular arrhythmias. Certain clinical parameters indicate a predilection for procedural failure or high arrhythmia recurrence rate. Untreated thyrotoxicosis, mitral valve disease, congestive heart failure, atrial fibrillation of more than one year's duration, and significant left atrial enlargement are all associated with a high recurrence rate in patients with atrial arrhythmias, and careful consideration of the procedure risk-benefit ratio should be analyzed in this group of patients.[19] Although acute success ranges from 70% to 90%, long-term maintenance of sinus rhythm is less impressive. Acute procedural failure has been linked to increased body size,[18] and in these patients intracardiac or transesophageal delivery of energy may be needed to achieve success. A number of studies suggest the chance of remaining in sinus rhythm at one year without antiarrhythmics is around 40% to 50% while use of serial antiarrhythmic therapy increases the prevalence of sinus rhythm at one year to 60% to 70%.[20]

The prevalence of cardioversion in the United States is difficult to ascertain but a sensible estimate is one procedure per month per cardiologist. Given 3000 cardiologists in the United States[7] and a conservative estimate of $1,000.00 per cardioversion, an annual rate of 36,000 procedures at an estimated cost of $36 million is reasonable.

CONTRAINDICATIONS

A number of relative contraindications to cardioversion exist. A patient in the nonfasting state is at risk for aspiration during administration of anesthesia. Electrolyte imbalance, especially hypokalemia, predisposes to the development of ventricular arrhythmias postcardioversion. Digitalis lowers the defibrillation threshold in the heart, and the delivery of DC current in a toxic state can have a proarrhythmic effect that is energy dependent. Prolonged periods of asystole have been described in the setting of digitalis excess, and serious ventricular tachyarrhythmias can develop.[3] There is no evidence that cardioversion during digitalis therapy, in the absence of toxicity, poses a significant hazard.[3,6]

Hemodynamically tolerated arrhythmias that are paroxysmal in nature are not indications for cardioversion because maintenance of sinus rhythm is the problem, not termination of the arrhythmia. Any tacharrhythmia associated with hemodynamic compromise is an indication for emergent cardioversion with the possible exception of digitalis-induced arrhythmias. Multifocal atrial tachycardia and sinus node dysfunction are associated with periods of bradyarrhythmia postcardioversion that may require further intervention.[6]

A number of possible special circumstances bear mention. Pregnancy is not a contraindication to cardioversion, although fetal monitoring during the procedure is recommended.[21] There is concern that the epicardial patches used in some implantable cardioverter-defibrillator systems insulate the heart and increase the number of shocks or the energy requirement for external cardioversion. Although laboratory studies suggest an increase in defibrillation threshold occurs,[22] a clinical trial comparing patients with epicardial ICD patches to a control group found no significant difference in number of episodes requiring more than one shock or the energy requirements for successful external defibrillation.[23] Knowledge of the position of the epicardial patches in these cases is helpful, and repositioning of the external defibrillator patches following procedural failure is reasonable. Cardioversion has been safely performed in patients with permanent pacemakers, but it is recommended to position the electrodes so the current of energy does not pass directly through the pulse generator.

COMPLICATIONS

In contrast to most special procedures in cardiology, cardioversion demands a minimum of technical skills but a maximum of cognitive skills. The latter assumes a thorough knowledge of indications, contraindications, complications (and their management), and adjunctive use of drug therapy. Any physician performing elective cardioversion should be competent to handle any sequelae of the procedure, including resultant arrhythmias or asystole.[6] Because several manufacturers produce equipment for performing cardioversion, it is important that the physician become thoroughly familiar with the device in use before attempting the procedure.

The overall incidence of complications with external cardioversion is low. The most common complication of cardioversion is minor burns to the skin at the site of the transcutaneous electrodes. The advent of self-adhesive electrode pads may decrease the incidence of thermal trauma and will decrease the incidence of inadvertent operator shock.[24] If traditional handheld paddles are to be used, a couplant between the interface of the paddles and the chest wall is necessary. Not only is the incidence of thermal injury decreased but the likelihood of successful cardioversion is increased, because transthoracic impedance is decreased dramatically with a couplant.[25] Flammable gels and ointments (NTG paste) need to be avoided at all cost.

Although elevation of circulating cardiac enzymes has been demonstrated post-cardioversion, true cardiac damage from cardioversion-defibrillation is unusual. A recent study used technetium-99m stannous pyrophosphate scans to examine the prevalence of myocardial injury in 25 patients postcardioversion.[26] No patient demonstrated radionuclide uptake in the myocardium, although several patients demonstrated uptake in the anterior chest wall. Serum creatine kinase was elevated postprocedure in several patients, and two patients had elevation of CPK-MB fractions. The enzyme elevations were felt to represent damage to skeletal muscle and not myocardial damage.

Cardiac arrhythmias postcardioversion are usually immediate and short-lived, although there are rare reports of symptomatic bradyarrhythmias occurring several minutes to hours after cardioversion. The vast majority of arrhythmias do not require any direct therapy but a history of coronary disease, antiarrhythmic medications, and preprocedural bradycardia all predispose to the development of postprocedure bradyarrhythmias, which may require treatment with either temporary pacing or chronotropic agents (atropine, isoproterenol). Central venous access before cardioversion in patients at high risk allows rapid placement of a temporary pacing wire if necessary, although newer devices are capable of transcutaneous pacing through the cardioversion patches. A small but significant incidence (<5%) of life-threatening ventricular tachyarrhythmias illustrates the need for vigilant monitoring postprocedure. In rare cases patients may demonstrate ST elevation postcardioversion, but this phenomenon is transient and not a harbinger of myocardial injury/ischemia, although ST elevation after cardioversion may be associated with a recrudescence of the primary arrhythmia.[27] Rarely, pulmonary edema can occur minutes to hours after cardioversion. This phenomenon is usually seen in patients with depressed LV function.

Recent studies have examined the benefit-risk ratio of antiarrhythmics to prevent atrial fibrillation after cardioversion. A metanalysis of quinidine therapy suggests maintenance of sinus rhythm is improved at the cost of a threefold increase in mortality compared with controls.[28] The CAST study did not involve cardioversion but showed an increased mortality in patients treated with class Ic antiarrhythmics who had coronary disease, frequent ventricular ectopy, and decreased LV function.[29] The risk of traditional antiarrhythmic therapy, especially in the setting of structural heart disease, needs to be judged on an individual basis. Antiarrhythmic agents with a lower incidence of proarrhythmia may increase the long-term maintenance of sinus rhythm with an acceptable risk profile. Amiodarone is such an antiarrhythmic and is especially effective in the treatment of atrial and ventricular arrhythmias.[30,31] Amiodarone depresses sinus node and AV node function,[32] and some data suggest it may raise defibrillation thresholds.[33,34] Given amiodarone's unique electrophysiologic effects, concern about its efficacy in external cardioversion is justified. In a nonrandomized study of patients taking amiodarone undergoing cardioversion,[35] there was no significant difference in acute cardioversion success rate, postprocedure bradyarrhythmias, or energy required for successful cardioversion compared to a control population taking no antiarrhythmics. Sotalol, another class-III antiarrhythmic with a low incidence of proarrhythmia, also shows promise in the treatment of recurrent atrial fibrillation. Other antiarrhythmic agents have been shown to increase defibrillation thresholds in experimental preparations but whether there is a clinical effect is unclear.[36,37]

The most devastating complication of external cardioversion is systemic embolization. Lown[38] reported an embolic rate of 1.2% in 456 patients not receiving anticoagulation who underwent cardioversion. In a nonrandomized study, Bjerkelund and Orning[39] reported a 5.3% incidence of stroke postcardioversion in nonanticoagulated patients compared to a 0.8% incidence in an anticoagulated population who were at higher risk for embolism than the nonanticoagulated patients. More recently, Mancini and Weinberg[40] analyzed embolic events after cardioversion for atrial fibrillation. They found no events in the group undergoing anticoagulant therapy, whereas 7% of the group without such therapy had embolic complications. Arnold et al[41] found an event rate of 1.3% in their experience of more than 450 cardioversions. All events occurred in patients who were not anticoagulated. No patient with atrial flutter had an embolic event regardless of anticoagulation status.

The mechanism of embolization is complex and probably is a combination of an increase in cerebral blood flow after conversion to sinus rhythm, an increase in humoral factors that may predispose to thrombus formation, and the return of mechanical atrial contraction several days to weeks after the return of organized electrical activity. Although randomized trials are lacking, it appears that anticoagulation before elective cardioversion of atrial fibrillation decreases the risk of embolic events. The duration of therapy before and after cardioversion is not as clearly defined. Assuming clot formation, organization, and adherence to the atrial wall takes several days to weeks, and atrial contractile activity does not maximize until weeks after cardioversion,[42] the generally accepted recommendations are that anticoagulation (PT 1.2 to 1.5x control, INR 2.0 to 3.0) be given for three weeks before cardioversion and four weeks after cardioversion. For atrial fibrillation of less than two days' duration, atrial flutter or supraventricular tachycardia, anticoagulation does not appear necessary unless other risk factors for embolism are present.[43]

Anticoagulation carries an inherent risk of complication in the form of bleeding. A number of randomized trials evaluating the efficacy of anticoagulation in nonrheumatic atrial fibrillation have recently become available and suggest a 2% per year risk for major bleeding and a 0.8% per year risk for fatal bleeding.[35] Although anticoagulation with cardioversion is of a shorter duration, there is certainly some risk of hemorrhage. Investigators have recently proposed using transesophageal echocardiography (TEE) to risk stratify patients for cardioversion.[44] If no evidence of atrial thrombus is seen at TEE, they suggest that cardioversion can be safely performed without prolonged anticoagulation. Larger, randomized trials are needed to confirm this hypothesis before this algorithm can be recommended for routine use. In patients who are at increased risk for bleeding complications, however, TEE may be a reasonable risk stratification before cardioversion. If no evidence for atrial "smoke" or thrombus exists, cardioversion without prolonged anticoagulation can be performed at relatively low risk for embolic event. If thrombus is seen at TEE, the risk of anticoagulation for a few weeks may be lower than the risk for embolic event and its potential catastrophic consequences.

External cardioversion is a relatively benign procedure that has a low incidence of complications. As with most interventional procedures, the true skill and art is in the selection of patients for the procedure. Proper preparation of equipment and staff, and an understanding of the potential complications is important in guaranteeing patient safety.

REFERENCES

1. Zipes D, Fischer J, King RM, et al. Termination of ventricular fibrillation in dogs by depolarizing a critical mass of myocardium. *Am J Cardiol.* 36:37–44, 1975.

2. Lown B, Amarasingham R, Neuman J. New method for terminating cardiac arrhythmias. *JAMA.* 182:548–555, 1962.

3. Lown BL, DeSilva RA. Cardioversion and defibrillation. In: Hurst JW, ed. *The Heart, Arteries and Veins.* New York, NY: McGraw-Hill; 1990 pp. 2095–2100.

4. Geddes LA. The use of the defibrillator. In: Karliner JS, Gregoratos G, eds. *Coronary Care.* New York, NY: Churchill Livingstone; 1981:

5. Mehra R, DeGroot P, Norenberg MS. Energy waveforms and lead systems for implantable defibrillators. In: Lüderitz B, Saksena S. *Interventional Electrophysiology.* New York, NY: Futura; 1991:

6. Yurchak PM, Williams SV, Achord JL, et al. Special sections: ACP/ACC/AHA task force statement: clinical competence in elective direct current (DC) cardioversion: a statement for physicians from the ACP/ACC/AHA task force on clinical privileges in cardiology. *J Amer Coll Cardiol.* 22:336–339, 1993.

7. Ewy GA. Optimal technique for electrical cardioversion of atrial fibrillation. *Circulation.* 86:1645–1647, 1992.

8. Lesser MF. Brief reports: safety and efficacy of in-office cardioversion for treatment of supraventricular arrhythmias. *Am J Cardiol.* 66:1267–1268, 1990.

9. Canesa R, Lema G, Urza J, et al. Anesthesia for elective cardioversion: a comparison of four anesthetic agents. *J CT Anesthesia.* 5:566–568, 1991.

10. Chambers W, Miles R, Stratbucker R. Human chest resistance during successive countershocks. *Med Instrum.* 12:53, 1978.

11. Winkle RA, Mead RH, Ruder MA, et al. Clinical investigation: effect of duration of ventricular fibrillation on defibrillation efficacy in humans. *Circulation.* 81:1477–1481, 1990.

12. Lyons A, Petrucelli RJ. *Medicine: An Illustrated History.* New York, NY: Abrams; 1987:

13. Hoffa M, Ludwig C. Einige neue versuche über herzbewegung. *Ztschr rat Med.* 9:107–144, 1850.

14. Prevost JL, Battelli F. Some effects of electric discharge on the hearts of animals. *Comptes Rendus Acad Sci.* 129:1267–1268, 1899.

15. Beck CS, Prilchard WH, Feil HS. Ventricular fibrillation of long duration abolished by electric shock. *JAMA.* 135:985–986, 1947.

16. Zoll PM, Linenthal AJ, Gibson W, et al. Termination of ventricular fibrillation in man by externally applied electric countershock. *N Engl J Med.* 254:727–732, 1956.

17. McKeown P, Croal S, Allen JD, et al. Clinical investigations: transesophageal cardioversion. *Am Heart J.* 125:396–404, 1956.

18. Levy S, Lauribe P, Dolla E, et al. Clinical trials: a randomized comparison of external and internal cardioversion of chronic atrial fibrillation. *Circulation.* 86:1415–1420, 1992.

19. Pai SM, Torres V. Atrial fibrillation: new management strategies. *Curr Probs Cardiol.* 18:233–300, 1993.

20. Van Gelder I, Crijns HJ, Van Gilst WH, et al. Arrhythmias and conduction disturbances: prediction of uneventful cardioversion and maintenance of sinus rhythm from direct-current electrical cardioversion and chronic atrial fibrillation and flutter. *Am J Cardiol.* 68:41–46, 1991.

21. Cullhed I. Cardioversion during pregnancy: a case report. *Acta Med Scand.* 214:169–172, 1983.

22. Lerman BB, Deale OC. Laboratory investigation: effect of epicardial patch electrodes on transthoracic defibrillation. *Circulation.* 81:1409–1414, 1990.

23. Pinski SL, Arnold AZ, Mick M, et al. Safety of external cardioversion/defibrillation in patients with internal defibrillation patches and no device. *PACE.* 14:7–12, 1991.

24. Kerber RE, Grayzal J, Hoyt R, et al. Self-adhesive, preapplied electrode pads for defibrillation and cardioversion. *J Am Coll Cardiol.* 3:815–820, 1984.

25. Sirna SJ, Ferguson DW, Charbonnier F, et al. Electrical cardioversion in humans: factors affecting transthoracic impedance. *Am J Cardiol.* 62:1048–1052, 1988.

26. Metcalfe MJ, Smith F, Jennings K, et al. Short reports: does cardioversion of atrial fibrillation result in myocardial damage? *Brit Med J.* 296:1364, 1988.

27. Van Gelder IC, Crijns HJ, Van Derl aarse A, et al. Clinical investigations: incidence and clinical significance of ST segment elevation after electrical cardioversion of atrial fibrillation and atrial flutter. *Am Heart J.* 121:51–56, 1991.

28. Coplen SE, Antman EM, Berlin JA, et al. Clinical investigation: efficacy and safety of quinidine therapy for maintenance of sinus rhythm after cardioversion: a metanalysis of randomized control trials. *Circulation.* 82:1106–1116, 1990.

29. Cardiac Arrhythmia Suppression Trial (CAST) Investigators. Preliminary report: effect of encainide and flecainide on mortality in a randomized trial of arrhythmia suppression after myocardial infarction. *N Engl J Med.* 321:406–412, 1989.

30. Horowitz LN, Spielman SR, Greenspan AM, et al. Use of amiodarone in the treatment of persistent and paroxysmal atrial fibrillation resistant to quinidine therapy. *J Am Coll Cardiol.* 6:1402–1406, 1985.

31. Herre JM, Sauve MJ, Malone P, et al. Long-term results of amiodarone therapy in patients with recurrent sustained ventricular tachycardia or ventricular fibrillation. *Am J Cardiol.* 13:442–449, 1989.

32. Zipes DP, Prystowsky EN, Heger JJ. Amiodarone: electrophysiologic actions, pharmacokinetics, and clinical effects. *J Am Coll Cardiol.* 3:1059–1071, 1984.

33. Troup PJ, Chapman DP, Olinger GN, et al. The implanted defibrillator: relation of defibrillator lead configuration and clinical variables to defibrillation threshold. *J Am Coll Cardiol.* 6:1315–1321, 1985.

34. Guarnieri T, Levine JH, Veltri EP, et al. Success of chronic defibrillation and the role of antiarrhythmic drugs with the automatic implantable cardioverter-defibrillator. *Am J Cardiol.* 60:1061–1064, 1987.

35. Sagrista SJ, Permanyer MG, Soler SJ. Clinical investigations: electrical cardioversion after amiodarone administration. *Am Heart J.* 123:1536–1542, 1992.

36. Hernandez R, Mann DE, Breckinridge S, et al. Experimental studies: effects of flecainide on defibrillation thresholds in the anesthetized dog. *J Amer Coll Cardiol.* 14:777–781, 1989.

37. Echt DS, Black JN, Barbey JT, et al. Laboratory investigation: evaluation of antiarrhythmic drugs on defibrillation energy requirements in dogs: sodium channel block and action potential prolongation. *Circulation.* 79:1106–1117, 1989.

38. Lown B. Electrical reversion of cardiac arrhythmias. *Br Heart J.* 29:469–489, 1967.

39. Bjerkelund CJ, Orning OM. The efficacy of anticoagulation therapy in preventing embolism related to direct current electrical conversion of atrial fibrillation. *Am J Cardiol.* 23:208–216, 1969.

40. Mancini GBJ, Weinberg DM. Cardioversion of atrial fibrillation: a retrospective analysis of the safety and value of anticoagulation. *Cardiovasc Rev Rep.* 11:18–23, 1990.

41. Arnold AZ, Mick MJ, Mazurek RP, et al. Reports on therapy: role of prophylactic anticoagulation for direct-current cardioversion in patients with atrial fibrillation or atrial flutter. *J Amer Coll Cardiol.* 19:851–855, 1992.

42. Manning WJ, Leeman DE, Gotch PJ, et al. Pulsed doppler evaluation of atrial mechanical function after elective cardioversion of atrial fibrillation. *J Am Coll Cardiol.* 13:617–623, 1989.

43. Laupacis A, Albers G, Dunn M, et al. Antithrombotic therapy in atrial fibrillation. *Chest.* 102:426S–433S, 1992.

44. Manning WJ, Silverman DI, Gordon SPF, et al. Cardioversion from atrial fibrillation without prolonged anticoagulation with use of transesophageal echocardiography to exclude the presence of atrial thrombi. *N Engl J Med.* 328:750–755, 1993.

— 12 —

Complications of Electrophysiologic Testing

Paul F. Walter, M.D.

HISTORY

Electrophysiological testing began 25 years ago with the recording of intracardiac signals from the region of the bundle of His.[1] Its clinical value quickly expanded to include location of atrioventricular (AV) blocks as well as better defining supraventricular and ventricular tachycardias.[2,3]

INDICATIONS

The study is useful in the diagnosis and treatment of patients who have intraventricular and AV conduction disturbances, sinus node dysfunction, supraventricular tachycardia, ventricular tachycardia, and unexplained syncope. Further advancement in techniques, including pacing techniques, permitted evaluations of sinus node dysfunction, AV blocks, and initiation of both supraventricular and ventricular arrhythmias.[3,4,5] Last year at Emory Hospital, more than 500 electrophysiologic tests were performed.

CONTRAINDICATIONS

Electrophysiological testing is not indicated when the detection of a cardiac arrhythmia will not enhance the patient's clinical course. Coagulation abnormalities, including an elevated prothrombin time, an elevated partial thromboplastin time, and thrombocytopenia in varying degrees, can be either an absolute or a relative contraindication depending on the degree of coagulopathy. Acute myocardial infarction, unstable angina, and ongoing myocardial ischemia would require stabilization and treatment of

112

the patient before contemplating electrophysiological evaluation of co-morbid rhythm disturbances or AV block.

DESCRIPTION OF THE PROCEDURE

Intracardiac electrophysiological testing provides a rational approach to the diagnosis and management of selected patients with tachyarrhythmias, bradyarrhythmias, and recurrent syncope. These studies have enhanced our understanding of the mechanisms of cardiac arrhythmias. Electrophysiological testing requires introducing multipolar electrocatheters into the venous and/or arterial systems. In most patients, the electrodes are positioned in the right atrium, the right ventricle, and across the tricuspid valve for His bundle recording. In selected patients, catheters are introduced into the left ventricle and coronary sinus. The distal two poles of a quadripolar catheter are used for intracardiac bipolar stimulation, and the proximal two poles for recording electrical activity.

COMPLICATIONS OF ELECTROPHYSIOLOGIC TESTING

Complications of electrophysiological testing can result from the intravascular catheterization procedure, the consequences of electrical stimulation of the heart, or the effects of antiarrhythmic drug therapy. Fortunately, electrophysiological studies can be done with a low risk, even in patients with life-threatening arrhythmias. An overall complication rate of less than 2% is readily achievable. The risk of a fatal arrhythmia is minimized by assiduous patient monitoring and the presence of skilled personnel with advanced life-support training. All patients should receive continuous electrocardiographic and oximetric monitoring and frequent sphygmomanometric blood pressure recording. Routine intraarterial pressure recording is not required. Provision for intracardiac pacing must always be available. The key maneuver in preventing a fatality is the prompt cardioversion of a hemodynamically unstable tachyarrhythmia. The availability of a second, backup defibrillator is recommended, as unexpected failure of an external cardioverter-defibrillator may occur.

Electrophysiological studies are quite safe; even the most sophisticated studies requiring use of multiple catheters are associated with a low mortality rate. The data from four major laboratories records only two deaths in 16650 electrophysiological studies.[6,7,8,9] In a survey of six university centers, five deaths occurred in 8545 electrophysiologic studies performed on 4015 patients (0.06%).[10] Two patients were in extremis at the time of study, and their death was imminent because of repeated ventricular tachyarrhythmia arrests. Neither patient could be resuscitated from electrically induced ventricular tachyarrhythmias. The remaining three deaths were unexpected and related to the procedure. Two patients died of refractory ventricular fibrillation, and one patient died from incessant ventricular tachycardia related to procainamide therapy. The patients at greatest risk of dying from the procedure generally have inducible rapid ventricular tachycardia in the setting of markedly decreased left ventricular systolic function or severe aortic outflow tract obstruction.

Complications Related to Catheterization Procedure

Complications related to the insertion and positioning of electrocatheters include deep venous thrombosis, pulmonary embolism, perforation of a cardiac chamber or coronary sinus, arterial injury, hemorrhage, infection at catheter sites, systemic infections, pneumothorax, and systemic arterial embolism.

Venous thrombotic events may result from in-situ thrombosis at the catheter entry site or thromboembolism from the catheter. Major venous thrombosis occurs in approximately 0.5% of patients, half of whom develop pulmonary embolism.[9,10] In most patients, the thrombotic site is the femoral vein. Factors predisposing to venous thrombosis are older age, long periods of limited physical activity, congestive heart failure, and multiple electrophysiological procedures. There is no consensus as to the value of heparin in preventing this complication. Heparin is always given when catheters are placed in the left heart prophylactic anticoagulation with heparin is recommended in patients with previous venous disease and for patients undergoing prolonged right-sided studies. The appearance of venous thrombosis may be delayed for a week or more following the procedure.

Symptomatic cardiac perforation occurs in 0.2% of patients.[7] Perforation of the right ventricle is most common because of its thin wall. The coronary sinus is another potential site for perforation. Cardiac perforation is often heralded by pericarditic chest pain, hypotension, and other signs of pericardial tamponade. The diagnosis is best confirmed by echocardiography. Less than one half of patients with cardiac perforation require pericardial drainage. Open surgical repair is needed when tamponade cannot be relieved by pericardiocentesis, abundant clot formation in the pericardial space leads to cardiac compression, or bleeding persists from the perforation site. The incidence of right ventricular perforation may be lessened by choosing smaller, more flexible electrode catheters in older patients and by keeping the right ventricular catheter away from the right ventricular apex.

The femoral artery may be injured during femoral artery puncture and catheterization for left ventricular electrophysiologic studies or from inadvertent puncture of the femoral artery during femoral venous catheterization. These complications are reported in only 0.4% of studies.[10] Femoral artery damage may produce femoral artery thrombosis or pseudoaneurysm formation, requiring vascular surgical correction. At present, the need for left ventricular catheterization during a diagnostic electrophysiologic study is infrequent. Occasionally, left ventricular stimulation may be needed to initiate sustained monomorphic ventricular tachycardia in a patient with spontaneous ventricular tachycardia. The use of triple extra stimuli that are delivered at several right ventricular sites lessens the need for left ventricular stimulation.

Hemorrhage from puncture sites can be minimized by maintaining firm pressure on these sites for 10 to 20 minutes or until the area is dry. Bed rest for 3 to 6 hours is followed by minimal activity for 12 to 24 hours. Splendid nursing observation is vitally important in detecting delayed hemorrhage. Abdominal pain following catheterization should trigger a heightened awareness of the potential for retroperitoneal bleeding. The vigorous treatment of nausea is warranted because the strain of vomiting may dislodge the vascular plug and initiate bleeding.

Both infection at the catheter site and systemic infection (bacteremia) are rare complications.[6] Infectious complications are more common when antecubital venous cutdowns are used. The use of indwelling electrocatheters also increases the infection risk. Neither procedure is in current use.

The expected rate of pneumothorax with subclavian catheterization is 0.25%.[11] This route may facilitate catheter placement in the coronary sinus and was previously used for insertion of an indwelling right ventricular catheter for serial drug testing. Coronary sinus catheterization can also often be accomplished from the femoral vein when steerable catheters are used.

Arrhythmia Complications of Electrophysiological Testing

Because the usual purpose of the electrophysiological study is to elicit arrhythmias, sudden bradycardia or tachycardia may result. Such arrhythmias are not considered complications of the study unless they are not relevant to the patient's indication for study or they fail to respond to treatment. Mechanical irritation from catheters during placement can cause atrial and ventricular ectopic beats and right bundle branch block (with right ventricular catheterization). Patients with a previous history of atrial fibrillation are especially prone to the occurrence of atrial fibrillation during catheter manipulation. Atrial fibrillation precludes study of any other type of supraventricular tachycardia. In patients without previous spontaneous atrial fibrillation, this arrhythmia usually subsides in seconds to minutes. Catheter-induced right bundle branch block may initiate complete heart block in patients with preexisting left bundle branch block.[12] This usually appears during manipulation of the AV junctional catheter in pursuit of a His bundle electrogram. The site of block is distal to the His bundle recording site. Catheter-induced complete heart block is usually transient.

A precise anatomic cardiac diagnosis should be established before electrophysiological evaluation of patients with malignant ventricular arrhythmias. This evaluation should include an assessment of coronary artery anatomy and left ventricular function. Patients with severe aortic outflow tract obstruction or active myocardial ischemia need surgical correction of the outflow tract obstruction or myocardial revascularization before electrophysiological evaluation of ventricular tachycardia. One question should always be asked: If ventricular fibrillation results, will resuscitation be successful? For some patients with severe left ventricular dysfunction (a left ventricular ejection fraction less than 20%, the risk of precipitating irreversible hemodynamic collapse with the induced ventricular arrhythmia may outweigh any potential benefit.

A troublesome facet of programmed ventricular stimulation is the occasional induction of polymorphous ventricular tachycardia or ventricular fibrillation in subjects without a history of ventricular tachycardia or cardiac arrest. Such arrhythmic events are not fatal but electrical cardioversion may be required, a disconcerting event for both patient and physician. Although there is no failsafe means of preventing the induction of these nonspecific ventricular arrhythmias, their appearance can be decreased by following certain guidelines. Ventricular stimulation is best done with the current output adjusted to twice the diastolic threshold. A current output in excess of 5 mA is not recommended because of a greater likelihood of initiating ventricular fibrillation. The delivery of up to three extra stimuli produces the optimal sensitivity and specificity for the initiation of ventricular tachycardia. Rarely, four extra stimuli are needed to induce a sustained monomorphic ventricular tachycardia. Additional measures that limit the initiation of nonspecific ventricular tachyarrhythmias include (1) avoidance of premature beat coupling intervals of less than 180 μsec and (2) refraining from shortening the coupling interval of premature extra stimuli when excess latency appears or when the QRS complex width of the premature beat increases as compared to baseline.

Complications Related to Antiarrhythmic Therapy

Occasionally, programmed ventricular stimulation precipitates an incessant ventricular tachycardia. This usually occurs when patients are receiving oral or intravenous antiarrhythmic drugs. This complication developed in 3% of patients who underwent electrophysiologic studies to test the effectiveness of antiarrhythmic drugs. No episodes were fatal but vigorous supportive care was required. Systemic arterial hypotension may complicate intravenous antiarrhythmic drug infusion. The blood pressure can be normalized by decreasing the drug infusion rate, administering volume replacement, and giving an alpha adrenergic agonist.

Electrical cardioversion is required to terminate approximately 50% of induced ventricular tachyarrhythmias. Although ventricular arrhythmia induction followed by cardioversion can induce myocardial infarction, cerebral infarction, or systemic arterial emboli, these complications occur infrequently.

Miscellaneous Complications

Although angina pectoris rarely develops during the course of an electrophysiologic study, its presence may be the first clue to serious underlying coronary artery disease. Angina pectoris may be precipitated by anxiety, rapid pacing, tachyarrhythmias, or an isoproterenol infusion. Upon the appearance of angina pectoris, the study should be terminated, a 12-lead electrocardiogram obtained, and treatment given.

CONCLUSIONS

Diagnostic electrophysiological testing is safer now than in the early years of the discipline. Subclavian vein catheterization is less frequent, indwelling subclavian vein catheterization is no longer performed, and there is a marked reduction in serial antiarrhythmic drug studies per individual patient.

REFERENCES

1. Scherlag BJ, Lau SH, Helfant RH, et al. Catheter technique for recording His bundle activity in man. *Circulation*. 39:13–18, 1969.
2. Goldreyer BN, Bigger JT. Spontaneous & induced reentrant tachycardia. *Ann Internal Med*. 70:87–98, 1969.

3. Mason JW, Winkel RA. Electrode catheter arrhythmia induction in the selection and assessment of antiarrhythmia drug therapy for recurrent ventricular tachycardia. *Circulation* 58: 971–985, 1978.

4. Mandel WJ, Hayakawa H, Danzig R. et al. Evaluation of sinoatrial node function in man by overdrive suppression. *Circulation* 44:59–66, 1971.

5. Navula OS, Samet P, Javier RP. Significance of the Sinus node recovery time. *Circulation.* 45:140–158, 1972.

6. DiMarco JP, Garan H, Ruskin JN. Complications in patients undergoing cardiac electrophysiologic procedures. *Ann Intern Med.* 97:490, 1982.

7. Horowitz LN, Kay HR, Kutalek SP, Discigil KF, Webb CR, Greenspan AM, Spielman SR. Risks and complications of clinical cardiac electrophysiologic studies: a prospective analysis of 1000 consecutive patients. *J Amer Coll Cardiol* 9:1261, 1987.

8. Akhtar M. Technique of electrophysiological testing. In: Schlant RC, Alexander RW, eds. *The Heart.* New York, NY: McGraw-Hill; 873–891, 1994.

9. Josephson ME. Electrophysiologic investigation: technical aspects. In: Josephson ME. *Clinical Cardiac Electrophysiology.* Philadelphia, PA: Lea and Febiger; 5–21, 1993.

10. Horowitz LN. Safety of electrophysiologic studies. *Circulation.* 73:II–28, 1986.

11. Bernard RW, Stahl WM. Subclavian vein catheterization: a prospective study. *Ann Surg.* 173:184, 1971.

12. Akhtar M, Damato AN, Gilbert-Leed CJ, et al. Induction of iatrogenic electrocardiographic patterns during electrophysiologic studies. *Circulation* 56:60, 1977.

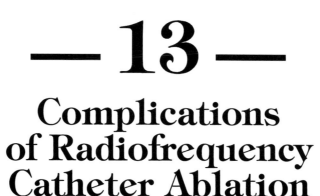

— 13 —

Complications of Radiofrequency Catheter Ablation

Terrence P. May, M.D.
Jonathan J. Langberg, M.D.

INDICATIONS

The goal of catheter ablation is controlled destruction of small areas of cardiac tissue critical for the initiation or perpetuation of arrhythmias. The introduction of radiofrequency energy has greatly enhanced the safety and effectiveness of ablation. This technique is now considered the treatment of choice for patients with recurrent paroxysmal supraventricular tachycardia due to AV nodal reentry or an extranodal accessory pathway.[1] Radiofrequency catheter ablation is also used to create complete AV block in order to palliate patients with drug-refractory atrial fibrillation.[2,3] Recently, radiofrequency ablation has been investigated for treatment of atrial tachycardia and flutter and for selected patients with ventricular tachycardia.[4–9]

CONTRAINDICATIONS

Groin complications and sequelae of perforation are more ominous in the setting of coagulation abnormalities, which should first be corrected. Concurrent infections should be treated before an elective ablation.

The most serious complications could arise from inaccurate interpretation of the

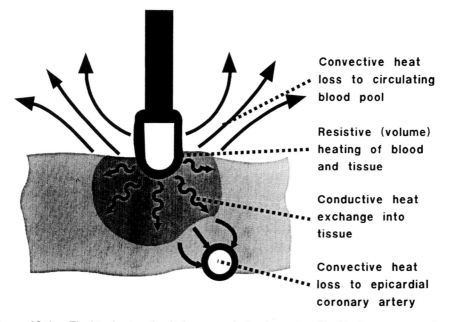

Convective heat loss to circulating blood pool

Resistive (volume) heating of blood and tissue

Conductive heat exchange into tissue

Convective heat loss to epicardial coronary artery

Figure 13.1. The biophysics of radiofrequency lesion formation. The black zone surrounding the distal electrode represents the region where current density is high enough to produce resistive heating. The majority of the lesion is formed by conduction of heat into the surrounding myocardium. Note that heat loss through convection produces relative sparing of the endocardium and coronary arteries. From Haines et al.[11] Reproduced with permission.

arrhythmia (either site or mechanism) or from incorrect placement of the ablation catheter. A thorough knowledge of the intracardiac structures and intracardiac electrograms is imperative.

TECHNIQUE OF RADIOFREQUENCY ABLATION

During radiofrequency ablation, current flows from the distal electrode at the tip of the catheter into the adjacent endocardium. This current accelerates ions in solution, resulting in resistive heating of the electrode-tissue interface. Heat is transferred to the surrounding myocardium by conduction, resulting in a spheroidal lesion 4 to 6 mm in diameter (Figure 13.1).[10] Histopathologic analysis of lesions reveals coagulative necrosis, with a well-demarcated border between necrotic and normal myocardium.[11]

Preliminary studies of patients treated with radiofrequency catheter ablation have been associated with a remarkably low incidence of adverse events. However, as with any invasive cardiovascular procedure, serious complications do occur. The purpose of this chapter will be to characterize the complications of radiofrequency catheter ablation. Data from a recent multicenter prospective trial (EP Technologies) will be described.[12] These results will be compared to the findings of a number of retrospective series from single institutions.

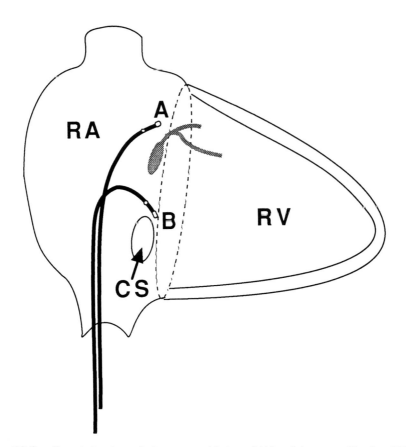

Figure 13.2.   Target sites for radiofrequency ablation of AV nodal reentry. The fast AV nodal pathway (A) is located near the apex of the triangle of Koch. The slow pathway (B) can be ablated posteriorly, near the ostium of the coronary sinus (CS). Note that fast-pathway target sites are closer to the specialized conduction system (gray), which accounts for the higher incidence of inadvertent AV block. RA = right atrium. RV = right ventricle.

COMPLICATIONS OF RADIOFREQUENCY CATHETER ABLATION FOR AV NODAL REENTRANT TACHYCARDIA

AV Block

AV nodal reentry is caused by a circus movement around the AV junction. During typical AV nodal reentry, antegrade conduction occurs over the "slow" AV nodal pathway, and retrograde conduction is via the "fast" pathway.[13] Fast pathway function is mediated by anterior atrial inputs to the AV node near the apex of the triangle of Koch, just proximal to the central fibrous body. The slow pathway is located posteriorally, near the ostium of the coronary sinus (Figure 13.2).

The first radiofrequency catheter ablation technique developed for treatment of AV nodal reentry targeted the fast pathway. During fast pathway ablation, sites are identified that are proximal and slightly anterior to the location of the maximal His

TABLE 13.1. Incidence of Permanent Atrioventricular Block Following Ablation of Atrioventricular Nodal Reentry Tachycardia: Anterior Versus Posterior Approach

Author	Year	Number of Patients	Anterior Approach	Posterior Approach
Calkins[22]	1991	46	1/46 (2%)	N/A
Chen[15]	1992	100	2/32 (6%)	0/68 (0%)
Haissaguerre[19]	1992	64	N/A	0/64 (0%)
Jackman[17]	1992	80	N/A	1/80 (1.3%)
Jazayeri[14]	1992	34	N/A	1/34 (3%)
Kay[18]	1992	49	4/19 (21%)	0/35 (0%)
Langberg[21]	1993	50	0/22 (0%)	1/28 (4.6%)
Lee[13]	1991	39	3/39 (8%)	N/A
Moulton[20]	1993	30	N/A	0/30
TOTAL			10/158 (6.3%)	3/309 (0.97%)

bundle electrogram recording. Although this technique is effective, it produces first-degree AV block, which occasionally is quite pronounced. More important, fast pathway ablation is associated with a significant risk of inadvertent high-grade AV block. This is likely due to the proximity between fast pathway target sites and the compact AV node and proximal His bundle.

The initial series of patients treated with fast-pathway ablation reported an incidence of complete AV block between 6% and 21%.[13–15] Although AV block usually occurs during the ablation session, its onset occasionally may be delayed by hours or days.

Langberg et al described a modification of the standard technique intended to reduce the incidence of complete AV block during fast-pathway ablation.[16] Rather than a fixed power output at each site, power was gradually incremented during each application. None of the 38 patients treated using titration of power output had AV block, compared with 9 out of 89 (10%) of historic controls who underwent fast pathway ablation using a fixed power output.

Slow-pathway function can be attenuated or eliminated using radiofrequency lesions made at the posteroseptal tricuspid annulus, adjacent to the ostium of the coronary sinus. Unlike fast-pathway ablation, these lesions are several centimeters from the distal AV node. Consequently, complete AV block is an infrequent event following slow-pathway ablation, with a reported incidence of 0% to 4.6% (Table 13.1).[14,17–22] The overall frequency of AV block in seven series was 3 out of 309 patients (1%). In a prospective multicenter trial, one case of AV block occurred in 52 patients treated with slow-pathway ablation.[12] In a recent study from the University of Michigan, 50 consecutive patients were randomly assigned to either an anterior (fast-pathway) or posterior (slow-pathway) approach for the treatment of typical AV nodal reentrant tachycardia.[21] One of the 28 patients treated with posterior lesions developed complete AV block.

In summary, radiofrequency AV nodal modification is an effective therapy for paroxysmal supraventricular tachycardia due to typical AV nodal reentry. However, inadvertent complete AV block occasionally complicates the procedure. (Figure 13.3)

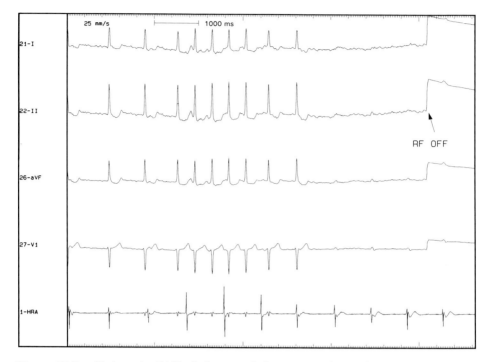

Figure 13.3. High-grade AV block during radiofrequency catheter ablation of the slow AV nodal pathway. There is an accelerated junctional rhythm with retrograde conduction during the first two beats of the tracing, which is common during successful slow pathway ablation. Next, the junctional rate increases with V-A dissocation, followed by high-grade AV block.

The incidence of AV block after anterior ablation (targeting the fast AV nodal pathway) is 5% to 10%. In contrast, slow-pathway ablation has a lower incidence of AV block of 1% to 4%, probably because of the greater distance between the target site and the distal AV node. Careful electrocardiographic monitoring and patient education concerning the importance of postprocedure bradycardia should increase early detection.

Tachyarrhythmias after AV Nodal Modification

New tachyarrhythmias sometimes occur after successful AV nodal modification. An increase in the frequency of atrial premature contractions and short runs of atrial tachycardia may be observed after therapy of AV node reentry. This is presumably due to abnormal automaticity at the atrial target site. The increase in atrial ectopy is transitory, with resolution within a few days to weeks.

After successful anterior (fast-pathway) ablation, a new paroxysmal supraventricular tachycardia is sometimes induced.[23] This arrhythmia is characterized by a short PR and a long RP interval, giving it the appearance of atypical AV nodal reentry. This new supraventricular tachycardia may be due to incomplete destruction of the fast AV nodal pathway, resulting in an increase in the retrograde (RP) conduction

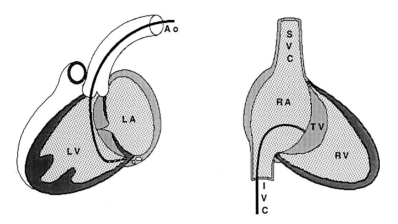

Figure 13.4. Techniques used to position radiofrequency ablation catheters at the sites of accessory pathways on the mitral and tricuspid annulus. Left-sided accessory pathways are often targeted using a retrograde approach. The ablation catheter is introduced into the femoral artery and advanced through the aortic valve into the left ventricle. It is positioned between the base of the mitral valve and left ventricular endocardium at the level of the annulus fibrosis. For right-sided accessory pathways, the ablation catheter is introduced into the femoral vein and positioned on the atrial side of the tricuspid annulus. Ao = aorta. IVC = inferior vena cava. LA = left atrium. LV = left ventricle. RA = right atrium. RV = right ventricle. SVC = superior vena cava. TV = tricuspid valve.

time during tachycardia. In other patients, elimination of the fast pathway unmasks a second, slower retrograde limb posteriorly that mediates atypical reentry.

Complications of Radiofrequency Catheter Ablation of Accessory Pathways

Accessory AV connections are strands of myocardium that traverse the AV groove. Typically, these pathways run subendocardially, adjacent to the annulus fibrosis, although they may also be subepicardial. Accessory pathways occur at all locations on both mitral and tricuspid annuli, with the possible exception of the aortic mitral continuity. Patients with accessory pathways often have recurrent paroxysmal supraventricular tachycardia. This is usually orthodromic reentry with antegrade conduction via the AV node and His-Purkinje system and retrograde conduction via the accessory pathway. Patients with rapid antegrade conduction over the accessory pathway may develop very fast ventricular response rates during atrial fibrillation. This is responsible for the approximately 0.5% incidence of sudden cardiac death in patients with Wolff-Parkinson-White syndrome.[24]

The approach to radiofrequency catheter ablation of accessory pathways is dependent on their location. A retrograde approach is often used for left-sided accessory pathways. The ablation catheter is introduced into the femoral artery and advanced through the aortic valve into the left ventricle. It is then positioned between the mitral valve and left ventricular endocardium at the level of the fibrous annulus (Figure 13.4). Recently, the transseptal approach has been increasingly used for left-sided accessory pathways. After transseptal puncture, a Mullins sheath is advanced into the left atrium. The ablation catheter is introduced via the sheath and positioned on the atrial side of the mitral annulus. For right-sided accessory pathways, the ablation catheter is inserted via the femoral or internal jugular veins and positioned on the atrial side of the tricuspid annulus.

The risks associated with radiofrequency catheter ablation of accessory pathways vary according to pathway location and the technique used to position the catheter at the target site. Ablation of septal pathways is associated with a risk of damage to the normal conduction system and AV block. Coronary and valvular complications may occur during ablation of left-sided accessory pathways using a retrograde approach. This would include coronary emboli, coronary dissection, and valve perforation. Myocardial ischemia occasionally complicates transseptal ablation, which may also produce tamponade due to perforation. Systemic emboli can occur with either technique.

Coronary Ischemia during Radiofrequency Catheter Ablation of Left-Sided Accessory Pathways

Investigators employing the retrograde approach and the transseptal approach have performed coronary angiography before and after ablation of left-sided accessory pathways.[25] These data show that the angiographic appearance of the coronary arteries is not affected by radiofrequency catheter ablation. Although subtle injury cannot be definitively excluded, it appears that the rapid blood flow in the epicardial coronary arteries produces marked convective cooling that protects them from thermal injury.

Ischemic complications of retrograde ablation occasionally result from inadvertent cannulation of the coronary ostia by the ablation catheter or from vasospasm due to ablation in proximity to the circumflex coronary artery. Ischemia has been produced by coronary air embolism during transseptal ablation.[26] (Figure 13.5) Myocardial infarction has been documented in 3 of 1073 accessory pathway ablations.[27–32] Two of these resulted from inadvertent radiofrequency application in the coronary artery when the catheter was believed to be positioned on the mitral annulus. In the third patient dissection of the left main artery caused an anteroseptal infarction 12 hours following ablation. This patient eventually required surgical repair of an expanding left main artery pseudoaneurysm.

Anginal chest pain and ST segment shifts developed following radiofrequency energy application in three additional patients. Vasospasm was suspected in each case because of normal emergent coronary angiograms, serial CK measurements, and the absence of ECG evolution indicative of a myocardial infarction. In a prospective multicenter trial, a small myocardial infarction was produced by inadvertent application of radiofrequency energy in the right coronary artery.[12] No other ischemic complications occurred in 143 patients having ablation of left-sided accessory pathways.

Valvular Complications of Accessory Pathway Ablation

Aortic insufficiency has resulted from the retrograde transaortic approach of accessory pathway ablation. The operator may choose to prolapse a loop of catheter formed

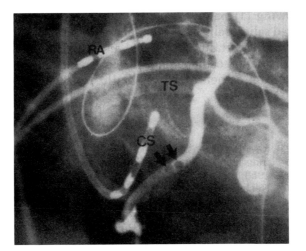

Figure 13.5. Air emboli complicating transseptal ablation of a left-sided accessory pathway. The two dark arrows show air bubbles and the distal circumflex coronary artery resulting in decreased flow distally. CS = electrode catheter in the coronary sinus. RA = right atrial electrode catheter. TS = transseptal sheath. From Lesh et al.[26] Reproduced with permission.

in the descending thoracic aorta or directly probe the aortic valve orifice with the steerable catheter. Because ablation catheters lack a lumen, these manipulations are performed without the benefit of guidewires or central pressure monitoring.

New aortic insufficiency was detected in postablation echocardiograms in 9 of 30 pediatric patients following the retrograde approach.[33] This has not been a common complication in a series of adults treated with radiofrequency ablation. If one considers only studies with 100% echocardiographic follow-up, 0 of 120 patients developed this complication.[28,30] If observations are extended to include series in which a majority of patients received echocardiographic follow-up, 1 of 387 patients developed mild aortic insufficiency.[27–30] This patient had a small leaflet perforation in a congenitally deformed valve. A recent case report described the occurrence of an aortic vegetation detected 20 hours after ablation of a left-sided accessory pathway.[34] (Figure 13.6) In a prospective multicenter trial of 257 accessory pathway ablations primarily using the retrograde transaortic approach, 2 patients developed mild aortic regurgitation.[12] If difficulty crossing the valve is anticipated because of aortic valve pathology, the transseptal approach should be employed for ablation of left-sided APs.

Thromboembolism

Histopathologic studies in animals after radiofrequency ablation have shown a thin (approximately 0.5 mm) layer of thrombus overlying the lesion.[35] However, studies of patients following ablation have shown a remarkably low incidence of mural thrombi. Using surface echocardiography, no thrombi were seen in several series of patients.[27–30] Goli et al performed transesophageal echocardiography in 95 patients after ablation of accessory pathways.[36] Although three small right atrial thrombi were identified, none of these were in proximity to the ablation site.

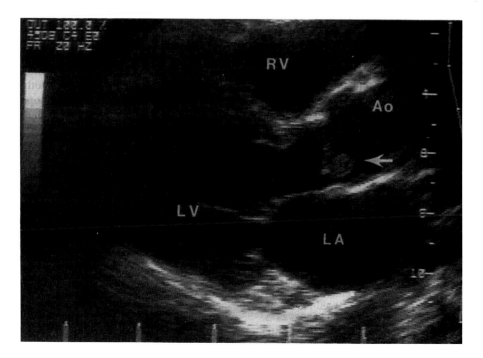

Figure 13.6. Parasternal long axis echocardiogram showing an aortic valve thrombus after retrograde ablation of a left-sided accessory pathway. The arrow points to a 5-mm echo-dense mass on the aortic leaflet. Ao = ascending aorta. LA = left atrium. LV = left ventricle. RV = right ventricle. From Raitt et al.[34] Reproduced with permission.

Embolic events rarely complicate left-sided ablation procedures. A transient neurologic deficit developed five days after successful accessory pathway ablation in one series of 250 patients.[27] Subsequent computed tomography was normal. One patient enrolled in a multicenter prospective trial sustained a hemispheric stroke following a protracted ablation procedure involving catheter exchanges through a long sheath in the aortic arch.[12] At our own institution, we have observed a patient who developed diplopia due to a third nerve palsy 8 hours following ablation. This resolved without residual symptoms and was felt to have been embolic in origin.

Other Complications of Ablation

Symptomatic arrhythmias during radiofrequency ablation have not been reported in previous series of AVNRT or accessory pathway ablation. Of the 458 patients enrolled in a prospective multicenter trial, 3 experienced ventricular tachycardias during radiofrequency application.[12] Two of the ventricular tachycardias were nonsustained, and the third degenerated into ventricular fibrillation that was promptly converted. A right-sided accessory pathway ablation failed because atrial fibrillation developed after each radiofrequency application. Only one other study has reported similar complications. Of 75 patients undergoing ablation, 2 developed ventricular fibrillation, and 1 developed atrial fibrillation during current delivery.[37] These arrhythmias occurred early in the authors' experience when impedance was not monitored in real time.

Continued current application after rapid impedance rise may lead to direct electrical stimulation of the endocardium. The relative rarity of such arrhythmias in the EPT trial, where impedance was monitored and radiofrequency automatically discontinued after rapid rise, supports this hypothesis.

The possibility of late arrhythmic complications has been evaluated in a number of studies. Follow-up Holter monitoring was performed at one and six months after ablation in the EPT trial. No new sustained tachyarrhythmias were detected.

Another series systematically evaluated Holter recordings following radiofrequency ablation. Ambulatory ECGs were recorded at one day, one week, and three months after ablation.[38] No sustained arrhythmias of any type occurred in the 35 patients studied. Premature ventricular contractions, ventricular couplets, and short (three- to six-beat) runs of ventricular tachycardia were statistically more common only in the first 24 hours following ablation. Thereafter, ventricular ectopy fell to baseline levels. These data are reassuring given the growing trend toward outpatient ablation, which has been safely performed in a select group of patients.

The possible chronic proarrhythmic effects of ventricular lesions produced during left-sided accessory pathway ablation has been studied. No clinical ventricular tachycardia occurred in 205 such patients during 9.8 ± 6.3 months of follow-up.[39] Of 33 patients who underwent repeat programmed ventricular stimulation four months after ablation, none had inducible monomorphic ventricular tachycardia. Similar data were reported in 59 patients using more aggressive ventricular stimulation protocols at one and three to six weeks after ablation.[38] Serial signal-averaged ECGs failed to demonstrate new late potentials following radiofrequency ablation.[40]

Bradycardia-dependent torsades de pointes has been reported following radiofrequency ablation of the AV junction.[41] We have seen this complication arise in patients with chronic atrial fibrillation with rapid ventricular response following His bundle ablation. Programming lower rate limits of permanent pacemakers implanted after the procedure to 80 to 90 per minute for 4 to 6 weeks should minimize the risk of life-threatening complications.

Radiation Risk

Calkins et al estimated the somatic and genetic risks of radiation exposure during radiofrequency ablation.[42] Dosimeters were placed on the anterior and posterior chest and the back in 35 patients undergoing ablation of accessory pathways. The mean duration of fluoroscopy exposure was 44 ± 40 minutes. The median radiation dose to the ninth vertebral body was 7.3 rem. The estimated increase in lifetime risk of a fatal malignancy as the result of this exposure was 0.1%, and the risk of a genetic defect was 20 per 1 million births. The amount of radiation received by the physician was well below occupational exposure guidelines established by the National Council on Radiation Protection and Measurements. More widespread use of pulsed fluoroscopy will decrease radiation exposure to patients and staff.

Perforation

Pericardial effusion and tamponade have rarely been reported to complicate catheter ablation.[28,29] This usually occurs in the anticoagulated patient as a result of diagnostic catheter perforation of the right ventricular wall. It has also been described after radiofrequency energy application in a branch of the coronary sinus.[29]

SUMMARY

Radiofrequency catheter ablation has revolutionized the field of cardiac electrophysiology. This technique is curative for the majority of patients with reentrant supraventricular tachycardia. It is also highly efficacious for therapy of selected patients with ventricular tachycardia, typical atrial flutter, and atrial tachycardia. Radiofrequency ablation of the bundle of His provides useful palliation of drug-refractory atrial fibrillation.

Serious complications during radiofrequency catheter ablation are infrequent but must be considered when evaluating prospective candidates for the procedure. Lesions are made in proximity to the specialized conduction system during ablation of AV node reentry and septal accessory pathways. This results in a risk of inadvertent AV block of approximately 1%. Ablation of left-sided accessory pathways is associated with a comparable incidence of serious adverse effects including valvular insufficiency, myocardial ischemia, and thromboembolism.

It is also important to remember that complications may arise as the result of vascular access or myocardial perforation, in similar frequency as diagnostic electrophysiology study (see chapter 12).

REFERENCES

1. Scheinman MM. Catheter ablation for cardiac arrhythmias, personnel and facilities. *PACE.* 15:715–721, 1992.
2. Langberg JJ, Chin MC, Rosenqvist M, Cockrell J, et al. Catheter ablation of the atrioventricular junction with radiofrequency energy. *Circulation.* 80:1527–1535, 1989.
3. Jackman WM, Wang X, Friday, KJ, Fitzgerald DM, Roman C, et al. Catheter ablation of atrioventricular junction using radiofrequency current in 17 patients. *Circulation.* 83:1562–1576, 1991.
4. Tracy CM, Swartz JF, Fletchter RD, et al. Radiofrequency catheter ablation of ectopic atrial tachycardia using paced activation sequence mapping. *JACC.* 21:910–917, 1993.
5. Feld GK, Fleck P, Chen P, et al. Radiofrequency catheter ablation of the treatment of human type 1 atrial flutter. *Circulation.* 86:1233–1240, 1992.
6. Klein LS, Shih H, Hackett K, et al. Radiofrequency catheter ablation of ventricular tachycardia in patients without structural heart disease. *Circulation.* 85:1666–1674, 1992.
7. Morady F, Harvey M, Kalbfleisch SJ, et al. Radiofrequency catheter ablation of ventricular tachycardia in patients with coronary disease. *Circulation.* 87:363–372, 1993.
8. Cohen TJ, Chien WW, Lurie KG, et al. Radiofrequency catheter ablation for treatment of bundle branch reentry tachycardia: results and long-term follow-up. *JACC* 18:1767–1773, 1991.
9. Kay GN, Chong F, Epstein AE, et al. Radiofrequency ablation for treatment of primary atrial tachycardias. *JACC.* 21:901–909, 1993.

10. Langberg JJ. Radiofrequency catheter ablation of AV nodal reentry: the anterior approach. *PACE* 16:615–622, 1993.

11. Haines DE. The biophysics of radiofrequency catheter ablation in the heart: the importance of temperature monitoring. *PACE.* 16(11):586–591, 1993.

12. Transcript of proceedings, Circulatory System Device Panel Meeting for the EPT-1000 Cardiac Ablation system. Miller Reporting Co., Washington, DC.; May 2, 1994. US Department of Health and Human Services, Public Health Service, Food and Drug Administration.

13. Lee MA, Morady F, Kadish A, et al. Catheter modification of the atrioventricular junction with radiofrequency energy for control of atrioventricular nodal reentry tachycardia. *Circulation.* 83:827–835, 1991.

14. Jazayeri MR, Hempe SL, Sra JS, et al. Selective transcatheter ablation of the fast and slow pathways using radiofrequency energy in patients with atrioventricular nodal reentry tachycardia. *Circulation.* 85:1318–1328, 1992.

15. Chen S, Chiang C, Tsang W, et al. Selective radiofrequency catheter ablation of fast and slow pathways in 100 patients with atrioventricular nodal reentrant tachycardia. *AHJ.* 125:1–10, 1993.

16. Langberg JJ, Harvey M, Calkins H, et al. Titration of power output during radiofrequency catheter ablation of atrioventricular nodal reentrant tachycardia. *PACE.* 16:465–470, 1993.

17. Jackman WM, Beckman KJ, McClelland JH, et al. Treatment of supraventricular tachycardia due to atrioventricular nodal reentry by radiofrequency catheter ablation of slow pathway conduction. *N Eng J Med.* 327:313–318, 1992.

18. Kay GN, Epstein AE, Dailey SM, et al. Selective radiofrequency ablation of the slow pathway for the treatment of atrioventricular nodal reentry tachycardia. *Circulation.* 85:1675–1688, 1992.

19. Haissaguerre M, Gaita F, Fischer B, et al. Elimination of atrioventricular nodal reentrant tachycardia using discrete slow potentials to guide application of radiofrequency energy. *Circulation.* 85:2162–2175, 1992.

20. Moulton K, Miller B, Scott J, et al. Radiofrequency catheter ablation for AV nodal reentry: a technique for rapid transection of the slow AV nodal pathway. *PACE.* 16:760–768, 1993.

21. Langberg JJ, Leon A, Borganelli M, et al. A randomized, prospective comparison of anterior and posterior approaches to radiofrequency catheter ablation of atrioventricular nodal reentry tachycardia. *Circulation.* 87:1551–1556, 1993.

22. Calkins J, Sousa J, El-Atassi R, Rosenheck S, et al. Diagnosis and cure of paroxysmal supraventricular tachycardia or the Wolff-Parkinson-White syndrome during a single electrophysiology test. *N Engl J Med.* 324:1612–1618, 1991.

23. Langberg JJ, Kim Y-N, Goyal R, Kou W, et al. Conversion of typical to "atypical" atrioventricular nodal reentrant tachycardia after radiofrequency catheter modification of the AV junction. *Am J Cardiol.* 85:565–573, 1992.

24. Klein GJ, Bashore TM, Sellers TD, Pritchett ELC, Smith WM, Gallagher JJ. Ventricular fibrillation in the Wolff-Parkinson-White syndrome. *N Engl J Med.* 301:1080–1085, 1979.

25. Solomon AJ, Tracy CM, Swartz JF, et al. Effect on coronary artery anatomy of radiofrequency catheter ablation of atrial insertion sites of accessory pathways. *JACC.* 21:1440–1444, 1993.

26. Lesh MD, Coggins DL, Ports TA. Coronary air embolism complicating transseptal radiofrequency ablation of left free-wall accessory pathways. *PACE.* 15:1105–1108, 1992.

27. Calkins H, Langberg JJ, Sousa J, et al. Radiofrequency catheter ablation of accessory atrioventricular connections in 250 patients. *Circulation.* 85:1337–1346, 1992.

28. Lesh MD, VanHare GF, Schamp DJ, et al. Curative percutaneous catheter ablation using radiofrequency energy in accessory pathways in all locations: results in 100 consecutive patients. *JACC.* 19:1303–1309, 1992.

29. Jackman WM, Wang Y, Friday KJ, et al. Catheter ablation of accessory atrioventricular pathways (Wolff-Parkinson-White syndrome) by radiofrequency current. *N Eng J Med.* 324:1605–1611, 1991.

30. Kuck KH, Schluter M. Radiofrequency catheter ablation of accessory pathways. *PACE.* 15:1380–1386, 1992.

31. Swartz JF, Tracy CM, Fletcher RD, et al. Radiofrequency endocardial catheter ablation of accessory pathway atrial insertion sites. *Circulation.* 87:487–499, 1993.

32. Lesh MD, Van Hare GF, Scheinman MM, et al. Comparison of the retrograde transaortic and transseptal methods for ablation of left free-wall accessory pathways. *JACC.* 22:542–549, 1993.

33. Minich L, Snider A, Dick M. Doppler detection of valvular regurgitation after radiofrequency ablation of accessory connections. *AJC.* 70:116–117, 1992.

34. Raitt MH, Schwaegler B, Pearlman AS, Poole JE, Bardy GH, Dolack GE, Kudenchuk PJ. Development of an aortic valve mass after radiofrequency catheter ablation. *PACE.* 16:2064–2066, 1993.

35. Jackman WM, Kuck KH, Nacarelli GV, Carmen L, Pitha J. Radiofrequency current directed across the mitral annulus with a bioplar epicardial-endocardial catheter electrode configuration in dogs. *Circulation.* 78:1288–1298, 1988.

36. Goli VD, Prasad R, Hamilton K, et al. Transesophageal echocardiographic evolution for mural thrombus following radiofrequency catheter ablation of accessory pathways. *PACE.* 140:1992–1997, 1991.

37. Leather RA, Leitch JW, Klein GJ, et al. Radiofrequency catheter ablation of accessory pathways: a learning experience. *AJC.* 68:1651–1655, 1991.

38. Chaing C, Chen S, Wang D, et al. Arrhythmogenicity of catheter ablation in supraventricular tachycardia. *Am Heart J* 125:388–95, 1993.

39. Twidale N, Beckman KJ, Hazlitt HA, et al. Radiofrequency catheter ablation of accessory pathways: are the ventricular lesions arrhythmogoenic? *Circulation.* (suppl 2):II-710, 1991. Abstract.

40. Hackett FK, Miles WM, Zipes DP, et al. Effect of radiofrequency catheter ablation for supraventricular tachycardia on the signal averaged electrocardiogram and programmed ventricular stimulation. *JACC.* 19(suppl A):183A, 1992. Abstract.

41. Calkins H, Niklason L, Sousa J, et al. Radiation exposure during radiofrequency catheter ablation of accessory atrioventricular connections. *Circulation.* 84:2376–2382, 1991.

42. Peters R, Wever E, Haver R, et al. Bradycardia-dependent QT prolongation and ventricular fibrillation following catheter ablation of the atrioventricular junction with radiofrequency energy. *PACE.* 17:108–112, 1994.

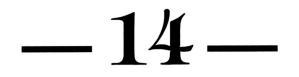

—14—

Implantation Complications of Permanent Cardiac Pacemakers

Robert S. Fishel, M.D.
Angel R. León, M.D.

INTRODUCTION

Although Hyman[1] is credited with designing the first pacemaker, Zoll[2] developed the high-voltage pacemaker in 1952. In 1958, Furman and Schwede developed the first long-term transvenous lead and the first implantable device was developed by Senning and Elmquist.[2] Last year approximately 130000 permanent cardiac pacemakers were implanted in the United States, and approximately 300000 new pacemakers were implanted worldwide. The number of pacer implants should continue to increase as the population ages, as developing countries acquire improving medical technology, and as existing pacing systems require generator replacement because of battery depletion. New indications for pacemakers, such as radiofrequency catheter ablation of the atrioventricular junction for control of atrial fibrillation,[3] rate responsive pacing to prevent atrial arrhythmia, and dual chamber pacing to decrease the outflow gradient in hypertrophic cardiomyopathy,[4] will further increase the number of implants.

Implantation of permanent cardiac pacemakers should be a relatively low-risk surgical procedure. However, cardiac pacemakers and defibrillators are usually implanted to treat potentially life-threatening disorders of cardiac conduction or automaticity and therefore, any complications affecting the performance of these devices has the potential to be lethal to the patient. The prompt recognition and treatment of implant-related complications are essential.

131

We classify complications of cardiac pacemaker implantation in this chapter as those arising within the first month of implantation and other complications that arise months to years later. The short-term complications can be further divided into those that arise as a direct result of the technique of obtaining access to the central circulation, and those that arise because of the presence of the implanted device itself.

INDICATIONS AND CONTRAINDICATIONS

Permanent pacing is indicated in those patients with severe symptomatic sinus bradycardia or AV block in whom the prognosis without pacing is poor (chronic complete heart block with slow ventricular response less than 40 beats per min, Mobitz type 2 block, symptomatic patients with bifascicular or intermittent third-degree block and a wide QRS, and asymptomatic patients with bifascicular block and a prolonged HV interval). Asymptomatic patients with sinus bradycardia or transient complete heart block with a narrow QRS are not considered candidates. The good prognosis with isolated first-degree AV block and Mobitz type I (Wenkebach) block also does not warrant permanent pacing.

Contraindications include patients with debilitating overall health, poor left ventricular function that will not be improved with pacing, dementia, and terminal cancer. Co-morbid infection and coagulation abnormalities may require treatment before permanent pacing.

SHORT-TERM PROCEDURE-RELATED COMPLICATIONS OF PERMANENT PACEMAKER IMPLANTATION

Numerous potentially serious complications may result from the implantation procedure itself. Certain complications are often reported and considered relatively common (Table 14.1), whereas other complications are rare, even bizarre (Table 14.2). The nature of implant-related complications can be traced to the type of surgical approach used to gain access into the central venous system and the heart. Unfortunately, few large prospective studies exist detailing the morbidity and mortality of pacemaker insertion. Older studies suggest operative and immediate postoperative mortality of pacemaker insertion to be approximately 1%.[5] Modern equipment and increasing experience with surgical techniques should decrease mortality and morbidity further. However, failure to recognize certain early complications would result in patient mortality and morbidity.

Pneumothorax

Pneumothorax has been reported to occur in 2.2% to 3.9% of attempts to access the subclavian vein.[6] This complication occurs much less frequently with internal jugular vein puncture and should not occur during cephalic vein cutdown.[7] The rate of pneumothorax formation seems to be in part dependent on the operator's

TABLE 14.1. Common Procedure-related Complications of Pacemaker Implantation

Electrocautery-induced injury
Inadvertent arterial cannulation
Lead/insulation damage
Lead dislocation
Myocardial puncture
Cardiac arrhythmia
Pacemaker pocket hematoma
Pacemaker pocket seroma
Pneumothorax
Hemothorax

experience.[6] It occurs more commonly in patients with hyperinflated lungs, such as can be seen in obstructive lung disease as well as in obese patients and patients with anatomic chest deformities. Evidence of the onset of pneumothorax includes aspiration of air during subclavian vein puncture, acute respiratory insufficiency, tracheal deviation, subcutaneous air, and hypotension. In most cases this complication is first discovered on the postoperative chest roentgenogram. If there is no respiratory embarrassment, the pneumothorax is judged to be less than 10%, and the apex of the lung has not dropped past the third intercostal space, then the patient may be observed with serial chest radiographs only.[8] The administration of oxygen theoretically accelerates the reabsorption of the extrapleural air. In the patient with respiratory insufficiency, a large or rapidly expanding pneumothorax, or hemodynamic compromise, insertion of a chest tube with continuous negative pressure relieves the pneumothorax by evacuating the extrapleural air. Related complications include hemothorax and hemopneumothorax formation (Figure 14.1). This complication results from laceration of the subclavian artery or the apex of the lung itself. Should hemothorax or

TABLE 14.2. Uncommon Procedure-related Complications of Pacemaker Implantation

Air embolism syndrome
Arterial venous fistula of the subclavian vein
Brachial plexus injury
Catheter embolism
Chordal rupture
Chylothorax
Coronary sinus contusion or thrombosis
Lymphatic fistula
Pericardial tamponade
Postcardiotomy syndrome
Proximal venous fragment embolism
Pulmonary artery lead fragment embolism
Tricuspid valve contusion/perforation

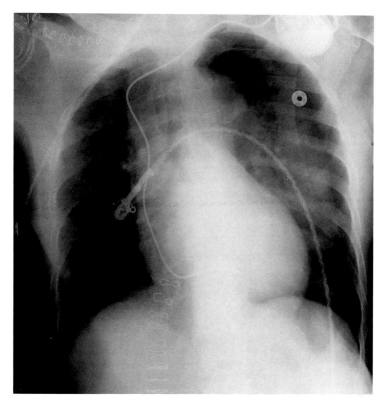

Figure 14.1.   Pneumothorax induced by pacemaker insertion.

hemopneumothorax formation be diagnosed, then prompt chest tube insertion is recommended given the inflammatory nature of intrapleural blood. To minimize the rate of this complication, the cephalic vein cutdown technique should be used whenever possible. Alternative techniques for venous access should always be considered in patients with distorted chest anatomy, coagulopathies, or obstructive lung disease.

Hematoma Formation

Pacemaker implantation often produces small amounts of incisional bleeding and local ecchymosis, which rarely have any consequence. Large hematoma in the pacemaker pocket, however, can have serious consequences. The hematoma may act as a nidus for infection, create pressure on the suture line leading to wound dehiscence, change the pacing thresholds of unipolar generators, or, rarely, disrupt the pacemaker header-lead connection. To avoid this complication, the patient should have a normal prothrombin and partial thromboplastin time at the time of pacemaker insertion. In addition, the use of antiplatelet drugs including aspirin should, if possible, be avoided for several days before implantation. Subcutaneous heparin should not be used for 24 hours before implantation. Intravenous heparin should be stopped 6 hours before the procedure. Anticoagulation should be withheld if possible for up to 48 hours after the surgery. Meticulous surgical technique and use of electrocautery during surgery can decrease the frequency of hematoma.

Usually only large (greater than 8 cm) or expanding hematomata following implantation require drainage. An expanding hematoma that retards wound healing or produces significant discomfort or neurovascular compromise to the patient needs to be evacuated. If leukocytosis or fever is associated with hematoma formation, or if the site is unusually tender or erythematous then the possibility of a pocket infection must be considered. Any drainage from the wound should be cultured, but needle aspiration of the hematoma is ill advised given the risk of introducing bacteria into the pacemaker pocket. Should infection be confirmed, then the pacing system should be explanted. In the absence of expansion, infection, or severe discomfort to the patient one should only observe the patient over time because most hematomata will eventually liquefy and reabsorb.

A seroma is collection of fluid that forms in the pacer pocket and surrounds the pacemaker. This is thought to arise as a result of an inflammatory response to either the surgery or the foreign body itself. Seromata usually require no treatment. Rarely a seroma or chronic hematoma produces enough discomfort to the patient to require percutaneous drainage. Percutaneous needle aspiration of fluid must be done in a strictly aseptic environment with care taken to avoid damage to the pacemaker or leads. Fluid obtained should be sent for cell counts and cultures to rule out an occult infection.

Inadvertent Arterial Cannulation

Unintentional entry into the subclavian artery results occasionally during attempts to gain venous access due to the proximity of the subclavian vein to the artery. Inadvertent entry into the common carotid during internal jugular puncture occurs less frequently. One can avoid undesired arterial entry by hydrating the patient well before attempts at central venous puncture, placing the patient in Trendelenberg's position to expand the vein, and by checking for pulsatile flow after needle puncture. Uncomplicated venous cannulation can rarely demonstrate pulsatile flow to a degree that can be mistaken for arterial cannulation. Exaggerated venous pulsatile flow occurs in patients with pulmonary hypertension and severe tricuspid insufficiency. Measurement of oxygen saturation in sampled blood, or injection of radiographic contrast material during fluoroscopic visualization, distinguishes between venous and arterial entry.

One should never insert an introducer or dilator into a vessel until the entry site has been clearly identified as a vein leading to the central circulation. Hematoma formation at the site of arterial puncture will occur if manual pressure is not maintained for a sufficient amount of time. Pseudoaneurysm formation should be considered should a pulsatile hematoma develop after inadvertent arterial cannulation. Subclavian artery laceration caused by advancement of an introducer or vigorous instrumentation can lead to hemothorax formation. Arterial-venous fistula development has been seen following inadvertent cannulation of the subclavian artery.[9,10] Other risks of arterial puncture include distal arterial embolism and retrograde arterial dissection.

Occasionally, arterial puncture goes unrecognized and the pacing lead enters into the left ventricle.[11] Cases detailing prolonged left ventricular pacing have been reported.[12] Because of the risk of stroke and arterial thromboembolism, one should remove any lead positioned in the left ventricle and reposition it in the right ventricle.

Myocardial Puncture

Perforation of the myocardium by advancing a pacemaker lead into the atrium or ventricle would at first consideration seem to be a relatively rare complication of pacemaker insertion. In fact, this complication probably occurs quite commonly but often goes unrecognized and unreported. Numerous case reports of myocardial perforation have been reported, and estimates of its frequency have ranged from 0.7% to 9% of all pacemaker implants.[5,13–15] Pleuropericardial pain, a high or rising stimulation threshold, a right bundle branch block morphology during pacing, a pericardial friction rub or clinical pericarditis, intercostal and diaphragmatic muscle stimulation, or cardiac tamponade temporally related to insertion of a pacing lead suggest perforation. However, most perforations produce no significant clinical sequelae.

When the surgeon notices lead penetration or perforation of the myocardium, the pacing lead should be removed immediately and repositioned elsewhere. Insertion of an active fixation lead into the intraventricular septum in the outflow tract avoids perforation of the thin right ventricular wall. One must always consider ventricular puncture with pericardial tamponade as a cause of acute hemodynamic compromise during pacemaker implantation.

Myocardial puncture by pacing leads rarely causes serious complications. When perforation causes a hemopericardium, serial echocardiograms, combined with blood pressure monitoring and the physical examination, will alert the physician of impending cardiac tamponade. Perforations of the right ventricle usually seal themselves owing to the relatively low systolic pressures generated by that chamber. Should the hemopericardium grow in size, or if signs of impending tamponade develop, one should perform pericardiocentesis to relieve or prevent tamponade. If possible, a drain should be left in place until the drainage has become serous and has decreased to less than about 5 cc per hour. In rare cases, open surgical repair of a punctured right ventricle with evacuation of the pericardial sac will be required.

Cardiac Arrhythmia

Mechanical irritation of atrial and ventricular myocardium produces arrhythmia. Non-sustained or hemodynamically insignificant arrhythmia from insertion of pacing leads should not be considered a complication of pacing system implants. More serious arrhythmia can occur. Atrial fibrillation is occasionally seen and can be precipitated by lead-induced atrial extrasystoles; it is often self-terminating. Persistent atrial fibrillation interferes with the determination of sensing and pacing thresholds through the atrial lead, and therefore requires pharmacological or electrical cardioversion. Manipulation of the ventricular lead produces ectopy, which may induce sustained ventricular tachycardia or fibrillation, particularly in patients with structural heart disease and ventricular dysfunction. Patients undergoing pacemaker placement should have anterior-posterior adhesive external defibrillation patches placed before the start of the procedure.

Patients undergo permanent pacemaker implantation for conduction system disease. During the procedure they are at risk for sinus bradycardia, sinus arrest, or atrioventricular block in the absence of temporary pacing. Increased vagal discharge due to the pain and anxiety associated with the procedure may produce or worsen bradycardia. Overdrive pacing during threshold testing can suppress the intrinsic rhythm and cause transient asystole upon termination of pacing. Insertion of the pacing lead into the right ventricle may cause asystole by traumatizing the bundle of His or right bundle branch, leading to complete atrioventricular block or mechanical disruption of a junctional escape mechanism. Patients with high-degree atrioventricular block or sinus arrest with unreliable escape rhythms should undergo insertion of a temporary pacing catheter before implantation of a permanent pacemaker. Careful continuous monitoring of the patient and prompt recognition of bradyarrhythmia or tachycardia are essential to safe permanent pacing system implantation.

Electrocautery Induced Injury

Electrocautery during pacing system implantation may produce significant problems. Contact between the electrocautery device and a pacing lead can injure the muscle in contact with the lead, induce ventricular fibrillation or damage the components of the pacing system.

Application of radiofrequency energy through a pacing lead into the myocardium produces a zone of thermal necrosis and scar. Fibrosis increases pacing thresholds. Transmission of current at the 200- to 500-kHz range as used in electrocautery may induce ventricular fibrillation. Electrocautery affects the myocardium either through direct contact with the pacing electrode, or via transmission by contact with the pacemaker generator of a unipolar pacing system.

Use of electrocautery near a pacemaker can significantly alter the functions of the pacemaker itself. Permanent damage, including loss of output due to instant battery depletion, can occur when radiofrequency current damages protective circuitry within the pulse generator. The pulse generator may be reprogrammed to new values. Most generators enter a "fall-back" mode. The characteristics of pacemakers in this mode vary among models and manufacturers, but most default to asynchronous pacing. The radiofrequency transmission from electrocautery may "fool" the sensing circuits of a pulse generator, producing inappropriate pacing inhibition and possibly asystole. Physicians should avoid the use of electrocautery near implanted pacing systems, especially unipolar generators that use a sensing dipole between the lead tip and the pulse generator. Far-field electrical interference, including electrocautery, affects the large sensing dipole of a unipolar pacing system much more than the small dipole of a bipolar sensing pulse generator.

Care must be taken to avoid contact between the cautery knife and implanted pacing leads during electrocautery. Use of bipolar electrocautery devices diminishes possible effects on implanted pacing systems.

Direct current defibrillation can damage a pacing system pulse generator.[16] All modern pacemakers contain a zener diode that protects circuits from DC current injury. However, when defibrillating a patient with a pacemaker, the current path should not be allowed to cross the pacemaker directly, and the defibrillator paddle should never be applied directly on top of a pacemaker.

Lead Dislodgment

Lead dislodgment occurs rarely but can be catastrophic in pacemaker-dependent patients. The incidence of lead dislodgment has been reported to be as high as 6.8%.[5] Current lead technologies reduce dislodgment to less than 2% of ventricular leads and less than 5% of atrial leads.[8] Signs of lead dislocation include increasing capture thresholds and failure to sense. The chest roentgenogram may demonstrate marked dislodgment of the lead to a different position; however, radiographs may miss microdislodgment. Treatment of this complication requires immediate reoperation with repositioning of the pacemaker lead.

Lead or Insulation Damage

Careless use of surgical instruments during the implantation procedure may damage the pacing electrode. The electrode itself may be cut by a scissors or scalpel or crushed by a clamp. The insulation material may be damaged or stripped by any sharp instrument or by rough handling. Signs of an occult electrode fracture include failure to capture, inappropriate sensing, or abnormally high lead impedance (greater than 1400 ohms). Signs of insulation damage include high pacing thresholds with an abnormally low impedance (less than 300 ohms). Damage to the outer insulating material may be repaired. Leads with damaged electrodes must be replaced. Careful handling of pacing leads reduces the probability of electrode or insulation damage.

The introduction of blood into the electrode lumen impacts the stylet within the lead. This often prevents any stylet from being advanced into the lead and results in the lead being entirely unusable. To avoid this complication, the implanting surgeon should frequently wash blood from his or her gloves before touching a stylet.

Rare Complications of Pacemaker Implantation

There are numerous uncommon complications of pacing system implants (Table 14.2). Contusions of cardiac structures from an advancing pacemaker lead have been reported. Leads introduced into the coronary sinus cause contusions or thrombosis of the sinus.[17,18] The tricusid valve may be damaged or perforated and the chordal structures may be traumatized.[19,20] Advancement of pacing leads through unrecognized septal defects may inadvertently position the electrode in the left side of the heart.[11,21] The presence of an unrecognized persistent left superior vena cava complicates lead insertion. Although the abnormal vena cava can be used as a route into the right side of the heart, it generally drains into the right atrium via the coronary sinus, a tortuous route that makes it quite difficult to properly position the lead.[22,23] Other rare complications, such as the postpericardiotomy syndrome or paradoxical embolism across patent foramina ovale, have also been reported.[24,25]

Distal embolization of a guidewire or lead fragment during the implantation procedure occurs usually because of carelessness. Usually, centrally embolized foreign bodies should be removed because of the high incidence of long-term complications.[26] The embolized catheter or lead may be removed percutaneously using various techniques including the Dormia basket.[27] It is best to try to avoid this complication by maintaining control of the proximal ends of any guidewires or pacing leads used.

SHORT-TERM COMPLICATIONS DUE TO THE PRESENCE OF A CARDIAC PACEMAKER OR LEADS

Infections

Infections occurring after pacemaker implantation represent one of the most serious avoidable complications seen with the procedure. Pocket infections predicate removal of the entire pacing system, a prolonged hospital stay for the patient, chronic antibiotic use, reoperation for subsequent permanent pacer placement, and the risks associated with any major infection including endocarditis, sepsis, and death. Infections involving implanted leads often cause endocarditis and thus have the potential to be equally serious. Implanting physicians should follow strict aseptic technique during the implantation procedure. Preoperative antibiotics have been shown to decrease the rate of infectious complications and should be administered whenever feasible.[28] No data support the routine use of postoperative antibiotics.

Persistent wound erythema, dehiscence, purulent drainage, or cellulitis suggest pacemaker pocket infection. Indolent infections can be difficult to detect and may only be manifest by pacemaker pocket erosion or adherence of the pacemaker to the skin.[8] Venous thrombosis, septicemia, and signs of systemic infection indicate lead infection.[29,30] Infected lead systems can frequently lead to valvular endocarditis.[31,32]

The microbiology of pacemaker pocket and lead infections tends to be similar to that seen in infections involving other permanently implanted devices such as prosthetic heart valves. *Staphylococcus aureus* and *Staphylococcus epidermidis* are frequently isolated. Less commonly, gram-negative organisms and fungi cause infection.[33]

Patients with infected pockets should receive intravenous antibiotic therapy guided by bacterial cultures with sensitivity testing. Conservative management of infections without pacing system explant may succeed.[34,35] However the majority of authors recommend complete removal of the pulse generator and leads.[36,37] We recommend removal of the entire system and a course of intravenous antibiotics administered before attempts at inserting a new system at a distant site.

Extracardiac Muscle Stimulation

Pulse generator output can occasionally stimulate the diaphragm, the intercostal, and the chest wall muscles. Unipolar pacing systems that use the pacemaker generator as the cathode stimulate extracardiac musculature more frequently than bipolar systems with a dipole localized to the distal pacing electrode. Pacing at maximal generator output after positioning the electrode within the heart detects extracardiac muscle stimulation. Repositioning the lead or using a bipolar electrode should eliminate the problem. When extracardiac muscle pacing occurs in a patient with a chronically implanted system, the one should determine stimulation thresholds for cardiac and extracardiac muscles. If there is an adequate safety margin between the two thresholds (twice the cardiac stimulation threshold), reprogramming the generator output between the two levels will correct the problem. However, when the cardiac stimulation threshold with a safety margin exceeds the extracardiac stimulation threshold, one should reposition or replace the electrode. Pacing system dysfunction with extracardiac muscle pacing long after implant suggests erosion of the electrode through the ventricle. Pectoral muscle stimulation by a unipolar pacing system suggests that noninsulated components of the pacemaker can contact skeletal muscle because of disruption of the insulation, or after manipulation of the generator flips it over within the pocket. Manually returning the pacemaker to its original position solves the latter problem. Insulation defects on the pulse generator that produce symptomatic pectoral muscle stimulation dictate replacement of the generator. Use of bipolar pacing systems and high-output testing at implant to detect diaphragmatic (ventricular leads) or phrenic nerve (right atrial leads) stimulation should eliminate extracardiac muscle stimulation.

Endless Loop Tachycardia

Patients with intact ventriculoatrial conduction and dual-chamber pacing systems can develop endless loop or pacemaker-mediated tachycardia (PMT). When retrograde activation of the atria follows ventricular pacing or a premature ventricular beat, the atrial sensing channel detects the atrial depolarization and follows with ventricular pacing after the appropriate atrioventricular delay. Perpetuation of this cycle causes PMT. The tachycardia occurs at the upper rate limit of the pacing system or the sum of the programmed atrioventricular delay plus the postventricular atrial refractory period. Extending the postventricular atrial refractory beyond the duration of ventriculoatrial conduction prevents the atrial channel from sensing atrial depolarization within this interval, the cycle cannot continue, and tachycardia cannot perpetuate.

Failure to Capture

Primary generator failure, faulty lead connections, electrode fracture, insulation failure, lead dislodgment, or myocardial perforation cause potentially catastrophic loss of capture. Interrogation of the pulse generator with determination of pacing threshold, pacing lead impedance, and sensing threshold helps identify the cause of capture loss. The chest roentgenogram should demonstrate obvious lead dislodgment, or electrode fractures; microdislodgment of the lead tip, or small lead fractures may go unrecognized by chest radiography. Up to 10% of patients develop progressively increasing pacing thresholds following initial implant due to fibrosis at the electrode-myocardium interface. High pacing thresholds lead to battery depletion, necessitating premature generator replacement. Repositioning the electrode at a site with better pacing thresholds relieves the problem. The diagnosis of chronically increasing pacing thresholds due to fibrosis should be made only after excluding the mechanical problems with the pacing system mentioned previously.

Oversensing and Undersensing Errors

Failure to sense intracardiac signals, or undersensing them, early after implant indicates an inadequate lead position due to either dislodgment or a poor initial position. Detection of artifact, extracardiac signals, or intracardiac events in an adjacent chamber by the pulse generator that inappropriately inhibit pacing (oversensing) can compromise the pacemaker-dependent patient. Oversensing most often occurs in unipolar pacing systems with their large sensing dipole, or "antenna," which detects far-field noise easier than bipolar systems with a short dipole. Oversensing also results when insulation defects develop in any type of pacing lead that exposes the electrode to ambient electrical interference. Pectoral muscle myopotentials that inhibit pacing in a unipolar pacing system are the most common example. In the absence of a mechanical defect within the lead, decreasing the gain of the sensing amplifier eliminates oversensing. One should be careful not to decrease the sensitivity excessively because that causes undersensing. Reversal of the atrial and ventricular lead connections into the pulse generator at the time of implant causes a form of inappropriate sensing. Reprogramming the pulse generator to asynchronous atrial pacing (AOO), which causes ventricular stimulation on the ECG, confirms this error.

Pacemaker Syndrome

Loss of atrioventricular synchrony or loss of the atrial contribution to cardiac output produces the symptom complex known as the pacemaker syndrome. During ventricular pacing the atria contract against a closed atrioventricular valve, or there may be ventriculoatrial conduction, producing suboptimal ventricular filling, particularly during exercise. Patients experience headaches, palpitations, early fatigue, upper body flushing, and a pounding awareness of ventricular pacing. Short of upgrading to a dual-chamber system, little can be done to alleviate symptoms. A 24-hour ECG analysis or event recorders help determine the circumstances under which the patient experiences the greatest symptoms. Most patients eventually adapt to some degree to the altered hemodynamics of single-chamber pacing. However, the young or active patient usually needs an upgrade to a dual-chamber unit with atrial tracking.

Pacemaker-AICD Interactions

Pacemakers may either inappropriately inhibit a defibrillator or trigger inappropriate therapy. Conversely, defibrillator discharges may reprogram pacemakers to undesired settings. Defibrillators respond to increases in the heart rate above a programmed threshold. If a rate-responsive pacemaker increases the patient's heart rate above the tachycardia detect rate, the defibrillator will deliver antitachycardia to a patient without ventricular tachycardia. Appropriate pacemaker programming eliminates the possibility of unnecessary tachycardia delivery by not exceeding the high rates required to activate the defibrillator (>150 per min). When a pacer emits pacing pulses in a patient with ventricular fibrillation, the pacing artifact may be large enough to inhibit the sensing circuitry of a defibrillator. Sensing circuits of all modern defibrillators use an automatic gain control that adjusts sensitivity to provide the best signal-to-noise ratio. The pacing artifact detected by the defibrillator may reset the gain control, "fool" the defibrillator (which interprets the spikes as an intrinsic rhythm), and decrease the sensitivity to a level above the fibrillatory potentials (which it interprets as noise). The patient remains in ventricular fibrillation; the defibrillator senses only the pacing spikes that inhibit therapy—with disastrous consequences. Unipolar pacing systems with large pacing artifacts more readily inhibit defibrillators than bipolar systems with small, local pacing artifacts. Pacing at the highest pacemaker pulse amplitude detects inappropriate inhibition of sensing at the time of defibrillator implant. One can avoid pacemaker-device interactions by explanting any unipolar pacing system at the time of defibrillator implant, placing the pacing lead at a distance from the defibrillator sensing lead, or lowering the pacing amplitude of the pacing generator.

Defibrillator discharges reprogram some pacing generators to "fall back" parameters. Some pacing generators pace asynchronously, others revert to unipolar pacing at full output. One should never use a pacing generator that reverts to unipolar pacing in a patient with an implantable defibrillator given the potentially disastrous consequences mentioned previously. Asynchronous pacing may theoretically induce arrhythmia, particularly in patients with defibrillators who are already at increased risk.

LONG-TERM COMPLICATIONS OF CARDIAC PACEMAKER INSERTION

Venous Thrombosis

Thrombosis at the entry site into the proximal central vein occurs frequently late after pacemaker implantation, but it can also happen in the early postoperative period.[38] Retrospective studies document abnormal venograms in 28% to 44% of patients after pacemaker implant, with total venous occlusion and collateral formation in 8% to 21% of all patients.[39–42] Symptomatic thrombosis of the upper extremities rarely occurs, probably because collateral venous channels form as the central venous thrombus slowly enlarges. Symptomatic thrombosis of the axillary or subclavian vein occurs in 1% to 3% of all patients.[43] Pain and swelling in the affected arm and dilation of collateralized superficial veins suggest venous occlusion. Occasionally painful thrombophlebitis appears.[44] If symptoms develop acutely, blood cultures should be obtained to rule out an occult infection. Treatment of symptomatic pacemaker-induced venous thrombosis includes rest and elevation of the affected extremity. For acute thrombi intravenous heparin therapy followed by systemic anticoagulation with warfarin may prevent progression. Thrombolytic therapy may benefit in patients with progressive or nonresolving subclavian vein thrombosis.[45,46]

Thrombi can grow and extend distally into the internal jugular vein, with further extension resulting into the cerebral venous sinuses,[47] or into the superior vena cava, producing superior vena cava obstruction.[48–51] Pulmonary thromboemboli in patients with pacemaker-induced superior vena cava syndrome occurs rarely.[52] Patients with superior vena cava obstruction should receive chronic oral anticoagulation with warfarin.

Pulmonary Embolism

Symptomatic pulmonary embolism complicates 0.6% to 3.5% of pacemaker implants.[53,54] One study documented asymptomatic pulmonary thromboembolism in 15% of patients.[55] A large right atrial thrombus can occasionally surround a pacing electrode, leading to a high mortality.[56,57] However, one should also consider underlying endocarditis in those patients. If possible, long-term systemic anticoagulation should be initiated in all patients with large atrial thrombi. One can consider thrombolytic therapy when tricuspid inflow obstruction can be demonstrated. Recurrent formation of thrombi dictates removal of the pacing lead.

Pacemaker Pocket Erosion

Pulse generators erode through the subcutaneous tissue and skin when implanted too superficially or when placed into an undersized pocket susceptible to tension after wound closure. Chronic friction on the generator contributes to pocket erosion. Revision of the pocket with reimplantation of the generator in the subpectoral space solves the problem of erosion. Skin flap reconstruction often provides an adequate alternative result. At the time of revision, cultures of the pocket should be obtained to rule out an indolent infection as a cause of the pocket erosion.

Twiddler's Syndrome

Continual manipulation of the pacemaker and its lead system twists or flips the generator or tangles or breaks the pacing leads. This tends to be seen in debilitated and mentally impaired patients and often occurs if there is a great deal of extra potential space available in the pacemaker pocket. A chest roentgenogram in a patient with twiddler's syndrome reveals severe coiling of the proximal pacing leads. Reversal of the orientation of the pulse generator header suggests flipping of the device within the pocket. Pacemaker revision for twiddler's syndrome should include submuscular reimplantation of the device and anchoring the header to adjacent connective tissue to prevent further manipulation.

RETAINED LEAD FRAGMENTS

Retained leads and lead fragments usually present no problem in the absence of infection. Retained leads can serve as a nidus for endocarditis, promote venous thrombosis, or migrate to other regions of the cardiovascular system. Documented infection of a retained pacing lead or its old pocket requires mandatory lead extraction.[58] Numerous removal techniques have been described, with perhaps the best technique using a locking stylet and a telescoping intravascular sheath, which allow traction and countertraction localized at the lead tip.[59] Complications of lead removal include myocardial rupture, lead fragmentation with distal embolization, and right ventricular inversion.[60]

Therapeutic and Diagnostic Medical Device Interactions

Ambient electromagnetic energy and radiofrequency affect pacing systems. Diagnostic radiography will not harm a pacemaker, but radiation therapy can permanently damage the circuitry. Proper shielding of the pulse generator in the patient undergoing radiation therapy protects the vulnerable components. One should avoid exposure of pulse generators to magnetic resonance imaging because the radiofrequency pulse used in these machines could cause the pacemaker to pace at rates above 3000 beats per min.[61] Other medical devices that may cause complications with implanted pacemakers include extracorporeal shock wave lithotriptors. As previously noted, electrocautery may cause pacemaker dysfunction even at a distance, and its use in surgical procedures should be as limited and kept at least 10 ft away from the pacing system.

Other Permanent Pacemaker Complications

Excessive cooling of a pulse generator reprograms the pulse generator to the "fallback" mode and provides false indications of battery failure. This should be suspected if abnormal pacing behavior is seen in a patient exposed to prolonged extreme cold or a pacemaker exposed to a cold environment before implant. Strong electromagnetic fields produced by power plants or arc welding can affect the pulse generator. A patient who survives being struck by lightning or other types of electrocution should undergo a complete evaluation of the pacing system. Microwave ovens have no discernible effect on the performance of modern pacemakers.

CONCLUSION

The development of permanent cardiac pacemakers represents one of the major medical and technological achievements of the 20th century. These devices have prolonged hundreds of thousands of lives and have increased the quality of life for countless numbers of patients. Implantation of these devices is generally safe. Recognition of the early and long-term complications associated with pacemaker implantation will continue to improve the benefits of this often lifesaving procedure.

REFERENCES

1. Hyman AS. Resuscitation of the stopped heart by intracardial therapy, II: experimental use as a cardiac pacemaker. *Arch Int Med.* 50:283–305, 1932.

2. Schecter DC. Background of clinical cardiac stimulation, VII: modern era of artificial cardiac pacemakers. *NY State J Med.* 72:1166–1191, 1972.

3. Kay GN, Epstein AE, Dailey SM, Plumb VJ. Role of radiofrequency ablation in the management of supraventricular arrhythmias: experience in 760 consecutive patients [see comments]. *J Cardiovasc Electrophysiol.* 4(4):371–389, 1993.

4. Fananapazir L, Cannon RO, Tripodi D, Panza JA. Impact of dual-chamber permanent pacing in patients with obstructive hypertrophic cardiomyopathy with symptoms refractory to verapamil and β-adrenergic blocker therapy. *Circulation.* 85(6):2149–2161, 1992.

5. Grogler FM, Frank G, Greven G, et al. Complications of permanent transvenous cardiac pacing. *J Thorac Cardiovasc Surg.* 69(6):895–904, 1975.

6. Sznajder JA, Zveibil FR, Bitterman H, Weiner P, Bursztein S. Central vein catheterization: failure and complication rates by three percutaneous methods. *Arch Intern Med.* 146:259–261, 1986.

7. Ong LS, Barold SS, Lederman M, Falkoff MD, Heinle RA. Cephalic vein guidewire technique for implantation of permanent pacemakers. *Am Heart J.* 114(4 pt 1):753–756, 1987.

8. Hayes DL. Pacemaker complications. In: Furman S, Hayes DL, Holmes DR, eds. *A Practice of Cardiac Pacing.* Mount Kisco, New York: Futura Publishing; 485–507, 1989.

9. Zullo MA, Wallerson DC, Lang S. Formation and spontaneous closure of an arteriovenous fistula after transvenous pacemaker placement. *Chest.* 100(2):572–574, 1991.

10. Kim HY, Heywood JT, Jacobson AK, Smith DC. Arteriovenous fistula: a complication of cardiac pacemaker lead placement and its management with percutaneous embolization. *Pace Pacing Clin Electrophysiol.* 16(12):2310–2312, 1993.

11. Winner SJ, Boon NA. Transvenous pacemaker electrodes placed unintentionally in the left ventricle: three cases. *Postgrad Med J.* 65(760):98–102, 1989.

12. Shmuely H, Erdman S, Strasberg B, et al. Seven years of left ventricular pacing due to malposition of pacing electrode. *Pace Pacing Clin Electrophysiol.* 15:369–372, 1992.

13. Parsonnet V. Passage of a pacemaker lead into the pericardial cavity: an unusual introducer complication. *Pace Pacing Clin Electrophysiol.* 16:80–81, 1993.

14. Sandler MA, Wertheimer JH, Kotler MN. Pericardial tamponade associated with pacemaker catheter manipulation. *Pace Pacing Clin Electrophysiol.* 12:1085–1088, 1989.

15. Rubenfire M, Anbe DT, Drake EH, Ormond RS. Clinical evaluation of myocardial perforation as a complication of permanent transvenous pacemakers. *Chest.* 63(2):185–188, 1973.

16. Alferness CA. Pacemaker damage due to external countershock in patients with implanted cardiac pacemakers. *PACE.* 5:146–150, 1982.

17. Hazan MB, Byrnes DA, Elmquist TH, Mazzara JT. Angiographic demonstration of coronary sinus thrombosis: a potential consequence of trauma to the coronary sinus. *Cathet Cardiovasc Diagn.* 8(4):405–408, 1982.

18. Chaithiraphan S, Goldberg E, Wolff W, Jootar P, Grossman W. Massive thrombosis of the coronary sinus as an unusual complication of transvenous pacemaker insertion in a patient with persistent left, and no right, superior vena cava. *J Am Geriatr Soc.* 22(2):79–85, 1974.

19. Christie JL, Keelan MHJ. Tricuspid valve perforation by a permanent pacing lead in a patient with cardiac amyloidosis: case report and brief literature review. *Pace Pacing Clin Electrophysiol.* 9:124–126, 1986.

20. Frandsen F, Oxhoj H, Nielsen B. Entrapment of a tined pacemaker electrode in the tricuspid valve: a case report. *Pace Pacing Clin Electrophysiol.* 13(9):1082–1083, 1990.

21. Erckelens FV, Sigmund M, Lambertz H, Kreis A, Reupcke C, Hanrath P. Asymptomatic

left ventricular malposition of a transvenous pacemaker lead through a sinus venosus defect: follow-up over 17 years. *PACE.* 14:989–993, 1991.

22. Gillmer DJ, Vythilingum S, Mitha AS. Problems encountered during insertion of permanent endocardial electrode. *Pace Pacing Clin Electrophysiol.* 4(2):212–215, 1981.

23. Zerbe F, Bornakowski J, Sarnowski W. Pacemaker electrode implantation in patients with persistent left superior vena cava. *Br Heart J.* 67(1):65–66, 1992.

24. Snow ME, Agatston AS, Kramer HC, Samet P. The postcardiotomy syndrome following transvenous pacemaker insertion. *Pace Pacing Clin Electrophysiol.* 10:934–936, 1987.

25. Silka MJ, Rice MJ. Paradoxic embolism due to altered hemodynamic sequencing transvenous pacing. *Pace Pacing Clin Electrophysiol.* 14:499–503, 1991.

26. Doering RB, Stemmer EA, Connolly JE. Complications of indwelling venous catheters. *Am J Surg.* 114:259–266, 1967.

27. Grabenwoeger F, Bardach G, Dock W, Pinterits F. Percutaneous extraction of centrally embolized foreign bodies: a report of 16 cases. *Br J Radiol.* 61(731):1014–1018, 1988.

28. Classen DC, Evans RS, Pestotnik SL, Horn SD, Menlove RL, Burke JP. The timing of prophylactic administration of antibiotics and the risk of surgical-wound infection [see comments]. *N Engl J Med.* 326(5):281–286, 1992.

29. Bluhm G, Julander I, Levander LM, Olin C. Septicaemia and endocarditis—uncommon but serious complications connected with permanent cardiac pacing. *Scand J Thorac Cardiovasc Surg.* 16(1):65–70, 1982.

30. Morgan G, Ginks W, Siddons H, Leatham A. Septicemia in patients with an endocardial pacemaker. *Am J Cardiol.* 44:221–224, 1979.

31. Teno LA, Bestetti RB, Oliveira WM, et al. Tricuspid endocarditis: a rare infectious complication of cardiac pacemaker in a patient with Chagas' disease—a case report. *Angiology.* 44(7):580–583, 1993.

32. Bryan CS, Sutton JP, Saunders DEJ, Longaker DW, Smith CW. Endocarditis related to transvenous pacemakers: syndromes and surgical implications. *J Thorac Cardiovasc Surg.* 75(5):758–762, 1978.

33. Davis JM, Moss AJ, Schenk EA. Tricuspid candida endocarditis complicating a permanently implanted transvenous pacemaker. *Am Heart J.* 77(6):818–821, 1969.

34. Dargan EL, Norman JC. Conservative management of infected pacemaker pulse generator sites. *Ann Thorac Surg.* 12:297, 1971.

35. Ruiter JH, Degener JE, Van MR, Bos R. Late purulent pacemaker pocket infection caused by *Staphylococcus epidermidis:* serious complications of in-situ management. *Pace Pacing Clin Electrophysiol.* 8(6):903–907, 1985.

36. Jara FM, Toledo-Pereya L, Lewis JWJ, Magilligan DJJ. The infected pacemaker pocket. *J Thorac Cardiovasc Surg.* 78:298, 1979.

37. Phibbs B, Marriott HJ. Complications of permanent transvenous pacing. *N Engl J Med.* 312(22):1428–1432, 1985.

38. Antonelli WM, Turgeman Y, Kaveh Z, Artoul S, Rosenfield T. Short-term thrombosis after transvenous permanent pacemaker insertion. *PACE.* 12:280–282, 1989.

39. Balau J, Buysch KH, Marx E, Seling A, Knieriem HJ. Thrombose der Vena subclavia nach transvenoser Schrittmacherimplantation. *Radiologie.* 11:50–53, 1972.

40. Marx E, Schulte HD, Balau J, Buysch KA. Phlebographische und klinische Früh- und Spätbefunde Bei Transvenos implanttierten Schrittmacherelektroden. *Z Kreislaufforsch.* 61:115–123, 1972.

41. Stoney WS, Addlestone RB, Alford WCJ, Burrus GR, Frist RA, Thomas CSJ. The incidence of venous thrombosis following long-term transvenous pacing. *Ann Thorac Surg.* 22:166–170, 1976.

42. Mitrovic V, Thormann J, Schlepper M, Neuss H. Thrombotic complications with pacemakers. *Int J Cardiol*. 2:363–374, 1983.

43. Spittell PC, Hayes DL. Venous complications after insertion of a transvenous pacemaker. *Mayo Clin Proc*. 67(3):258–265, 1992.

44. Swinton NWJ, Edgett JW, Hall RJ. Primary subclavian vein thrombosis. *Circulation*. 38:737–745, 1968.

45. Bradof J, Sands MJJ, Lakin PC. Symptomatic venous thrombosis of the upper extremity complicating permanent transvenous pacing: reversal with streptokinase infusion. *Am Heart J* 104:1112–1113, 1982.

46. Rubenstein M, Creger WP. Successful streptokinase therapy for catheter-induced subclavian vein thrombosis. *Arch Intern Med*. 1980;140:1370–1371.

47. Girard DE, Reuler JB, Mayer BS, Nardone DA, Jendrzejewski J. Cerebral venous sinus thrombosis due to indwelling transvenous pacemaker catheter. *Arch Neurol*. 37(2):113–114, 1980.

48. Chamorro H, Rao G, Wholey MH. Superior vena cava syndrome: a complication of transvenous pacemaker implantation. *Radiology*. 126:377–378, 1978.

49. Youngson GG, McKenzie FN, Nichol PM. Superior vena cava syndrome: case report. A complication of permanent transvenous endocardial cardiac pacing requiring surgical correction. *Am Heart J*. 99(4):503–505, 1980.

50. Krug H, Zerbe F. Major venous thrombosis: a complication of transvenous electrodes. *Br Heart J*. 44(2):158–161, 1980.

51. Blackburn T, Dunn M. Pacemaker-induced superior vena cava syndrome: consideration of management. *Am Heart J*. 116(3):893–896, 1988.

52. Kaulbach MG, Krukonis EE. Pacemaker electrode-induced thrombosis in the superior vena cava with pulmonary embolism: a complication of pervenous pacing. *Am J Cardiol*. 26:205–207, 1970.

53. Friendman SA, Berger N, Cerruti MM, Kosmoski J. Venous thrombosis and permanent cardiac pacing. *Am Heart J*. 85:531, 1985.

54. Bernstein V, Rotem CE, Peretz DI. Permanent pacemakers: 8-year follow-up study. Incidence and management of congestive cardiac failure and perforations. *Ann Intern Med*. 74(3):361–369, 1971.

55. Seeger W, Scherer K. Asymptomatic pulmonary embolism following pacemaker. *Pace Pacing Clin Electrophysiol*. 9(2):196–199, 1986.

56. London AR, Runge PJ, Balsam RF, Bishop MB, Bousvaros G. Large right atrial surrounding thrombi permanent transvenous pacemakers. *Circulation*. 40(5):661–664, 1969.

57. Nicolosi GL, Charmet PA, Zanuttini D. Large right atrial thrombosis. Rare complication during permanent transvenous endocardial pacing. *Br Heart J*. 43(2):199–201, 1980.

58. Byrd CL, Schwartz SJ, Hedin N. Lead extraction: indications and techniques. *Cardiol Clin*. 10(4):735–748, 1992.

59. Fearnot NE, Smith HJ, Goode LB, Byrd CL, Wilkoff BL, Sellers TD. Intravascular lead extraction using locking stylets, sheaths, and other techniques. *Pace Pacing Clin Electrophysiol*. 13:1864–1870, 1990.

60. Garcia JA, Botana ACM, Gutierrez CJM, Galban RC, Alvarez DI, Navarro PF. Myocardial rupture after pulling out a tined atrial electrode with continuous traction. *Pace Pacing Clin Electrophysiol*. 15(1):5–8, 1992.

61. Hayes DL, Vlietstra RE. Pacemaker malfunction. *Ann Intern Med*. 119:828–835, 1993.

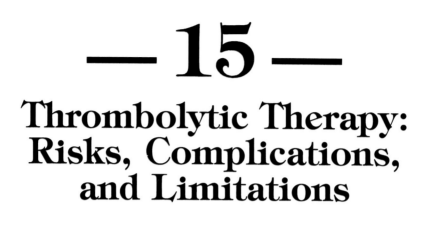

— 15 —

Thrombolytic Therapy: Risks, Complications, and Limitations

Laurence S. Sperling, M.D.
David A. Cutler, M.D.
Marschall S. Runge, M.D., Ph.D.

INTRODUCTION

Thrombolytic therapy is considered the standard of care for treatment of acute myocardial infarction in the appropriate clinical setting.[1] Over the past decade, randomized clinical trials have collectively demonstrated a 20% to 30% reduction in mortality with the administration of thrombolytic and adjunctive agents.[2-8] The efficacy and benefit of thrombolysis in evolving myocardial infarction has been clearly confirmed, and accumulating data suggest a beneficial role in the treatment of peripheral arterial occlusion, pulmonary embolism, deep venous thrombosis, and perhaps thrombotic stroke. These trials also delineate the various risks, complications, and limitations of this pharmacologic intervention. Many of the adverse effects of thrombolytic therapy are better understood by considering the basic mechanisms of thrombosis and thrombolysis, the dynamic nature of the vessel wall, and the delicate balance of the clotting cascade.

This chapter summarizes: (1) the basic mechanisms of thrombolysis and the agents used clinically; (2) related biology of the vessel wall and pathophysiology of thrombosis; (3) potential risks and the importance of individual risk-benefit evaluation; (4) complications of thrombolytic agents; and (5) current limitations of therapy.

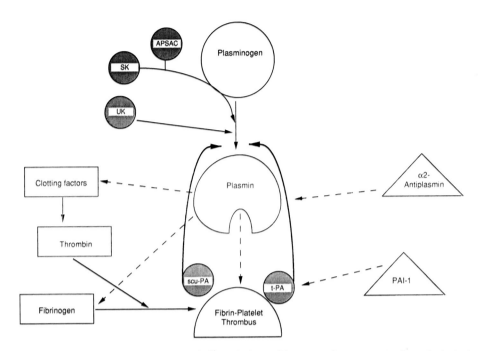

Figure 15.1. Basic mechanisms of thrombolysis. The central enzyme in thrombolysis is plasmin. Plasminogen activators (shaded circles) promote conversion of plasminogen to plasmin, which causes lysis of vascular thrombi. Tissue-plasminogen activator (t-PA) and single-chain urokinase plasminogen activator (scu-PA) are relatively fibrin-specific, whereas urokinase (UK), streptokinase (SK), and anisoylated plasminogen-streptokinase activator complex (APSAC) are relatively nonspecific. Several of plasmin's nonspecific actions are depicted, such as degradation of clotting factors and circulating fibrinogen. Plasmin also degrades von Willebrand's factor, complement components, and platelet membrane glycoproteins (not illustrated). Endogenous inhibitors of this process (represented by triangles), such as α_2-antiplasmin and plasminogen activator-1 (PAI-1), are important counterregulatory proteins. Dashed lines denote inhibition or lytic activity.

BASIC MECHANISMS OF THROMBOLYSIS—AGENTS USED

Basic Mechanisms of Thrombolysis-Thrombosis

The central enzyme in thrombolysis is plasmin (Figure 15.1), which is a serine protease generated by the action of plasminogen activators on plasminogen. Fibrin, the end product of the coagulation cascade and structural frame for thrombus formation, is plasmin's favored substrate. However, plasmin also has nonspecific actions. It degrades coagulation factors V and VIII, circulating fibrinogen,[9] von Willebrand's factor, components of the complement pathway, and platelet membrane glycoproteins.[10] Usually, there is very little active circulating plasmin because of the tightly controlled counterbalancing system to fibrinolysis. Plasmin is rapidly inactivated by a specific inhibitor, α_2-antiplasmin, and nonspecific inactivators such as macroglobulin.[11] Specific inhibitors of plasminogen activators have also been identified, including plasminogen activator inhibitor 1 (PAI-1), which appears to bind directly to the activator's catalytic domain.[9]

Under normal circumstances there exists a homeostasis between procoagulant and fibrinolytic mechanisms at the level of the vessel wall where patency is maintained. The intact endothelial cell monolayer is thought to play a critical role in preserving this balance. Disruption of vessel wall integrity initiates a "response-to-injury" cascade of events[12] involving platelets, cytokines, and plasmin inhibitors, which can acutely precipitate thrombus formation. Often this process is episodic. Although this response is necessary for wound-healing, disruption of the vessel wall can precipitate the formation of pathologic thrombi.

Thrombolytic Agents

In 1912 Herrick[13] described a clinical syndrome associated with blockage of the coronary arteries and noted that acute thrombotic occlusion was likely responsible. It was subsequently demonstrated by DeWood[14] that thrombus was present early in the majority of obstructive coronary lesions in patients with acute transmural infarction and that its formation was often at a site of a fissured or ruptured atherosclerotic plaque.[15] Based on these observations, it was reasoned that lysis of the occluding thrombus would be beneficial. In fact, in 1958 the first clinical attempt to use a thrombolytic agent in acute myocardial infarction was made based on this rationale.[16]

The class of agents known as thrombolytics are plasminogen activators (Table 15.1). Although none currently available are truly fibrin-specific, it is instructive to group them into two classes. The more fibrin-specific agents are tissue plasminogen activator (t-PA) and single-chain urokinase plasminogen activator (scu-PA). The non-fibrin-specific agents are urokinase (UK), streptokinase (SK), and anistreplase (anisoylated plasminogen-streptokinase activator complex, or APSAC). In addition to fibrin-specificity these agents differ with respect to half-life, antigenicity, mechanism of action, and cost.[10]

t-PA and scu-PA are endogenous human proteins produced by a number of tissues, including vascular endothelial cells. Together they are critical for the maintenance of local vascular patency. Initially t-PA was isolated from the Bowes melanoma cell line and scu-PA from transformed human kidney cells. Today, both are produced by recombinant DNA techniques.[17] They are similar in that both have short in-vivo plasma half-lives (approximately five minutes), are hepatically cleared from the circulation, and display relative fibrin selectivity.[10] Although scu-PA is not currently available for clinical use in the United States, its clinical efficacy is equivalent to t-PA in European trials.

Relative fibrin selectivity, which mechanistically is different in t-PA and scu-PA, imparts both advantages and disadvantages to these agents. Advantages include a higher early patency rate,[19–20] reduced systemic fibrinolytic effects, and the theoretical probability of fewer hemorrhagic complications. However, the lack of fibrinogen depletion may be related to a higher rate of subsequent reocclusion seen with fibrin selective agents.[21–22] Additionally, for reasons not fully understood, when t-PA is given at current clinical dosages the incidence of bleeding may, in fact, be higher.

Streptokinase is a single-chain polypeptide produced by group C beta hemolytic streptococci. Urokinase is a double-chain enzyme initially isolated from human urine and subsequently from renal parenchymal cell cultures. Neither is fibrin-specific and

TABLE 15.1. Thrombolytic Agents

Agents	Clinical Indications	Plasma Half-Life (min)	Dosing Regimen
Streptokinase	Q-wave myocardial infarct (MI)	20	MI: 1.5 million U over 60 minutes
	Pulmonary Embolism (PE)		PE: 0.25 to 0.50 million U bolus followed by 100000 U/hr infusion
	Deep Venous Thrombosis (DVT)		
APSAC	Q-wave MI	90	Single 30-mg bolus
t-PA*	Q-wave MI	5	Standard: 10-mg bolus; 50 mg over 1st hour; 20 mg over next 2 hours
	PE		Accelerated: 15-mg bolus; 0.75 mg/kg over 1st 30 min; 0.50 mg/kg over next 60 min
			*IV heparin is required adjunct
Urokinase	Q-wave MI (not in U.S.)	20	MI (Europe): 2 to 3 million U bolus over 90 min
	PE		PE: 4400U/kg bolus over 10 min followed by 4400U/kg/hr for 12 to 24 hr
	Arterial Occlusion (peripheral)		
	DVT		

each has a different mechanism of action. Urokinase directly cleaves plasminogen, whereas streptokinase must first bind to plasminogen in a 1:1 ratio, causing molecular-conformational alterations that lead to formation of an active enzyme complex.[9] This complex has been generated in vitro and chemically modified to form anistreplase (APSAC) which is enzymatically inactive until deacylation occurs upon binding to fibrin. This modification results in modestly increased fibrin-specificity and a prolonged plasma half-life (approximately 90 minutes for APSAC compared with 20 minutes for UK and SK) which permits administration as a single dose injection.[23] UK and SK both lack clot selectivity and therefore both consume a large proportion of fibrinogen and cause the release of more plasmin than can be inhibited by α_2-antiplasmin in the plasma. While SK and APSAC are used for therapy of acute myocardial infarction in the United States, UK has been limited here to treatment of peripheral arterial occlusion, venous thrombosis, pulmonary embolism and for intracoronary administration during some angioplasty procedures complicated by thrombus.

The active components of both SK and APSAC are foreign bacterial proteins to which many patients have preformed antibodies.[24] A consequence of this antigenicity is the potential for immunologically based side effects that will be discussed in further detail later in the chapter. In contrast, the other available thrombolytic agents are human-derived proteins, and thus are not significantly antigenic.

BENEFITS AND RISKS OF THROMBOLYTIC THERAPY

The clinical benefits of thrombolysis have been well documented. Nonetheless, as with all medical interventions, treatment poses potential risks. Thrombolytic therapy is most effective when adjuncts such as aspirin and heparin (with t-PA) are concomitantly administered.[4-7] Therefore, the possible benefits and risks may, in fact, be additive or even synergistic. In choosing a treatment strategy for an individual patient one must assess the overall net clinical benefit, weighing the efficacy of treatment against the risk of potential complications for that particular patient. This comparison is important because in many cases individuals considered to be at the highest risk for complications (eg, the elderly) also stand to gain the most from treatment.

Careful selection of patients for thrombolysis can maximize the net clinical benefit. Recent clinical trials, independently and collectively, indicate that thrombolytic treatment is potentially beneficial for many subsets of patients previously excluded such as the elderly,[8,25] patients presenting later than 6 hours after symptom onset,[25] and patients who have had cardiopulmonary resuscitation.[26-27] Absolute benefit appears to be greatest in patients with anterior ST elevation, although all patients with ST elevation or left bundle branch block consistent with acute infarction probably benefit.[25] However, there is no significant benefit and, in fact, increased morbidity when thrombolytic therapy is given to patients presenting with ST depression or other EKG abnormalities.[25]

The most important risk of treatment is bleeding. An initial explanation suggested an association between the generation of a systemic "lytic state,"[28] created by the depletion of fibrinogen and coagulation factors, and bleeding complications. As the overall risks of systemic bleeding complications appear similar comparing fibrin-specific and nonspecific agents this theory has fallen into disfavor.[5] The major risk factors for systemic bleeding are the use of invasive procedures, major surgery or trauma in the previous six weeks, and a history of a significant bleeding diathesis.[29] The most feared bleeding complication is the potential for intracranial hemorrhage. Major risk factors for intracranial hemorrhage include previous neurosurgery, age, hypertension, recent head trauma or stroke, and a known intracranial tumor.[29] It has been shown, however that the increased risk of intracranial bleeding following thrombolytic therapy is more than balanced by a decreased risk of embolic or thrombotic stroke.[30]

COMPLICATIONS

Overall, thrombolysis has proven to be a relatively safe and effective intervention. Most complications of this therapy are not life-threatening or severely disabling. Im-

TABLE 15.2. Complications of Thrombolytic Therapy—Approximate Risks

Complication	Approximate Risk	Reference Nos.
Intracranial Hemorrhage	0.3% to 0.9%	5, 7, 8
Noncerebral Bleeding (severe)		
with invasive procedures	12% to 15%	41
without invasive procedures	0.5% to 1.1%	8, 25, 41
Allergic/Immunologic (SK + APSAC)		
anaphylaxis	0.1% to 0.6%	3, 4, 7, 8
minor reactions	2.5% to 5.8%	3, 4, 7, 8
Hypotension (severe)	SK: 4.4% to 6.8%	5, 6, 7
	APSAC: 7.2%	7
	t-PA: 2.0% to 4.3%	5, 6, 7
Myocardial Rupture	? 0.5%	25

portantly, proper patient selection and knowledge of risk factors for potential complications may minimize adverse events. Despite this, recognition and awareness of possible clinical complications is vital. Known complications include intracranial hemorrhage, systemic bleeding, immunologically related side effects, hypotension, myocardial rupture, and reperfusion arrhythmias (Tables 15.2 and 15.3). The thrombolytic clinical trials conducted thus far are significantly heterogeneous in study design, dosing regimens, adjunctive schemes, and specific definitions of negative outcomes.

TABLE 15.3. Complications of Thrombolytic Therapy—Risk Factors*

Complication	Risk Factors
Intracerebral hemorrhage	Recent head trauma, stroke, or neurosurgery
	Known intracranial tumor
	Hx of cerebrovascular disease
	Severe refractory hypertension
	Age > 75
	? small body mass
Noncerebral bleeding	Recent surgery, biopsy, or trauma
	Hx of recent GI/GU bleeding
	Bleeding diathesis
	Invasive procedures
	Pericarditis or aortic dissection
	? prolonged CPR
	? small body mass
Allergic/immunologic	Treatment with SK or APSAC in past 6 to 9 months
	? recent streptococcal infection
Hypotension	Rate of thrombolytic infusion too fast
Myocardial rupture	? > 12 hours from symptom onset
	? elderly

*Modified from Califf et al. *Am J Cardiol.* 1992;69:12A–20A. (Ref 29) with permission of publisher and author

Therefore, definite large-scale comparisons between thrombolytic agents are difficult, even with respect to rates of complication.

Intracranial hemorrhage is the most serious potential complication of thrombolytic therapy. It is important to note that stroke was reported to complicate 2.5% of acute myocardial infarctions before the thrombolytic era[31–32] and was more common before routine use of aspirin and heparin. Most strokes were of embolic etiology, and intracranial hemorrhage was highly uncommon. Since the administration of thrombolytics, the overall incidence of stroke with myocardial infarction appears to be declining, and the distribution of stroke subtype has shifted to include various types of intracranial hemorrhage.[33] Fortunately, intracranial bleeding is a rare complication.

Recent trials and collaborative overviews are better defining the incidence and risk factors for intracranial hemorrhage. The Fibrinolytic Therapy Trialist's (FTT) Collaborative Group[25] reviewed and compiled data from nine major thrombolytic trials conducted between 1984 and 1992. They reported a small but significant excess of 3.9 strokes per 1000 patients given thrombolytic agents. All of this excess appeared on days 0 to 1, and was largely attributable to cerebral hemorrhage. The overall reported risk of intracerebral hemorrhage was 0.4%. Likewise, recent trials have reported a 0.3% to 0.9% rate of intracerebral bleeding.[5,7–8]

There are data from several trials that suggest that intracranial bleeding is more common with t-PA. Data from the GUSTO Trial[8] demonstrates an excess of 2 hemorrhagic strokes per 1000 patients treated with accelerated t-PA as compared with SK. The incidence of stroke in t-PA–treated patients was 1.55%, with a 0.78% incidence of hemmorhagic stroke or hemorrhagic conversion. In the SK-treated patients incidence of stroke was 1.22% to 1.40% (subcutaneous vs IV heparin), with a 0.53% to 0.59% incidence of hemorrhagic stroke or conversion. Similarly, ISIS-3[7] reported a greater incidence of cerebral hemorrhage in patients treated with t-PA (0.7%) as compared with APSAC (0.6%) or SK (0.3%).

The small, but statistically significant, excess incidence of intracranial hemorrhage related to t-PA suggests that an underlying mechanism for intracranial hemorrhage may be lysis of protective, hemostatic plugs[34] in the central nervous system. These may be at the sites of preexisting atherosclerotic plaque or amyloid deposition. Both depletion of clotting factors and loss of vascular integrity may contribute to increased intracranial bleeding risks.[35] There is concern that elderly patients may have more silent defects in vascular integrity,[36–37] and therefore are more likely to have intracranial bleeding complications.[38–39] In support of this hypothesis, both the GUSTO Trial[8] and the FTT Collaborative Group[25] data show an excess risk of hemorrhagic stroke or stroke of any type in treated patients over the age of 75. However, the overall net benefit of thrombolysis was similar in both older and younger patients.[8,25] Although a significant incremental elevation in blood pressure may contribute to the risk of intracerebral hemorrhage,[38–40] and is currently viewed as a substantial relative contraindication for therapy,[29] there may be overall net benefit with treatment following medical lowering of hypertension.[25] However, lowering of an elevated blood pressure before thrombolysis has not been shown to decrease the rise of ICH.

Not surprisingly, the most common complication of thrombolytic therapy is peripheral or systemic bleeding. Hemorrhagic complications can be separated into two major categories: those related to the use of invasive procedures, and those that occur spontaneously. For the most part, bleeding complications are minor and easily managed. Despite this, major bleeds (those requiring blood transfusion or that are life-threatening) have been reported to occur with an incidence of approximately

0.5% to 1.1% in noninvasive clinical trials.[8,25,41] However, the determination and definition of what constitutes significant bleeding varies among studies. Adjunctive agents such as heparin and aspirin may also contribute to the severity of bleeding.[2,7,42]

The most significant risk factor for hemorrhagic complications is the use of invasive procedures. A review by Fennerty et al[41] reported that the incidence of major bleeding was 12% to 15% in trials involving early invasive procedures, compared with 0.8% in noninvasive protocols. Major bleeding was often associated with early cardiac catheterization, and minor bleeding with venipuncture sites. Other procedures reported to increase risk of significant bleeding related to recent thrombolysis include intraaortic balloon-pump placement, coronary artery bypass surgery, and coronary angioplasty.[37] Obviously, these interventions are not definitely contraindicated following thrombolytic administration, nor is thrombolytic therapy contraindicated following these interventions, although they should be used judiciously and cautiously.

In addition to invasive procedures, important risk factors for systemic bleeding complications include recent major surgery or trauma, gastrointestinal or genitourinary bleeding within the previous six months, and a history of a bleeding diathesis.[29] Underlying aortic dissection or pericarditis may also lead to catastrophic complications.[43] The risk attributed to recent cardiopulmonary resuscitation may be overestimated or even absent.[26-27] The FTT Collaborative Group[25] reported a 1.1% incidence of major noncerebral bleeding in such patients treated with thrombolytics, and an associated 7.3 per 1000 excess of bleeds over those not treated. No statistically significant increase in stroke risk was seen among subgroups studied, including elderly patients, females, and those who presented with a high blood pressure or history of diabetes. There may be associated excess bleeding in those with smaller body size; thus weight-adjusted dosing regimens should be considered.[44] There is no substantial difference in bleeding risk between fibrin-specific and nonspecific agents. The GUSTO Trial[8] found t-PA and SK similar in terms of incidence of severe or life-threatening bleeding. Unfortunately, there are no biochemical or hematological assays that are clinically useful for the prediction of bleeding complications.[44]

Management of bleeding complications depends on the severity and site (Table 15.4). Minor bleeding related to a puncture site will often resolve after manual compression. Serious bleeding, on the other hand, demands discontinuation of heparin and antiplatelet drugs, transfusion of red cells when the hematocrit falls below 25%, and administration of cryoprecipitate to replace fibrinogen and factor VIII.[29,45] Epsilon-aminocaproic acid (Amicar), which actively counters fibrinolysis, should be used only as a last resort, as it may initiate refractory thrombosis.[29]

Allergic and immunologic complications have been almost exclusively associated with the foreign streptococcal proteins in SK or its chemically modified analog, APSAC.[46-47] These complications can be divided into immediate, IgE-mediated reactions including anaphylaxis, urticaria, and bronchospasm, and the delayed, IgG-mediated reactions including serum sickness, fever, and arthralgia. Overall, the allergic complications are minor, although the possibility of anaphylaxis should not be ignored.

Anaphylactic shock has been reported in 0.1% to 0.6% of patients receiving either SK or APSAC.[3-4,7-8] Many patients have preformed antistreptococcal antibodies,[24] creating the potential for an immediate, IgE-mediated reaction. Skin testing with small doses of intradermal SK has been suggested as a good predictor of immediate, allergic responses[48] and is recommended.[46] Pretreatment with steroids has not proven effective in preventing severe, anaphylactic immune reactions.[3,49] If anaphylaxis is

TABLE 15.4. Complications of Thrombolytic Therapy—Management

Complication	Management
Intracranial hemorrhage	Supportive
	Discontinue thrombolytic infusion and anticoagulant therapy
	Hyperventilation, mannitol if severe
Noncerebral bleeding	Manual compression
	Discontinue thrombolytic infusion and anticoagulant therapy
	Red cell transfusion
	Cryoprecipitate
	Epsilon-aminocaproic acid if severe
Anaphylaxis	?? steroid pretreatment
	Discontinue thrombolytic infusion
	Intravenous fluids
	Subcutaneous epinephrine
Hypotension	Slow rate of thrombolytic infusion
	Intravenous fluids
	Trendelenberg's position
Myocardial rupture	Supportive
	Emergent surgical repair

suspected the thrombolytic agent should be discontinued, intravenous fluids administered, and, if absolutely necessary, epinephrine may be given subcutaneously.[29]

Minor allergic reactions have been reported to occur with a frequency of 2.5% to 5.8%. Delayed reactions are usually mild and self-limited, although acute immune-complex-mediated renal failure,[50] leukocytoclastic vasculitis,[51] and Guillain-Barré syndrome[52] have been reported. Since persistence of an IgG response has been demonstrated,[53] current recommendations for repeat administration of both SK and APSAC include retreatment within 48 hours of original dosing, or after a 6- to 9-month interval.[10]

Fever and hypotension are relatively frequent minor complications of SK and APSAC administration. An average systolic blood pressure decrement of 35 mm Hg has been well documented[54] in patients administered SK, and a similar decrease in systolic pressure has been reported with APSAC.[38] A correlation has been demonstrated between increased speed of SK infusion and marked hypotension.[54] The frequency of severe hypotension reported with SK is 4.4% to 6.8%[5,7] as compared with 7.2% with APSAC[7] and 2.0% to 4.3% with t-PA.[5,7] The incidence of febrile reaction is as high as 30%. Possible mechanisms for thrombolytic-related hypotension include systemic plasmin generation leading to conversion of kallikrein to the endogenous vasodilator bradykinin, activation of the complement pathway, and endothelial cell prostacyclin release.[54] The SK agents additionally may have antigen induced hypotension and fever although prophylaxis or treatment with corticosteroids usually remedies this response. Hypotension can be easily managed by discontinuing or slowing the thrombolytic infusion, administering intravenous fluid, and placing the patient in Trendelenberg's position. In less than 5% of cases vasopressors may be required.[29]

Importantly, the onset of hypotension in a patient with acute myocardial infarction may be related to problems other than the minor thrombolytic complication discussed previously. Severe left ventricular compromise, acute hemorrhage, anaphylaxis, the Bezold-Jarisch reflex (hypotension due to vagal-mediated bradycardia), and possible right ventricular involvement should be considered, depending on the thrombolytic agent given, in addition to electrocardiographic and clinical findings.

An increased frequency of myocardial rupture during the first 24 hours following thrombolytic administration has been reported.[55–56] Although this issue remains somewhat controversial,[57] this early excess appears to increase with delay in time from symptom onset to thrombolysis,[55–56] and is supported by ISIS-2 data where a 0.5% incidence of cardiac rupture on days 0 to 1 was noted with SK as compared with 0.3% in controls.[25] Rupture may occur as a result of dissection of necrotic myocardium to the epicardium by hemorrhagic infarction.[29] However, there is speculation that reperfusion injury consisting of leukocyte and free oxygen radical toxicity may also be a contributing factor.[58] Deaths secondary to cardiac rupture may contribute to the "early hazard" of thrombolysis demonstrated repeatedly in placebo-controlled trials.[25]

Arrhythmias may be a marker of reperfusion, but reperfusion arrhythmias are probably not a true complication of thrombolysis. Although malignant arrhythmias are not uncommon in the setting of acute myocardial infarction, the issue of specific reperfusion arrythmias remains highly questionable. Arrhythmias such as accelerated idioventricular rhythm and ventricular tachycardia occurring during thrombolytic treatment have been used as a possible nonangiographic marker of reperfusion.[59] Experimental data have suggested these arrythmias might be related to the effect of toxic free radicals on the myocardium.[60] Other data, though, suggest that the human heart is less susceptible to reperfusion arrythmias than the animal heart, and that arrhythmic events are not reliable indicators of clinical reperfusion.[61–62]

LIMITATIONS

Despite enormous impact on the treatment of acute myocardial infarction, thrombolytic agents have not yet achieved maximal safety and efficacy.[63] Clinical trials, in addition to basic science investigation, continue to define and improve upon current limitations. These include the risk of severe bleeding complications, ineffective reperfusion, the potential for rethrombosis, and the incompletely explained excess of deaths during the first 24 hours of therapy referred to as "early hazard."

The risk of severe bleeding complications has been previously discussed. Agents with relative fibrin-specificity have not yet minimized this problem. This may be partly due to the fact that currently administered doses and dosing regimens are based on an end point of coronary patency.[63] To achieve an adequate frequency of recanalization, a degree of nonspecific plasmin activity inevitably occurs. If severe hemorrhage solely arises from sites such as the cerebral vasculature or gastrointestinal mucosa where protective, hemostatic plugs are disrupted, then the property of fibrin-specificity is irrelevant. The ability of an agent to distinguish fresh thrombus from older clot and recently activated, fibrin-bound platelets from those that are quiescent may be beneficial.

Suboptimal reperfusion and arterial rethrombosis continue to limit the efficacy of thrombolysis. The recent GUSTO angiographic substudy[20] supports the open-artery hypothesis[64] that rapid restoration of normal flow to an infarct-related artery preserves functioning myocardium and decreases mortality. Many patients treated with thrombolytic agents, though, do not achieve the normal, TIMI grade-3 flow, which appears to correlate with most favorable outcome.[65] In fact, only 54% achieved TIMI grade-3 flow with the accelerated t-PA regimen at 90 minutes in the GUSTO substudy.[20] It appears that, unfortunately, angiographic patency rates reported previously in clinical trials do not necessarily equate to adequate reperfusion.[20,66–67] Even in successfully reperfused vessels there seems to be a period of cyclic flow believed related to platelet aggregation and thrombin activation.[68,69] Reports indicate that this cyclic flow may precipitate subsequent ischemia and reocclusion.[70]

Reocclusion/rethrombosis is not an infrequent sequela, occurring early in 5% to 13% of those treated.[22,63] It represents an unfavorable event associated with a marked increase in mortality and decrease in ejection fraction.[71] It has been suggested that the reocclusion rate may be higher in patients treated with t-PA,[20,22,72] as there is less systemic fibrinogen depletion. This may have been due to the length of infusion in earlier trials. More recently, the GUSTO substudy[20] found no statistical difference between patients treated with SK and those treated with accelerated t-PA. It is believed that thrombolysis initiates a paradoxical phenomenon of increased local thrombin generation, possibly elaborated from the dissolving clot, which leads to increased platelet aggregation and subsequent rethrombosis.[73–74] Data suggest aspirin may delay or diminish reocclusion.[2] More importantly, intravenous heparin is required to decrease the incidence of reocclusion when t-PA is administered.[75–77]

An excess of deaths in the first 24 hours has been consistently demonstrated with thrombolytic therapy in placebo-controlled trials.[25,78–79] This early hazard was initially demonstrated by GISSI-1 data where an excess in deaths during the first 6 hours was largely attributed to heart failure and electromechanical dissociation.[79] Early hazard has subsequently been confirmed with all currently available agents. The FTT Collaborative Group[25] reported a 26% excess of deaths during days 0 to 1 (2.4% vs 1.9% in controls), especially among patients presenting more than 12 hours from symptom onset, patients over the age of 75, and patients with a systolic blood pressure greater than 175 mm Hg. In all groups, though, this was outweighed by a substantial mortality benefit from days 2 to 35. Therefore, an early hazard does not diminish the overall net clinical benefit. Thus far, the causes for this early hazard remain unclear. It may, in part, be related to a combined excess of early deaths from hemorrhagic stroke[25] and myocardial rupture,[55–56] although it has been suggested that it may also be due to some form of reperfusion injury.[80] It should be noted that no mortality benefit has been shown for patients presenting with cardiogenic shock, possibly related to inadequate flow to the infarct related artery or the high mortality seen in this group.

CONCLUSION

The thrombolytic era has been a great advance in the treatment of acute myocardial infarction and various other thrombotic events. The benefits of thrombolytic agents are now well recognized. Significant risks, complications, and limitations of currently available thrombolytic agents have been identified. Recently, the risk factors for specific complications have been better defined, and it has been demonstrated that careful assessment and selection of patients can improve net clinical benefit. Still, deficiencies in both safety and efficacy are notable. The potential for severe bleeding complications, suboptimal reperfusion, reocclusion, and an early hazard remain important limitations. Underutilization of this potentially lifesaving therapy continues to be another major limitation. These and other concerns may ultimately be minimized with the development of novel thrombolytic agents, more selective antithrombins, more specific platelet inhibitors, and further investigation of the basic mechanisms of thrombosis.

REFERENCES

1. Braunwald E. Myocardial reperfusion, limitation of infarct size, reduction of left ventricular dysfunction, and improved survival—should the paradigm be expanded? *Circulation.* 79: 441–444, 1989.
2. Yusuf S, Collins R, Peto R, et al. Intravenous and intracoronary fibrinolytic therapy in acute myocardial infarction: overview of results on mortality, reinfarction, and side-effects from 33 randomized controlled trials. *Eur Heart J.* 6:556–585, 1985.
3. Gruppo Italiano per lo studio della streptochinari nell infarcto miocardio (GISSI). Effectiveness of intravenous thrombolytic treatment in acute myocardial infarction. *Lancet.* 1:397–402, 1986.
4. ISIS-2 (Second International Study of Infarct Survival) Collaborative Group. Randomized trial of intravenous streptokinase, oral aspirin, both, or neither among 17 187 cases of suspected acute myocardial infarction: ISIS-2. *Lancet.* 2:349–360, 1988.
5. Gruppo Italiano per lo studio della sopravvivenza nell infarcto miocardio. GISSI-2: a factorial randomized trial of alteplase versus streptokinase and heparin versus no heparin among 12 490 patients with acute myocardial infarction. *Lancet.* 336:65–71, 1990.
6. The International Study Group. In-hospital mortality and clinical course of 20 891 patients with suspected acute myocardial infarction randomized between alteplase and streptokinase with or without heparin. *Lancet.* 336:71–75, 1990.
7. ISIS-3 (Third International Study of Infarct Survival) Collaborative Group. ISIS-3: a randomized comparison of streptokinase vs tissue plasminogen activator vs anistreplase and of aspirin plus heparin vs aspirin alone among 41 299 cases of suspected acute myocardial infarction. *Lancet.* 339:753–770, 1993.
8. The Gusto Investigators. An international randomized trial comparing four thrombolytic strategies for acute myocardial infarction. *N Eng J Med.* 329:673–682, 1993.
9. Runge MS, Quertermous T, Haber E. Plasminogen activators: the old and the new. *Circulation.* 79:217–223, 1989.
10. Kessler CM. The pharmacology of aspirin, heparin, coumarin, and thrombolytic agents: implications for thrombolytic use in cardiopulmonary disease. *Chest.* 99(4 suppl):975–1125, 1991.
11. Nazari J, Davison R, Kaplan K, Fintel D. Adverse reactions to thrombolytic agents: implications for coronary reperfusion following myocardial infarction. *Med Tox Adv Drug Exp.* 2(4):274–286, 1987.
12. Ross R. The pathogenesis of atherosclerosis: a perspective for the 1990s. *Nature.* 362: 801–809, 1993.
13. Herrick JB. Clinical features of sudden obstruction of the coronary arteries. *JAMA.* 59: 2015–2020, 1912.
14. DeWood MA, Spores J, Notske R, et al. Prevalence of total coronary occlusion during the early hours of transmural infarction. *N Eng J Med.* 303:897–902, 1980.
15. Davies MJ, Thomas AC. Plaque fissuring—the cause of acute myocardial infarction, sudden ischemic death, and crescendo angina. *Br Heart J.* 53:363–373, 1985.

16. Fletcher AP, Alkjaersig N, Smyrniotis FE, Sherry S. The treatment of patients suffering from early myocardial infarction with massive and prolonged streptokinase therapy. *Trans Assoc Am Physicians.* 71:287–296, 1958.

17. Pennica D, Holmes WE, et al. Cloning and expression of human tissue–type plasminogen activator cDNA in *E. coli. Nature.* 301:214–221, 1983.

18. Van de Werf F, Nobuhara M, Collen D. Coronary thrombolysis with human single-chain urokinase-type plasminogen activator in patients with acute myocardial infarction. *Ann Int Med.* 104:345–348, 1986.

19. Topol EJ et al. Thrombolysis with recombinant tissue plasminogen activator in atherosclerotic thrombotic occlusion. *J Am Coll Cardiol.* 5:85–91, 1985.

20. The GUSTO Angiographic Investigators. The effect of tissue plasminogen activator, streptokinase, or both on coronary-artery patency, ventricular function, and survival after acute myocardial infarction. *N Engl J Med.* 329:1615–1622, 1993.

21. Stump DC et al, TAMI Study Group. Pharmacodynamics of thrombolysis with recombinant tissue-type plasminogen activator: correlation with characteristics of and clinical outcomes in patients with acute myocardial infarction. *Circulation.* 80:1222–1230, 1989.

22. Granger CB, Califf RM, Topol EJ. Thrombolytic therapy for acute myocardial infarction: a review. *Drugs.* 44:293–325, 1992.

23. Monk JP, Heel RC. Anisoylated plasminogen streptokinase activator complex (APSAC): a review of its mechanism of action, clinical pharmacology, and therapeutic use in acute myocardial infarction. *Drugs.* 34:25–49, 1987.

24. Fears R et al. Monitoring of streptokinase resistance titre in acute myocardial infarction patients up to 30 months after giving streptokinase or anistreplase and related studies to measure specific antistreptokinase IgG. *Br Heart J.* 68:167–170, 1992.

25. Fibrinolytic Therapy Trialist's Collaborative Group. Indications for fibrinolytic therapy in suspected acute myocardial infarction: collaborative overview of early mortality and major morbidity results from all randomized trials of more than 1000 patients. *Lancet.* 343:311–322, 1994.

26. Tenaglia AN et al. Thrombolytic therapy in patients requiring cardiopulmonary resuscitation. *Am J Cardiol.* 68:1015–1019, 1991.

27. Scholz KH et al. Frequency of complications of cardiopulmonary resuscitation after thrombolysis during acute myocardial infarction. *Am J Cardiol.* 69:724–728, 1992.

28. Collen D. On the regulation and control of fibrinolysis. *Thromb Haemost.* 43:77–89, 1980.

29. Califf RM, Fortin DF, Tenaglia AN, Sane DC. Clinical risks of thrombolytic therapy. *Am J Cardiol.* 69:12A–20A, 1992.

30. Sloan MA. Thrombolysis and stroke: past and future. *Arch Neurol.* 44:748–768, 1987.

31. Thompson PL, Robinson JS. Stroke after acute myocardial infarction: relation to infarct size. *Br Med J.* 2:457–459, 1978.

32. Komrad MS, Coffey CE, Coffey MS, McKinnis R, Massey EW, Califf RM. Myocardial infarction and stroke. *Neurology.* 34:1403–1409, 1984.

33. Sloan MA, Gore JM. Ischemic stroke and intracranial hemorrhage following thrombolytic therapy for acute myocardial infarction: a risk-benefit analysis. *Am J Cardiol.* 69:21A–38A, 1992.

34. Cairns JA, Collins R, Fuster V, Passamani ER. Coronary thrombolysis. *Chest.* 95(2 suppl):73s–87s, 1989.

35. Marder VJ. Relevance of changes in blood fibrinolytic and coagulation parameters during thrombolytic therapy. *Am J Med.* 83:15–19, 1987.

36. O'Connor CM et al. Stroke and acute myocardial infarction in the thrombolytic era: clinical correlates and long-term prognosis. *J Am Coll Cardiol.* 16:533–540, 1990.

37. Califf RM et al, TAMI Study Group. Hemorrhagic complications associated with the use of intravenous tissue plasminogen activator in the treatment of acute myocardial infarction. *Am J Med.* 85:353–359, 1988.

38. Anderson JL, Karagounis L, Allen A, Bradford MJ, Pryot TA. Age and systolic hypertension are risk factors for intracranial hemorrhage after thrombolysis. *Circulation.* 82(suppl):III–431, 1990.

39. Chaitman BR et al for the TIMI Investigators. The use of tissue-type plasminogen activator for acute myocardial infarction in the elderly: results from the TIMI Phase I open-label studies, and the TIMI Phase II pilot study. *J Am Coll Cardiol.* 14:1159–1165, 1989.

40. Althouse RH, Weaver WD, Kennedy JW. Transient elevation of diastolic blood pressure in acute myocardial infarction: a contraindication to thrombolytic therapy. *Circulation.* 76(suppl):IV–306, 1987.

41. Fennerty AG, Levine MN, Hirsh J. Hemorrhagic complications of thrombolytic therapy in the treatment of myocardial infarction and venous thromboembolism. *Chest.* 95(suppl 2):885–975, 1989.

42. Bovill E et al. Hemorrhagic events during therapy with recombinant tissue-type plasminogen activator, heparin, and aspirin for acute myocardial infarction. *Ann Int Med.* 115:256–265, 1991.

43. Blankenship JC, Almquist AK. Cardiovascular complications of thrombolytic therapy in patients with a mistaken diagnosis of acute myocardial infarction. *J Am Coll Cardiol.* 14:1579–1582, 1989.

44. Tracy RP, Bovill EG. Fibrinolytic parameters and hemostatic monitoring: identifying and predicting patients at risk for major hemorrhagic events. *Am J Cardiol.* 69:52A–59A, 1992.

45. Sane DC, Califf RM, Topol EJ, Stump DC, Mark DB, Greenberg CS. Bleeding during thrombolytic therapy for acute myocardial infarction: mechanisms and management. *Ann Int Med.* 111:1010–1022, 1989.

46. McGrath K, Patterson R. Immunology of streptokinase in human subjects. *Cl Exp Imm.* 62:421–426, 1985.

47. McGrath KG, Zeffren B, Alexander J, Kaplan K, Patterson R. Allergic reactions to streptokinase consistent with anaphylactic or antigen-antibody complex–mediated damage. *J All Cl Imm.* 76:453–457, 1985.

48. Dykewicz MS et al. Identification of patients at risk for anaphylaxis due to streptokinase. *Arch Int Med.* 146:305–307, 1986.

49. McGrath KG, Patterson R. Anaphylactic reactivity to streptokinase. *JAMA.* 252:1314–1317, 1986.

50. Murray N, Lyons J, Chappell M. Crescentric glomerulonephritis: a possible complication of streptokinase treatment for myocardial infarction. *Br Heart J.* 56:483–485, 1986.

51. Noel J et al. Serum sickness–like illness and leukocytoclastic vasculitis following intracoronary arterial streptokinase. *Am Heart J.* 113:395–397, 1987.

52. Leaf DA et al. Streptokinase and the Guillain-Barré syndrome. *Ann Int Med.* 100:617, 1984.

53. Jalihal S, Morris GK. Antistreptokinase titres after intravenous streptokinase. *Lancet.* 335:184–185, 1990.

54. Lew AS, Laramee P, Cercek B, Shah PK, Ganz W. The hypotensive effect of intravenous streptokinase in patients with acute myocardial infarction. *Circulation.* 72:1321–1326, 1985.

55. Honan MB et al. Cardiac rupture, mortality, and the timing of thrombolytic therapy: a metanalysis. *J Am Coll Cardiol.* 16:359–367, 1990.

56. Loukinen KL, O'Neill W, Laufer N, Lew A, Timmis GC. Myocardial rupture complicating tissue plasminogen activator therapy of acute myocardial infarction. *J Am Coll Cardiol.* 13:94, 1989.

57. Massel DR. How sound is the evidence that thrombolysis increases the risk of cardiac rupture? *Br Heart J.* 69:284–287, 1993.

58. Bell D, Jackson M, Nicoll JJ, Miller A, Dawes J. Inflammatory response, neutrophil activation, and free radical production after acute myocardial infarction: effect of thrombolytic treatment. *Br Heart J.* 63:82–87, 1990.

59. Miller FC et al. Ventricular arrhythmias during reperfusion. *Am Heart J.* 112:928–932, 1986.

60. Vandeplassche G et al. Singlet oxygen and myocardial injury: ultrastructural, cytochemical, and electrocardiographic consequences of photoactivation of rose bengal. *J Mol Cell Cardiol.* 22:287–301, 1990.

61. Opie LH. Reperfusion injury and its pharmacologic modification. *Circulation.* 80:1049–1062, 1989.

62. Fox KAA. Reperfusion injury: laboratory phenomenon or clinical reality? *Cardiovasc Res.* 26:656–659, 1992.

63. Collen D. Designing thrombolytic agents: focus on safety and efficacy. *Am J Cardiol.* 69:71A–81A, 1992.

64. Belenkie I et al. Importance of effective, early, and sustained reperfusion during acute myocardial infarction. *Am J Cardiol.* 63:912–916, 1989.

65. Chesebro JH, Knatterud G, Roberts R, et al. Thrombolysis in myocardial infarction (TIMI) trial, phase 1: a comparison between intravenous tissue plasminogen activator and intravenous streptokinase: clinical findings through hospital discharge. *Circulation.* 76:142–154, 1987.

66. Karagounis L et al. Does thrombolysis in myocardial infarction (TIMI) perfusion grade 2 represent a mostly patent artery or a mostly occluded artery? enzymatic and electrocardiographic evidence from the TEAM-2 study. *J Am Coll Cardiol.* 19:1–10, 1992.

67. Vogt A et al. Impact of early perfusion status of the infarct-related artery after thrombolysis for acute myocardial infarction on short-term mortality: a retrospective analysis of four German multicenter studies. *J Am Coll Cardiol.* 21:1391–1395, 1993.

68. Golino P et al. Mediation of reocclusion by thromboxane A_2 and serotonin after thrombolysis with tissue-type plasminogen activator in a canine preparation of coronary thrombosis. *Circulation.* 77:678–684, 1988.

69. Eidt JF et al. Thrombin is an important mediator of platelet aggregation in stenosed canine coronary arteries with endothelial injury. *J Clin Invest.* 84:18–27, 1992.

70. Dellborg M, Topol EJ, Swedberg K. Dynamic QRS complex and ST segment vectorcardiographic monitoring can identify vessel patency in patients with acute myocardial infarction treated with reperfusion therapy. *Am Heart J.* 122:943–948, 1991.

71. Ohman Em et al, TAMI Study Group. Consequences of reocclusion following successful reperfusion therapy in acute myocardial infarction. *Circulation.* 82:781–791, 1990.

72. Gold HK et al. Acute coronary reocclusion after thrombolysis with recombinant tissue-type plasminogen activator: prevention by a maintenance infusion. *Circulation.* 73:347–352, 1986.

73. Aronson DL, Chang P, Kessler CM. Platelet-dependent thrombin generation after in-vitro fibrinolytic treatment. *Circulation.* 85:1706–1712, 1992.

74. Anderson HV, Willerson JT. Thrombolysis in acute myocardial infarction. *N Eng J Med.* 329:703–708, 1993.

75. Bleich SD et al. Effect of heparin on coronary arterial patency after thrombolysis with tissue plasminogen activator in acute myocardial infarction. *Am J Cardiol.* 66:1412–1417, 1990.

76. Hsia J et al. A comparison between heparin and low-dose aspirin as adjunctive therapy with tissue plasminogen activator for acute myocardial infarction. *N Eng J Med.* 323:1433–1437, 1990.

77. de Bono DP et al. Effect of early intravenous heparin on coronary patency, infarct size, and bleeding complications after alteplase thrombolysis: results of a randomized double blind European Cooperative Study Group trial. *Br Heart J.* 67:122–128, 1992.

78. Lincoff AM, Topol EJ. The illusion of reperfusion. Does anyone achieve optimal reperfusion during acute myocardial infarction? *Circulation.* 87:1792–1805, 1993.

79. Mauri F et al. In-hospital causes of death in patients admitted to the GISSI study. *G Ital Cardiol.* 17:37–44, 1987.

80. Braunwald E, Kloner RA. Myocardial reperfusion: a double-edged sword? *J Clin Invest.* 76:1713–1719, 1985.

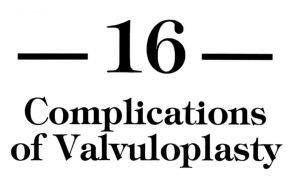

— 16 —

Complications of Valvuloplasty

Peter C. Block, M.D.

HISTORY OF MITRAL BALLOON VALVULOPLASTY

Percutaneous Mitral Balloon Valvotomy (PMV) is an alternative to surgery for selected patients with mitral stenosis. The procedure evolved from balloon valvuloplasty for patients with pulmonic valve stenosis, was introduced by Kan et al[1] and was refined by Inoue[2] and Lock.[3]

TECHNIQUE OF MITRAL BALLOON VALVULOPLASTY

There are many variations of the technique such as the double balloon technique,[4-7] the retrograde arterial technique,[8] the combined retrograde and transseptal technique,[9] and single balloon technology.[2] The results are similar, and it appears there is little advantage of one technique over the others except for operator experience and confidence. Most operators use the transseptal antegrade approach. Using the standard transseptal technique, the atrial septum is punctured in the area of the fossa ovalis from the right femoral vein using a modified Brockenbrough needle. A sheath is placed across the atrial septum and systemic anticoagulation is achieved by giving 100 units/kg body weight of heparin. The mitral valve is crossed either with a floating 7 French balloon wedge catheter (Arrow International, Reading, Pennsylvania) or by the dilating balloon itself, which is partially inflated (Inoue technique). When the double balloon technique is used, two guidewires are placed across the stenotic mitral valve with their tips either in the left ventricular apex, the distal aorta, or a combination of the two. Balloon catheters are advanced over the wire guides. Once in position the balloon or balloons are inflated briefly and deflated, causing splitting of the mitral commissures. Following balloon deflation and removal a post-PMV mitral gradient and cardiac outputs are measured to allow calculation of the final mitral valve area for comparison with values attained during previous cardiac catheterization. Left ventricular cineangiography in the right anterior oblique projection or echocardiography are used to evaluate mitral regurgitation. Hemostasis of the venous puncture is achieved by direct compression of the femoral vein. Patients usually leave the hospital within 24 hours.

INDICATIONS/CONTRAINDICATIONS/PATIENT SELECTION

PMV relieves mitral stenosis by splitting of fused commissures. Because the mechanism of PMV is similar to that of surgical commissurotomy, the baseline pathoanatomy of the mitral valve is critical to predict outcome. Two-dimensional and Doppler echocardiography examination identify which patients are appropriate for PMV. Valve rigidity, thickening, the amount of valve calcification, and the extent of subvalvular stenosis all should be evaluated pre-PMV. An echocardiographic "score" has been developed for each of these four characteristics. The arithmetical sum is obtained, and if the score is less than 8 the patient is generally a good candidate for PMV. Some patients with higher echocardiographic scores can have good results with PMV. However, if the echocardiographic score is greater than 11, PMV should be undertaken only if mitral valve replacement is contraindicated. Patients with severe valve thickening, rigidity, and calcification and severe subvalvular fibrosis are not satisfactory candidates.

Evidence of left atrial thrombus, severe mitral valve calcification, a recent embolic event (within 3 months), or evidence of calcification within the mitral commissures are contraindications for PMV. Patients with atrial fibrillation should receive anticoagulant therapy for 2 to 3 months before PMV. If there is a question of left atrial thrombus by transthoracic echocardiography, a transesophageal echocardiogram should be performed. If left atrial thrombus is seen, PMV should be delayed. After 2 to 3 additional months of anticoagulation, a repeat transesophageal echocardiogram should be done to document dissolution of thrombus before the procedure is attempted.

COMPLICATIONS OF PMV

Perforations of the iliac vein or inferior vena cava may occur with any right ventricular catheterization but are rare if the transseptal sheath is advanced over a guidewire. Most complications of PMV are due to sequelae of transseptal puncture or balloon inflation (See Table 16.1).

Perforation of the right atrium or posterior wall of the left atrium during transseptal catheterization occurs in 1% to 6% of patients undergoing PMV (Figure 16.1). In an anticoagulated patient, blood slowly accumulates in the pericardial space leading to cardiac tamponade (usually during the midportion or toward the end of the procedure). The aorta can be entered from the right atrium if the transseptal needle puncture is too superior and anterior (Figure 16.1). Systemic arterial pressure measured

TABLE 16.1. Complications of Percutaneous Mitral Balloon Valvotomy

	Number of Patients	Mortality	Embolism/ Stroke	Severe Mitral Regurgitation (4+)	Atrial Septal Defect	Tamponade	Left Ventricular Perforation
MGH	570	0.5%	1%	1.4%	16%	1%	0.00%
Loma Linda	238	1%	1%	1%	2%	1.2%	1.2%
Beth Israel	146	1.7%	1.7%	1.7%	19%	3%	0.8%
M Heart	74	2.7%	4%	2%	18%	6%	2%
Mayo Clinic	120	1%	1%	1.5%		2%	1%

MGH   = Massachusetts General Hospital
M Heart = Multiple Hospital East Atlantic Restenosis Trial Group
From: Topol. *Textbook of Interventional Cardiology*, 2nd ed., vol. 2. Philadelphia PA: W.B. Saunders & Co.; 1994:1201.
Reproduced with permission

from within the transseptal needle indicates that this complication has occurred. Occasionally the needle can be withdrawn without sequelae. However, the pericardium extends around the base of the aorta. If the intraaortic position of the needle is not appreciated and the dilator is advanced, the result is usually catastrophic, sudden tamponade. The posterior wall of the left atrium can be traversed by either the tip of transseptal needle or the dilator as they are advanced across the atrial septum or by a guidewire as attempts are made to cross the stenotic mitral valve (Figure 16.1). The combination of hypotension, diminished cardiac pulsation under fluoroscopy, and symptoms of low cardiac output should alert the operator to the presence of tamponade. Since emergency pericardiocentesis performed in the catheterization laboratory is the best initial therapy, PMV should be undertaken with a pericardiocentesis set ready to be opened should tamponade occur.

Mortality can also occur from right ventricular failure in patients with severe pulmonary hypertension. If severe pulmonary vascular disease is present, brief periods of hypotension or rhythm abnormality can cause right ventricular dilation and failure. Immediate institution of inotropic support is the correct treatment.

Perforation of the left ventricular apex can occur either from guidewire manipulation or from the balloon catheter tip itself. Partial ventricular perforation produces a dissecting hematoma in the myocardium, which may reach the pericardial space. This complication is usually accompanied by chest pain, transient rhythm disturbances, and hypotension. If hemorrhage is severe, pericardial blood can be drained by a pigtail catheter inserted into the pericardial space. The blood may be returned directly to the femoral vein to minimize red cell loss. Even if successfully treated with pericardiocentesis, surgery should be performed in the event of ventricular perforation to avoid late rebleeding. If mitral stenosis has not been completely relieved, a mitral valve repair/commissurotomy can also be performed after the ventricular perforation is repaired.

Systemic embolism (1% to 4%), the development of severe mitral regurgitation with congestive heart failure (<2%), and left-to-right shunting through the iatrogenically created atrial communication (approximately 15%) are mechanical complications of balloon inflation.

Systemic embolism including stroke may be caused either by dislodgement of a left atrial thrombus by transseptal puncture or manipulation of balloon catheters or

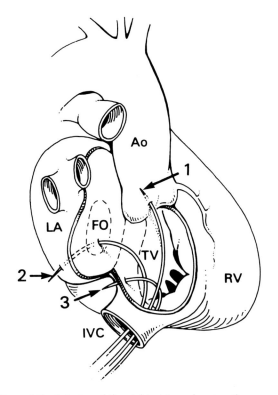

Figure 16.1A. View of the interior of the right atrium showing three possible complications of transseptal puncture:
1. Puncture of the aortic root
2. Puncture through the foramen ovale and the posterior left atrial wall into the pericardial space
3. Puncture of the posterior right atrial wall into the pericardial space.
Ao = aorta
LA = left atrium
FO = foramen ovale
TV = tricuspid valve
RV = right ventricle
IVC = inferior vena cava

guidewires in the left atrium. Debris is rarely dislodged from the mitral valve itself. Catheters and guidewires in the left atrium may enter the left atrial appendage. This is the most common site for left atrial thrombus, especially in patients with atrial fibrillation. Anticoagulation should be initiated after the transseptal puncture has been safely performed to minimize clot formation on catheters and guidewires.

Some increase in mitral regurgitation occurs in 45% of patients who have had PMV.[10] In most patients the amount of increase is mild $(1+/4+)$. An increase of more than two grades occurs in less than 15% of patients. Severe mitral regurgitation $(4+/4+)$ is usually the result of rupture of the chordae tendineae cordis or tearing of a mitral leaflet (usually the anterior leaflet) and occurs in less than 2% of patients.

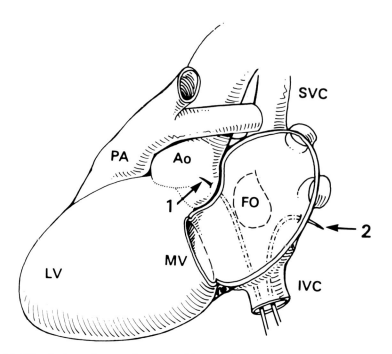

Figure 16.1B.   Left atrial view of two possible complications of transseptal puncture:
1. The needle tip is rotated anteriorly and too superiorly. The aorta is entered.
2. The needle is rotated too far posteriorly and punctures the right atrial posterior wall.
PA   = pulmonary artery
Ao   = aorta
LV   = left ventricle
MV   = mitral valve
FO   = foramen ovale
SVC = superior vena cava
IVC = inferior vena cava

There are two causes for iatrogenic mitral regurgitation: selection of too large a balloon size and incorrect positioning of the dilating balloon. A ratio of effective balloon dilating area divided by the body surface area of the patient of > 3.9 cm^2/m^2 is a predictor of an undesirable increase in mitral regurgitation.[10] It is important that the balloon tip (or tips) be passed through the center of the mitral orifice to avoid trans-chordal passage. This is best achieved by crossing the valve with an inflated floating balloon catheter or a partially inflated dilating balloon (Inoue technique). Full inflation of a dilating balloon in the intrachordal apparatus may cause chordal rupture or tearing of a mitral leaflet. Mitral regurgitation is well tolerated, and most patients remain free of symptoms. However, elective mitral valve replacement may be necessary if congestive heart failure occurs as a result of the procedure. In some patients mitral regurgitation decreases at 6-month follow-up catheterization.[10] Reversible mitral valve stretching, commissural fibrosis, or reversal of transient papillary muscle insufficiency caused by balloon trauma may explain this phenomenon.

Less than 20% of patients undergoing PMV develop left-to-right shunting through the atrial septal puncture site.[11] In 80% of these patients the pulmonary-to-systemic blood flow ratio is $< 2:1$. Predictors of significant post-PMV shunting are older age, lower cardiac output, a higher NYHA class before PMV, presence of mitral valve calcification and higher echocardiographic score.[11] Sixty percent of the defects close within 6 months. However, if persistent left-to-right shunting is noted after PMV and the patient undergoes cardiac surgery at a later date because of an unsatisfactory result, the surgeon should be prepared to close the atrial septal defect at the time of surgery.

PERCUTANEOUS BALLOON AORTIC VALVULOPLASTY (PBAV)

History

Although the results of early studies of PBAV were promising,[12,13] follow-up studies of PBAV have shown a high rate of restenosis within one year.[14–18] PBAV is useful, therefore, only in the treatment of selected patients with symptomatic aortic stenosis who are not operative candidates or who have another severe pathology that does not allow aortic valve surgery. An occasional patient with cardiogenic shock due to aortic stenosis can be transiently improved by PBAV as a "bridge" to cardiac surgery.[19]

Technique

Most PBAV is performed retrograde from the right or left femoral artery. A diagnostic catheter is passed retrograde across the stenotic aortic valve into the left ventricle, and a 0.038-in stiff transfer guidewire is advanced through the catheter and coiled at the apex of the left ventricle. This minimizes ventricular ectopy and the chances of ventricular perforation. The catheter is removed, leaving the guidewire in place across the stenotic aortic valve, and a dilating balloon catheter (usually between 15 and 23 mm in diameter) is advanced antegrade over the guidewire. The size of the dilating balloon catheter should be large enough to produce transient hypotension with full inflation. This indicates that the aortic annulus has been completely filled by the inflated balloon catheter. It is best to use increasing balloon sizes until transient hypotension occurs—usually beginning with a 15- or 18-mm balloon. "Oversizing" the balloon may cause complications. Multiple inflations of the balloon are performed. At the end of the procedure repeat hemodynamic measurements are obtained and the final aortic valve area is calculated. An antegrade transseptal technique can be used, if severe aortoiliac disease is present, that does not allow passage of the balloon catheters or placement of the transfer guidewire across the aortic valve.[20] Severe tortuosity of the iliac vessels or the presence of an abdominal aortic aneurysm may also preclude retrograde catheterization. If an antegrade approach is used, a transseptal catheterization is performed from the right femoral vein. The transseptal sheath is placed with its tip in the left atrium and a floating balloon catheter passed through the sheath, across the mitral valve, and out the aortic valve. A 0.035 or 0.038 mm soft guidewire is placed through the floating balloon catheter so that its tip lies either in the ascending or (preferably) in the descending aorta. Dilating balloon catheters are then passed antegrade over the guidewire once the floating balloon catheter has been removed and the guidewire left in place. Full inflation of the dilating balloon catheter within the stenotic aortic valve should produce transient hypotension. Repeat hemodynamic measurements are performed after the dilating balloon is removed from across the aortic valve.

Selection of Patients for PBAV

Clinical and hemodynamic improvement is short-lived after PBAV in most patients with degenerative aortic calcific stenosis. This limits the use of PBAV to patients who are not surgical candidates. There are three groups of patients:

1. Patients who are not surgical candidates but are incapacitated by symptoms of aortic stenosis.
2. Patients with calcific aortic stenosis who require urgent surgery for other organ dysfunction (GI bleeding, neoplasm, etc). PBAV may be done to transiently improve the hemodynamic status so that other organ surgery can be performed safely. The patient can then be referred for cardiac surgery at a later date.[21]
3. Patients with heart failure and cardiogenic shock due to aortic stenosis. This rare group of patients may benefit from PBAV so that cardiac surgery can be undertaken at a later date in a safer setting. The use of PBAV as a "bridge" to surgery under these circumstances should be limited to patients who are in severe cardiogenic shock and need pressor support.[19]

Contraindications for PBAV

1. Any patient who is a cardiac surgery candidate (because the results are so short-lived).
2. Patients with unicommissural congenital aortic stenosis. The aortic valve will usually be torn during the procedure, resulting in severe aortic regurgitation.
3. Patients with occlusive coronary disease may not tolerate the hypotension associated with balloon inflation in the aortic outflow tract.
4. Patients with more than 2+ aortic regurgitation.

Complications of PBAV (Table 16.2)

There are two groups of complications of PBAV: those resulting from balloon inflation within the aortic valve (central), and those resulting from vascular complications (peripheral).

Central Complications

Aortic regurgitation of a severe degree can occur, usually due to avulsion of an aortic valve leaflet.[22] Although rare, tearing of the aortic outflow tract may cause paravalvu-

TABLE 16.2. Incidence of Complications Produced by PBAV

Center	In-Hospital Mortality	Vascular Injury	Embolus/ Stroke	Severe AI	Tamponade	MI
MGH (n = 308)	5.0%	9%	2.0%		0.3%	0.5%
Rouen (n = 284)	4.0%	13%	2.0%	2%	1.0%	0.5%
Beth Israel (n = 205)	4.5%	10%	0 %	1%	1.5%	0.5%
Mansfield Registry	4.9%	11%	2.2%	1%	1.8%	0.2%

AI = Aortic insufficiency
MI = Myocardial infarction
n = number
From: Topol. *Textbook of Interventional Cardiology*, 2nd ed., vol. 2. Philadelphia PA: W.B. Saunders & Co.; 1994:1195. Reproduced with permission.

lar regurgitation into the left ventricle.[23] Peripheral embolism and transient rhythm disturbances (including heart block) may also occur. Rhythm disturbances are usually self-limited and rarely cause hemodynamic deterioration. If high-degree heart block occurs, the placement of a temporary pacemaker may be necessary. Tearing of the aortic outflow tract and pericardial tamponade may occur if the balloon used is too large. For this reason smaller balloons (15 to 18 mm) should be used initially in patients with lesser body surface areas. Upsizing of balloons should be done until transient hypotension occurs with full balloon inflation.

Peripheral Complications

The most common complications are vascular. Blood loss, either locally at the femoral site or in the retroperitoneal space, due to vascular tearing by the large sheath or passage of the balloon catheters can occur. The need for prolonged compression of the femoral entry site may cause thrombus formation near the site of vascular entry with resultant limb ischemia. These complications should be promptly recognized and treated by vascular surgery.

REFERENCES

1. Kan JS, White RI, Jr, Mitchell SE, Gardner TJ. Percutaneous balloon valvuloplasty: a new method for treating congenital pulmonary-valve stenosis. *N Engl J Med.* 307:540–542, 1982.

2. Inoue K, Owaki T, Nakamura T, Kitamura F, Miyamoto N. Clinical application of transvenous mitral commissurotomy by a new balloon catheter. *J Thorac Cardiovasc Surg.* 87:394–402, 1984.

3. Lock JE, Khalilullah M, Shrivastava S, Bahl V, Keane JF. Percutaneous catheter commissurotomy in rheumatic mitral stenosis. *N Engl J Med.* 313:1515–1518, 1985.

4. Palacios IF, Block PC, Brandi S, Blanco P, Casal H, Pulido JI, Munoz S, D'Empaire G, Ortega MA, Jacobs M, Vlahakes G. Percutaneous balloon valvotomy for patients with severe mitral stenosis. *Circulation.* 75:778–784, 1987.

5. McKay RG, Lock JE, Safian RD, Come PC, Diver DJ, Baim DS, Berman AD, Warren SE, Mandell VE, Royal HD, Grossman W. Balloon dilatation of mitral stenosis in adult

patients: postmortem and percutaneous mitral valvuloplasty studies. *J Am Coll Cardiol.* 9:723–731, 1987.

6. Al Zaibag M, Ribeiro PA, Al Kasab S, Fagih MR. Percutaneous balloon mitral valvotomy for rheumatic mitral valve stenosis. *Lancet.* I:757–761, 1986.

7. McKay RE, Kawanishi DT, Rahimtoola SH. Catheter balloon valvuloplasty of the mitral valve in adults using a double-balloon technique: early hemodynamic results. *JAMA.* 257:1753–1761, 1987.

8. Stefanadis C, Stratos C, Kallikazaros I, Tsiamis E, Vlachopoulos C, Foussas S, Sideris A, Toutouzas P. Acute complications after retrograde nontransseptal balloon mitral valvuloplasty. *Circulation.* 88, 4(suppl):P1351, 1993.

9. Babic UU, Pejcic P, Djurisic Z, Vucinic M, Grujici SM. Percutaneous transarterial balloon valvuloplasty for mitral valve stenosis. *Am J Cardiol.* 57:1101–1104, 1986.

10. Roth RB, Block PC, Balacios IF. Mitral regurgitation after percutaneous mitral valvuloplasty. predictors and follow-up. *Circulation.* 78:1947A, 1988.

11. Palacios IF, Block PC. Atrial septal defect during percutaneous mitral balloon valvotomy (PMV): immediate results and follow-up. *Circulation.* 78:2114A, 1988.

12. Letac B, Cribier A, Koning R, Bellefleur J-P. Results of percutaneous transluminal valvuloplasty in 218 adults with valvular aortic stenosis. *Am J Cardiol.* 62:598–605, 1988.

13. Cribier A, Scroudi N, Besland J, Savin T, Rocha P, Letac B. Percutaneous transterminal valvuloplasty of acquired aortic stenosis in elderly patients: an alternative to valve replacement? *Lancet.* I:63–67, 1986.

14. Leonard BM, McKay LL, Ransil BJ, Diver DJ, Safian RD, McKay RG. Hemodynamic results and clinical follow-up in patients undergoing repeat balloon aortic valvuloplasty. *J Am Coll Cardiol.* 13:148A, 1989.

15. Block PC, Palacios IF: Clinical and hemodynamic follow-up after percutaneous aortic valvuloplasty in the elderly. *Am J Cardiol.* 62:760–763, 1988.

16. Litvack F, Jakubowski AT, Buchbinder NA, Eigler N. Lack of sustained clinical improvement in an elderly population after percutaneous aortic valvuloplasty. *Am J Cardiol.* 62:270–275, 1988.

17. O'Neill WW: Predictors of long-term survival after percutaneous aortic valvuloplasty. *J Am Coll Cardiol.* 17:193–198, 1991.

18. Block PC. Aortic valvuloplasty—a valid alternative? (editorial). *N Engl J Med.* 319:169–171, 1988.

19. Moreno PR, Jang I, Palacios I. Does percutaneous balloon valvuloplasty have a role in patients with cardiogenic shock and critical aortic stenosis? *JACC.* 21;2:215A, 1993.

20. Block PC, Palacios IF. Comparison of hemodynamic results of anterograde versus retrograde percutaneous balloon aortic valvuloplasty. *Am J Cardiol.* 60:659–662, 1987.

21. Roth RB, Palacios IF, Block PC. Percutaneous aortic balloon valvuloplasty: its role in the management of patients with aortic stenosis requiring major noncardiac surgery. *J Am Coll Cardiol.* 13:1039–1041, 1989.

22. Lewin RF, Dorros G, King JF, Seifert PE, Schmahl TM, Auer JE. Aortic annular tear after valvuloplasty: the role of aortic annulus echocardiographic measurement. *Cathet Cardiovasc Diagn.* 16:123–129, 1989.

23. Dean LS, Chandler JW, Saenz CB, Baxley WA, Bulle TM. Severe aortic regurgitation complicating percutaneous aortic valve valvuloplasty. *Cath Cardiovasc Diagn.* 16:130–132, 1989.

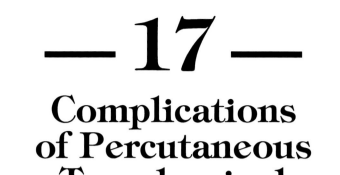

— 17 —

Complications
of Percutaneous
Transluminal
Coronary Angioplasty

John S. Douglas, Jr., M.D.

DESCRIPTION OF PROCEDURE

Percutaneous transluminal coronary angioplasty (PTCA) is a widely applied, nonsurgical technique for relief of myocardial ischemia caused by focal coronary artery and graft stenoses or occlusions. Percutaneous coronary angioplasty is commonly performed from the femoral approach using preformed guide catheters to selectively intubate native coronary arteries and bypass grafts. Guide catheters serve as conduits through which steerable guidewires, balloon catheters, and nonballoon devices are passed to reach and relieve occlusive coronary lesions. The choice of interventional strategy, whether a balloon dilatation catheter or new device such as atherectomy or laser, is based on lesion and patient characteristics and operator experience. At Emory University Hospital, approximately 80% of patients who underwent PTCA in 1993 were treated with balloon dilatation catheters alone and the remainder with atherectomy, laser, or stents (with or without adjunctive balloon dilatation). Improved technology has permitted a dramatic broadening of indications for percutaneous coronary angioplasty, but not without attendant complications, some of which are rather device-specific.

HISTORY OF THE PROCEDURE

The first percutaneous coronary angioplasty was performed in 1977 by Andreas Gruentzig, who used a crude nonsteerable balloon catheter to dilate a high-grade

173

proximal left anterior descending coronary artery stenosis. Gruentzig initially envisioned balloon angioplasty as a treatment for single, discrete, proximal lesions, but distal sites and multivessel disease were approached with increasing frequency following the introduction of steerable over-the-wire balloon catheters in 1983. In the decade that followed, angioplasty techniques were refined and applied worldwide, and the use of percutaneous revascularization surpassed surgical revascularization in the United States. In 1990 the first nonballoon technique for percutaneous myocardial revascularization, directional atherectomy, received U.S. Federal Drug Administration approval and by 1994 lasers, stents, rotational atherectomy, and transluminal extraction atherectomy devices had been approved for coronary use. PTCA procedures are currently performed in more than 500000 patients annually worldwide, and sales of angioplasty-related equipment exceed one billion dollars.

INDICATIONS

PTCA is indicated for relief of clinically important myocardial ischemia (symptomatic or asymptomatic) that is attributable to coronary artery or graft lesions amenable to percutaneous strategies. Selection for percutaneous intervention should be based on a careful analysis of multiple factors including the probability of a successful procedure, complications, and likelihood of long-term benefit compared to medical or surgical therapy. Although contemporary balloon angioplasty has demonstrated favorable success rates in some complex lesions, newer devices have been particularly effective in the treatment of bulky lesions, ostial sites, bifurcations, calcified lesions, and localized dissections. The choice of interventional strategies has become increasingly difficult because of the constantly evolving technology, paucity of comparative studies, economic constraints, and the varied level of experience of interventional cardiologists. PTCA is generally accepted as the treatment of choice for single vessel disease. The subsets of patients with multivessel disease, which are best treated with PTCA compared to surgery, is still being investigated.

CONTRAINDICATIONS

Percutaneous coronary angioplasty should not be carried out when in the opinion of the operator the risk of the procedure outweighs the potential gain. Contraindications include unprotected left main coronary lesions in patients who are candidates for surgical revascularization, diffuse degenerative vein graft disease, and inability to use heparin anticoagulation during and following the procedure.

COMPLICATIONS OF PTCA

Although the outcome of percutaneous coronary angioplasty cannot be reliably predicted in an individual patient, clinical and anatomic factors play an important role in determining the probability of favorable or adverse outcome. Operator experience and available technology are also important. The major acute complications of PTCA are coronary occlusion, myocardial infarction, need for emergency bypass surgery, and death. In the first National Heart, Lung, and Blood Institute (NHLBI) registry published in 1983, myocardial infarction occurred in 5.5% of cases, bypass surgery was needed in 6.6% and mortality was 0.9%.[1] In the 1985 to 1986 NHLBI registry, more difficult patients were attempted with a higher procedural success rate, 88% versus 67%, and lower rates of myocardial infarction and bypass surgery (4.3% and 3.4% respectively) and similar mortality, 1%.[2] In 10785 consecutive patients who underwent PTCA at Emory University between 1980 and 1991, angiographic success was achieved in 90% of cases, 0.8% experienced Q-wave myocardial infarction, emergency surgery was needed in 2.1%, and 0.3% of patients died in-hospital.[3] Evolving technology and operator experience have permitted maintenance of low rates of major complications in the 1990s as patients with unfavorable anatomy for balloon angioplasty have been increasingly selected for nonballoon intervention. In many cases, failures of standard angioplasty have been effectively managed with perfusion balloons, directional atherectomy, or stents without resorting to emergency bypass surgery. Emerging, however, has been a heightened awareness of the complications related to nonsurgical "bailout" of angioplasty failures, especially bleeding, local vascular problems, and subacute coronary occlusion.

Predictors of Major Complications

There are a number of clinical factors associated with an increased risk of major complications during or after PTCA. These include unstable angina, acute myocardial infarction, advanced age, and female sex. A uniform definition of unstable angina has not been used in published studies, but patients undergoing angioplasty within about 2 weeks of angina acceleration have a 10% to 12% risk of major complications compared with a 5% risk in patients stabilized for more than 2 weeks or in stable patients.[4–7] Stabilization of patients taking heparin and aspirin is recommended; however, the optimal time for intervention balancing economic and clinical factors has not been determined.[8] At Emory University, patients with unstable angina are often stabilized for 2 to 3 days with heparin, aspirin, and intravenous nitroglycerin before intervention with the hope of minimizing lesion-associated thrombus. By using this strategy of watchful waiting and by avoiding intervention in the presence of angiographically obvious thrombus (Figure 17.1), quite satisfactory angioplasty results have been obtained in this difficult patient subgroup. Preliminary data reporting the results of thrombolytic therapy in unstable angina patients do not support routine use of this strategy.[9–10]

In the most experienced hands, direct PTCA for the treatment of acute myocardial infarction has a success rate of 93%, and an in-hospital mortality of 7.2%; 12% of patients require repeat PTCA because of reocclusion.[11] Early infarct vessel patency is clearly higher with PTCA than with intravenous thrombolytic therapy. Recent randomized trials comparing direct PTCA with intravenous thrombolytic therapy have confirmed the value of direct PTCA, which has its greatest benefit in those with large infarctions and cardiogenic shock.[12,13] In contradistinction, the use of immediate PTCA after thrombolytic therapy led to unexpectedly poor outcomes, and most oper-

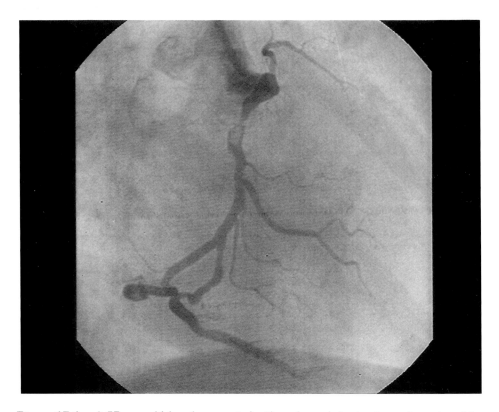

Figure 17.1. A 57 year old female presented with prolonged chest pain, and was found to have severe stenosis of the right coronary artery with a large thrombus just distal to the lesion (Figure 2, RAO view). Because of the presence of thrombus, the patient was observed for 6 days on intravenous heparin, nitroglycerin, and aspirin. Repeat coronary arteriography revealed complete clearing of thrombus, and balloon angioplasty was performed successfully with an excellent angiographic result and discharge of the patient the following day. In our experience, spontaneous thrombolysis is common when intravenous heparin is maintained for 5–7 days, and this strategy allows one to avoid the complications associated with balloon angioplasty in the presence of thrombus.

ators reserve PTCA in the presence of thrombolytic agents for those patients with suspected failure of reperfusion or clinical evidence of reocclusion. Surprisingly, more frequent intraprocedural complications (arrhythmias, heart block, hypotension) were reported for rescue angioplasty of the right coronary artery as compared with the left anterior descending coronary artery, warranting a cautionary note.[14]

A number of angiographic variables have been shown to be predictive of the outcome of balloon angioplasty. Because acute coronary occlusion is the more serious complication of PTCA, most estimates of adverse outcome relate to the probability of acute occlusion and its potential consequences. The following factors are associated with an increased risk of acute occlusion: lesion length, bend or branch point stenosis, lesion-associated thrombus, multiple stenoses in the vessel dilated, multivessel disease, and ostial right coronary lesion.[15] Estimates of the consequence of acute occlusion must consider the amount of myocardium in jeopardy, left ventricular function,

TABLE 17.1. Lesion-Specific Characteristics of Type A, B, and C Lesions

Type A Lesions (High Success, >85%; Low Risk)

- Discrete (<10 mm length)
- Concentric
- Readily accessible
- Nonangulated segment, <45°
- Smooth contour

- Little or no calcification
- Less than totally occlusive
- Nonostial in location
- No major branch involvement
- Absence of thrombus

Type B Lesions (Moderate Success, 60 to 85%; Moderate Risk)

- Tubular (10 to 20 mm length)
- Eccentric
- Moderate tortuosity of proximal segment
- Moderately angulated segment, >45°, <90°
- Irregular contour

- Moderate to heavy calcification
- Total occlusions <3 months
- Ostial in location
- Bifurcation lesions requiring double guidewires
- Some thrombus present

Type C Lesions (Low Success, <60%; High Risk)

- Diffuse (>2 cm length)
- Excessive tortuosity of proximal segment
- Extremely angulated segments >90°

- Total occlusions >3 months old
- Inability to protect major side branches
- Degenerated vein grafts with friable lesions

From the ACC/AHA Task Force Report: Guidelines for percutaneous transluminal coronary angioplasty. *J Am Coll Cardiol.* 12:529, 1988. Reproduced by permission of the American College of Cardiology.

and the ability to rapidly intervene surgically.[16] Coronary arteriography and left ventriculography therefore provide the best preprocedural assessment of the risk of PTCA. The American College of Cardiology/American Heart Association (ACC/AHA) classification uses lesion characteristics to estimate procedural results (Table 17.1). The validity of this classification in predicting outcome of balloon angioplasty was confirmed using patient experiences from 1986 to 1989 and a subclassification of B lesions into B1 and B2 lesions was recommended.[17,18]

Recent reports suggest, however, that the technology and operator experience level present in the 1990s may reduce the predictive value of the ACC/AHA classification. In reviewing their 1991 experience, the MAPS study group reported procedural success in 97% of type A lesions, 94% of type B1 lesions, 73% of type B2 lesions, and 68% of type C lesions.[19] Multivariate analysis found chronic total occlusions, long lesions, bend lesions, proximal tortuosity, calcification, and bifurcation lesions to be independent predictors of failure. Operators at the San Francisco Heart Institute reporting results of procedures in 1990 and 1991 noted procedural success in 99% of type A lesion, 92% of type B lesions, and 90% of type C lesions.[4] Multivariate analysis found chronic total occlusion, unprotected bifurcation lesions, long lesions, and thrombus to be the only independent predictors of failure. In addition to reduced success rates, angioplasty of chronic total occlusions has been associated with significant complications. Myler et al reported 333 procedures with a 6% incidence of acute closure, 4% with myocardial infarction, and 2.4% requiring emergency bypass surgery.[20] Long lesions are associated with an increased risk of coronary dissection, presumably related to the diffuse atherosclerotic disease present. In observational trials, results of rotational atherectomy and excimer laser angioplasty have been quite favorable in long lesions. Although the presence of lesion-associated thrombus has been a predictor of ischemic complications, therapy has not been standardized. In our hands, aggressive antiplatelet therapy and prolonged heparinization has been used successfully,[21] but ischemic complications were not completely obviated, and in many patients clinical instability mandates intervention in the presence of thrombus. In this case, intracoronary thrombolytic agents are commonly used. Whether the use of new antiplatelet or antithrombin agents will prove more effective in these patients remains to be determined. In a multicenter study of balloon angioplasty for right coronary artery ostial stenosis, Topol et al reported a 9.5% incidence of emergency coronary bypass surgery.[21] Unfavorable outcome with balloon angioplasty in patients in this subgroup has led most operators to favor directional or rotational atherectomy or laser angioplasty.

Procedural factors have also been shown to play an important role in determining the outcome of PTCA. In a randomized trial at Emory University Hospital, balloon oversizing (balloon-to-artery ratio of 1.13) resulted in a 2.5-fold increase in ischemic complications compared with balloon-to-artery ratio of 0.93. A recently published randomized trial comparing standard with long (15-minute) balloon inflations suggested that long inflations were associated with an improved outcome in type B2, irregular, and thrombus-containing lesions.[22] Adequacy of heparin anticoagulation has been shown to be an important determinant of procedural success and complications. However, the optimal degree of anticoagulation and how it should be measured has not been established.[23]

Management of Major Complications

Fortunately, the majority of acute closures occur during or immediately following coronary angioplasty. Those that occur after the patient has left the laboratory usually do so within 4 hours, upon discontinuation of heparin, or in association with hypotension related to hypovolemia or vasovagal reactions. These temporally associated events provide potentially important clues to situations that should be avoided (hypovolemia, inadequate anticoagulation) and also suggest the possible value of a brief period of observation following the last balloon inflation. In one report of 1000 consecutive patients observed for 10 minutes, repeat dilatation was required in 7% of cases; subsequent acute closure was virtually nonexistent.[24] In the early experience with coronary angioplasty, most patients with severe dissection or abrupt closure underwent urgent coronary bypass surgery; however, with the advent of steerable catheter systems, it became apparent that repeat PTCA was successful in approximately one half of patients.

The treatment sequence that an angioplasty operator follows in the management of acute closure is determined by the magnitude of myocardial ischemia and the angiographic identification of its cause. Localized dissection with intimal flap formation, elastic recoil, thrombus formation, or coronary artery spasm may be present. In our experience, coronary artery dissection (Figure 17.2) is the most common finding, although thrombotic occlusion may occur in patients with unstable angina or lesion-associated thrombus. Intracoronary nitroglycerin is administered in virtually all patients, and adequacy of anticoagulation is ensured by measuring ACT or by empiric administration of additional heparin. Hypotension is aggressively treated with volume expansion and, if necessary, intraaortic balloon pumping and vasoconstrictors. In the presence of coronary dissection, prolonged inflations of 10 to 20 minutes with a perfusion balloon are commonly effective if the entire length of the dissection can be spanned. In an occasional patient, prolonged inflations for several hours may be effective when shorter inflations are not. If the length of dissection exceeds the length of available perfusion balloons, a sufficiently long conventional balloon is chosen and inflation is maintained to the limit of patient tolerance.

To assess the potential value of intracoronary stents and perfusion balloon technology in the treatment of acute closure after PTCA at Emory University, the outcome of 166 patients with acute closure before the availability of these devices was compared to a later group of 156 patients who experienced acute closure during the availability of these devices. The later group had fewer Q-wave myocardial infarctions (9.1% versus 20%, P = 0.005), lower peak creatine phosphokinase levels, and less coronary artery bypass grafting (30% versus 39%, P = 0.02).[25] However, only 47% of the later group were actually treated with intracoronary stent or perfusion balloon. In a matched case control study comparing intracoronary stenting for abrupt closure with earlier conventional therapy, a more dramatic decrease in bypass surgery was reported (4.9% versus 18%, P = 0.02); however, the incidence of Q-wave myocardial infarction was nearly the same in the two groups (20% versus 32%, P = NS).[26] If, in the management of the abrupt closure patient, an adequate result cannot be obtained with prolonged balloon inflations, coronary stenting or directional atherectomy should be considered.[27] Patients selected for directional atherectomy are those with quite focal intimal flaps or elastic recoil. If intracoronary thrombus is present, intracoronary urokinase (250000 to 500000 units) combined with balloon dilatation and followed by several days of heparin therapy may be effective. In patients with refractory closure, early surgical intervention is desirable. In patients with successful restoration of flow but nonideal angiographic results, intraaortic balloon pumping may play a role in maintaining patency in the subsequent 24 to 48 hours.

Major complications are more frequent in older patients undergoing PTCA, and this is probably related to the presence of more diffuse disease, calcified lesions, and co-morbidity. Among 10785 consecutive patients who underwent elective PTCA at Emory University, in-hospital mortality occurred in 0.04% of patients less than age 50, but in 0.1%, 0.3%, 0.6%, and 4.3% of patients in their 50s, 60s, 70s, and 80s, respectively. Thus, most of the increased risk occurred in those over age 80. Women develop coronary disease later in life, and in many but not all studies, women have been reported to have higher risk with PTCA. At Emory University, comparison of PTCA outcome in women and men revealed that in-hospital mortality was higher in women (0.7% versus 0.1%, P < 0.0001), but female sex was not a multivariate correlate of long-term survival.

When emergency coronary bypass surgery is required because of persisting ischemia or important vessel instability, myocardial infarction and mortality rates are higher and revascularization less complete than that achieved in elective surgery.[28] Mortality rates have been reported to range from 0% to 19%, and Q-wave infarction occurred in 8% to 57% of reported patients. Although some operators have suggested that excellent PTCA results can be obtained without on-site surgical backup,[29] this practice cannot be recommended currently in the United States where ample surgically supported angioplasty centers exist.

In a thorough analysis of complications of PTCA, Bredlau reported the following minor complications: side branch occlusion (1.4%), ventricular arrhythmia requiring DC shock (1.5%), emergency recatheterization (0.8%), femoral artery repair (0.6%), transfusion requirement (0.3%), coronary embolus (0.1%), cardiac tamponade (0.1%), and stroke (0.03%).[30] In recent years, vascular complications have been noted with increasing frequency, and these complications account for significant morbidity and in some cases mortality. This increased complication rate has been attributed to the use of larger guide catheters required by new coronary angioplasty devices and by the increased postprocedure use of heparin. In a recent analysis of more than 1400 patients undergoing balloon or new device angioplasty, vascular complications developed in 5.9% of patients. Vascular complications were defined as formation of a pseudoaneurysm, arteriovenous fistula, retroperitoneal hematoma, or groin hematoma associated with a > 15 point hematocrit drop or the need for surgical repair. Vascular complications developed more frequently after intracoronary stenting (14.0%) and transluminal extraction atherectomy (12.5%) than after balloon angioplasty (3.2%) (odds ratios, 4.9 and 4.2).[31] Management is the same as described when complications occur as a result of cardiac catheterization.

Similarly, with the advent of new intracoronary devices, coronary artery perforation (Figure 17.3) has been noted more frequently. In a recent report, perforation occurred in 0.2% of balloon angioplasties, but higher rates were observed with directional atherectomy (0.6%), rotational atherectomy (1.3%), extraction atherectomy (2.0%), and excimer laser angioplasty (1.6%).[32] Cardiac tamponade occurred in two thirds of patients who developed free perforation. Mortality in these patients was 14%; 75% required emergency coronary bypass surgery, and one third sustained Q-wave myocardial infarction. Prompt recognition and use of an occluding balloon is essential to limit morbidity and mortality associated with this complication.

SUMMARY

As percutaneous revascularization strategies have evolved, new and heretofore infrequent complications have emerged. It is incumbent on both clinical and interventional cardiologists that they become completely familiar with these complications, their recognition and management. It is the special responsibility of the interventional cardiologist to plan his approach so as to maximize the opportunity for success while holding complications to an absolute minimum.

Figure 17.2. Balloon angioplasty of a lesion in the distal right coronary artery was complicated by dissection of the proximal vessel, apparently due to guide catheter trauma (A, LAO view). Shortly after the dissection became apparent, chest pain occurred associated with dramatic inferior ST segment elevation and stasis of contrast media in the distal vessel (B). Because of ongoing ischemia and associated hypotension, a 3.5 mm Cook balloon-mounted stent was quickly inserted and the stent deployed by balloon inflation

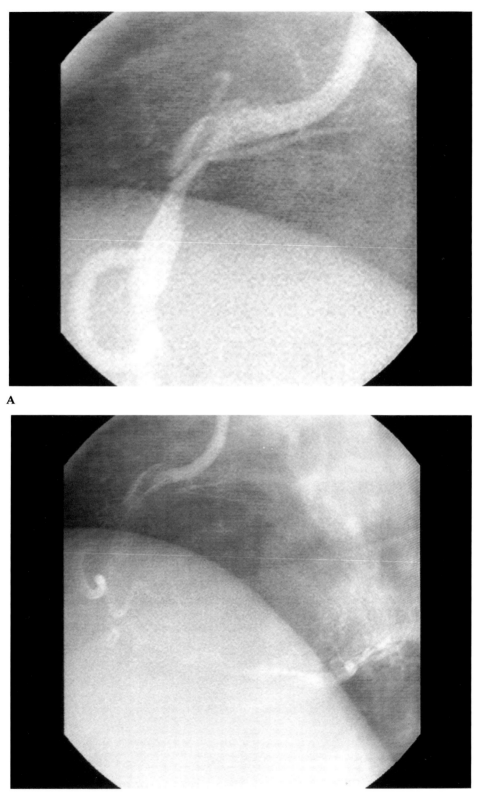

A

B

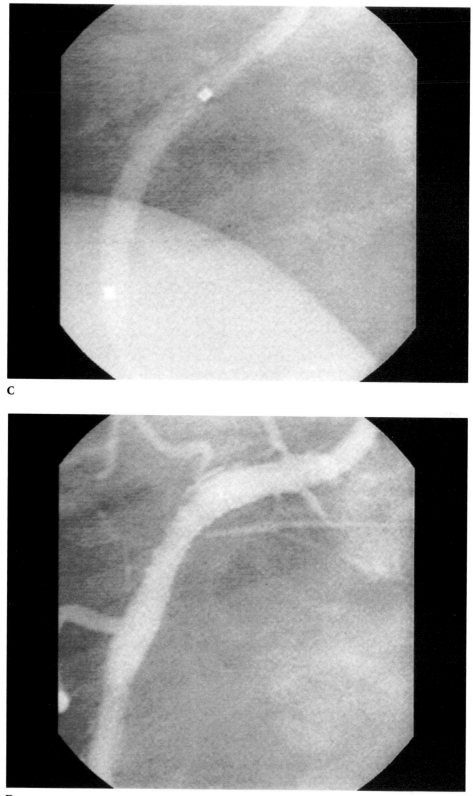

C

D

182

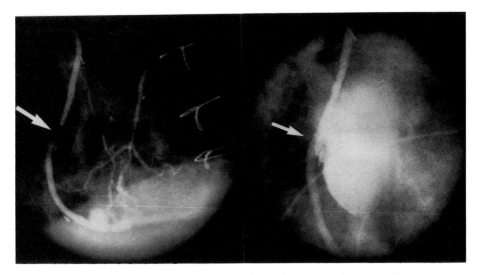

Figure 17.3. A 71 year old male developed unstable angina 9 years following coronary bypass surgery. High grade focal stenosis was found in the saphenous vein graft to the posterior descending coronary artery (left panel). Grafts to the left coronary artery were patent. Balloon angioplasty was attempted with a 2.5 mm balloon, with very little improvement. A 3 mm balloon was inserted, but a significant stenosis persisted following balloon deflation. Following inflation of a 3.5 mm balloon to 10 atmospheres, vein graft rupture occurred with development of a large expanding hematoma (B) and inferior myocardial ischemia. A perfusion balloon was inserted without success in sealing the perforation. The perforation was closed surgically, and a saphenous vein graft was placed to the posterior descending coronary artery. The procedure was complicated by development of a Q wave myocardial infarction. Reproduced with permission from Douglas, JS Jr: In: Topol, EJ (ed) Text book of Interventional Cardiology, Second Edition. WB Saunders, Philadelphia, PA, 1994 pp. 339–354.

REFERENCES

1. Cowley JM, Dorros G, Kelsey SF, et al. Acute coronary events associated with percutaneous transluminal coronary angioplasty. *Am J Cardiol.* 53:12C–16C, 1983.
2. Detre K, Holubkov R, Kelsey S, et al. Percutaneous transluminal coronary angioplasty in 1985–1986 and 1977–1981. *N Engl J Med.* 318:265–270, 1988.
3. Cardiac Data Bank, Emory University.
4. Myler RK, Shaw RE, Stertzer SH, et al. Lesion morphology and coronary angioplasty: current experience and analysis. *J Am Coll Cardiol.* 19:1641–1642, 1992.
5. de Feyter PJ, Serruys PW, Wijns W, et al. Emergency PTCA in unstable angina pectoris refractory to optimal medical treatment. *N Engl J Med.* 313:342–346, 1985.
6. de Feyter PJ, Serruys PW, Soward A, et al. Coronary angioplasty for early postinfarction unstable angina. *Circulation.* 74:1365–1370, 1986.

Figure 17.2. (C). An excellent angiographic result was obtained (D). The patient was anticoagulated with Coumadin and discharged home in good condition without the need for emergency bypass surgery.

7. Black AJ, Brown CS, Feres F, et al. Coronary angioplasty and the spectrum of unstable angina pectoris: what determines increased risk? *Circulation*. Abstract. 78:(suppl 2):II–8, 1988.

8. Theroux P, Ouimet H, McCans J, et al. Aspirin, heparin, or both to treat acute unstable angina. *N Engl J Med*. 319:1105–1111, 1988.

9. Ambrose JA, Torre SR, Sharma SK, et al. Adjuvant urokinase for PTCA in unstable angina: final angiographic results of TAUSA pilot study. *Circulation*. Abstract. 84(suppl 2):II–590, 1991.

10. Ambrose JA, Sharma S, Torre S, et al. Thrombolysis and angioplasty in unstable angina (TAUSA) trial. *Circulation*. 88:I–208, 1993.

11. O'Keefe JH, Rutherford BD, McConahay DR, et al. Early and late results of coronary angioplasty without antecedent thrombolytic therapy for acute myocardial infarction. *Am J Cardiol*. 64:1221–1230, 1989.

12. Grines CL, Browne KF, Marco J, et al. A comparison of immediate angioplasty with thrombolytic therapy for acute myocardial infarction. *N Engl J Med*. 328:673–679, 1993.

13. Gacioch GM, Ellis SG, Lee L, et al. Cardiogenic shock complicating acute myocardial infarction: the use of coronary angioplasty and the integration of the support devices into patient management. *J Am Coll Cardiol*. 19:647–653, 1992.

14. Abbottsmith CW, Topol EJ, George BS, et al. Fate of patients with acute myocardial infarction with patency of the infarct-related vessel achieved with successful thrombolysis versus rescue angioplasty. *J Am Coll Cardiol*. 16:770–778, 1990.

15. Ellis SG, Roubin GS, King SB III, et al. Angiographic and clinical predictors of acute closure after native vessel coronary angioplasty. *Circulation*. 77:372–379, 1988.

16. Ellis SG, Roubin GS, King SB III, et al. In-hospital cardiac mortality following acute closure after percutaneous transluminal coronary angioplasty—analysis of risk factors from 8207 procedures. *J Am Coll Cardiol*. 11:211–216, 1988.

17. Cragg DR, Friedman HZ, Almany SL, et al. Early hospital discharge after percutaneous transluminal coronary angioplasty. *Am J Cardiol*. 64:1270–1274, 1989.

18. Ellis SG, Vandormael MG, Cowley MJ, et al. Coronary morphologic and clinical determinants of procedural outcome with angioplasty for multivessel coronary disease. *Circulation*. 82:1193–1203, 1990.

19. Ellis SG, Cowley MJ, Whitlow PL, et al. Percutaneous transluminal coronary revascularization in 1986–87 and 1991–1992 improved results with initial experience using integrated technologies. *JAMA*. (submitted for publication).

20. Andreae GE, Myler RK, Clark DA, et al. Acute complications following coronary angioplasty of totally occluded vessels. *Circulation*. 76(suppl 4):IV–400, 1987.

21. Topol EJ, Ellis SG, Fishman J, et al. Multicenter study of percutaneous transluminal angioplasty for right coronary artery ostial stenosis. *J Am Coll Cardiol*. 9:1214–1218, 1987.

22. Kereiakes DJ, Knudtson ML, Ohman EM, et al. Prolonged dilatation improves initial results during PTCA of complex coronary stenoses: results from a randomized trial. *J Am Coll Cardiol*. 21:290A, 1993.

23. Harrington RA, Leimberger JD, Berdan L, et al. The ACT Index: a method for stratifying likelihood of success and risk of acute complications in coronary intervention. *Circulation*. 88:I–208, 1993.

24. Satler, LF, Leon MB, Kent KM, et al. Strategies for acute occlusion after coronary angioplasty. *J Am Coll Cardiol*. 19:936–938, 1992.

25. Scott NA, Weintraub WS, Carlin SF, et al. Recent changes in the management and outcome of acute closure after percutaneous transluminal coronary angioplasty. *Am J Cardiol*. 71:1159–1163, 1993.

26. Lincoff AM, Topol EJ, Chapekis AT, et al. Intracoronary stenting compared with conventional therapy for abrupt closure complicating coronary angioplasty: a matched case-control study. *J Am Coll Cardiol.* 21:866–875, 1993.

27. Hearn JA, King SB III, Douglas JS, Jr, et al. Clinical and angiographic outcomes after coronary artery stenting for acute or threatened closure after percutaneous transluminal coronary angioplasty. *Circulation.* 88:2086–2096, 1993.

28. Talley JD, Weintraub WS, Roubin GS, et al. Failed elective percutaneous transluminal coronary angioplasty requiring coronary artery bypass surgery. In-hospital and late clinical outcome at 5 years. *Circulation.* 82:1203, 1990.

29. Reifart N, Schwarz F, Preusler W, et al. Results of PTCA in more than 5000 patients without surgical standby in the same center. *J Am Coll Cardiol.* 19(suppl A):229A, 1992. Abstract.

30. Bredlau CE, Roubin GS, Leimgruber PP, et al. In-hospital morbidity and mortality in patients undergoing elective coronary angioplasty. *Circulation.* 72:1044–1052, 1985.

31. Popma JJ, Satler LF, Pichard AD, et al. Vascular complications after balloon and new device angioplasty. *Circulation.* 88:1569–1578, 1993.

32. Ellis SG, Arnold AZ, Raymond RE, et al. Increased coronary perfusion in the new device era: incidence, classification, management, and outcome. *Circulation.* Abstract. 86:I–787, 1992.

— 18 —

Complications of Laser Coronary Angioplasty

John A. Bittl, M.D.
Pedro Estella, M.D.
George S. Abela, M.D.

The mechanism of vessel dilatation in balloon angioplasty involves intimal fissuring, limited penetration into the subintimal space, and occasionally deep dissection into the media. Although it was hoped that laser angioplasty would precisely ablate atheromatous plaque and produce lesser degrees of vessel disruption than balloon angioplasty, complications such as vessel dissection and perforation continue to occur despite an improved understanding of laser-tissue interactions and refinements in laser catheter design. The purpose of this chapter is to review the improvements in laser coronary angioplasty during the past 10 years. The paper will emphasize the incidence, mechanisms, and treatment of complications of laser angioplasty and discuss the current indications and contraindications for laser angioplasty.

HISTORY OF CORONARY LASER ANGIOPLASTY

Continuous-wave Systems

Continuous-wave (cw) laser systems were the first to be used for laser angioplasty, because these systems were already well established in other clinical applications such as ophthalmology, dermatology, and general surgery. Most cw systems could be readily coupled to standard optical fibers for intravascular delivery of laser energy via catheters, but most continuous wave systems involved the use of stiff fibers and lacked thermal feedback control. Overheating resulted in a superficial zone of charring and a subjacent zone of polymorphous vacuoles, findings consistent with thermal injury,[1] and underheating led to mechanical recanalization without plaque ablation. To reduce the extent of thermal injury to surrounding arterial tissue, the output of continuous-wave lasers was modified by techniques such as "chopping" to reduce the amount of thermal injury by allowing the heat to dissipate between pulses. These methods eventually proved to be inferior to the alternative approach of using pulsed laser systems operating in the ultraviolet (190 to 388 nm) or deep infrared (10,600 nm) regions of the electromagnetic spectrum. Whereas several studies have shown that the continuous wave argon laser at 448 nm has a tissue penetration depth of approximately 2.0 mm, the excimer laser at 308 nm has a shallow penetration of only 50 μm. In addition, the bare laser fibers used in prototype systems were not as suitable for revascularization when compared with the over-the-wire, flexible, multifiber laser catheters currently available, which permit the laser energy to be aimed in a coaxial fashion, thus reducing the likelihood of vessel perforation.

Continuous-wave Laser Systems and Bare Optical Fibers

The first attempts at laser angioplasty involved the use of bare optical fibers delivering laser radiation to peripheral arterial stenoses from either an argon or a neodymium: yttrium-aluminum-garnet (Nd:YAG) continuous wave laser.[2,3] Vessel perforation was observed in 2 of 16 patients,[4] which halted further investigation of laser angioplasty performed with bare optical fiber systems.

Thermal-based Angioplasty Systems

In the early investigations with laser angioplasty, the mechanism responsible for tissue removal was thought to be photothermal ablation. A system was then developed to reduce the risk of vessel perforation and yet allow thermal ablation by placing a blunt, olive-shaped metal cap at the tip of the rigid optical fiber. Thermal probe angioplasty, or "hot-tip" laser angioplasty, was used successfully to treat occlusions in the straight segments of the superficial femoral artery and, in anecdotal cases, in the coronary arteries. Most of the successes with thermal probe angioplasty were attributed to the inherent stiffness of the catheter that in many cases led to subintimal passage, dissection, and perforation,[5] and ultimately resulted in nearly complete abandonment of the procedure.

A hybrid laser system was developed to allow 20% of the laser beam to exit from the metal tip, conditioning the plaque before contact with the metal tip. The remaining 80% of laser energy was used to heat the metal tip of the probe. The system used a continuous-wave laser generator. Initial reports described the use of the hybrid probe in treating total peripheral occlusions of native arteries and prosthetic grafts.[6] In one randomized study, no significant difference was seen between the hybrid probe with conventional guidewire technique for recanalizing total femoral or iliac occlusions,[7] limiting the appeal of the system. In other studies, calcified plaque was found to deflect the probe and lead to vessel perforation (Figure 18.1).

Laser Balloon Angioplasty Systems

The combination of conventional coronary angioplasty with cw laser energy to heat vascular tissue was used in at least two systems. One system used a modified coronary

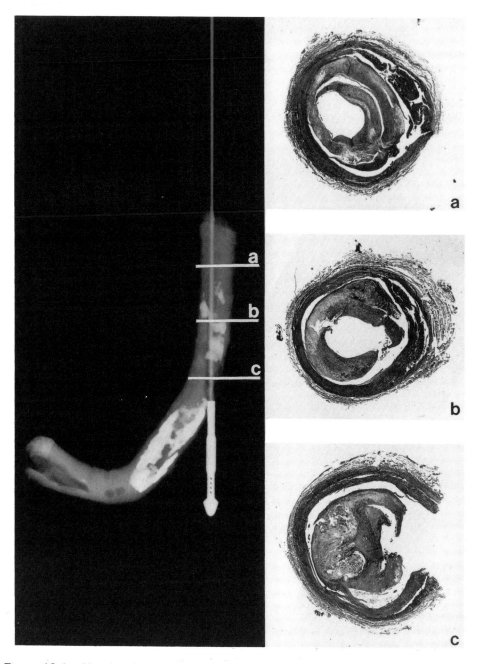

Figure 18.1.   Vessel perforation with a thermal probe. Plain radiograph of a densely calcified artery treated with thermal probe angioplasty causing a perforation at a temperature of 250°C (left). This illustrates the relation of the hybrid probe to the calcific deposit and suggests deflection of the probe by the "hard" calcific plaque, resulting in perforation. Histologic cross sections corresponding to three anatomic sites (right a, b, c) show the increasing density and calcification of the plaque from section a to section c, where perforation occurred (Masson's trichrome, magnification 15X). (Published with permission of authors and publisher.[47])

angioplasty catheter and a special helical heating element energized by a cw Nd:YAG laser. This was used to "weld" dissection flaps in the setting of abrupt vessel closure,[8] but restenosis rates consistently >50% limited the appeal of the procedure.[9]

Another system used the balloon-centering approach in treating total or subtotal occlusion when conventional guidewires were unable to cross the lesion. In the treatment of coronary artery disease, success was achieved in 51 of the 67 lesions (76%).[10] Limitations of the technique included the need for relatively straight arterial segments and the incidence of vessel perforation.

Pulsed Laser Systems

Pulsed Dye Laser for Thrombus Ablation

A pulsed dye laser system has undergone early clinical trials for selective intracoronary thrombus ablation in patients with acute myocardial infarction. The system incorporates a pulsed dye laser operating at 480 nm, a novel catheter system using contrast medium to transmit the energy to the intracoronary thrombus, and energy levels below the threshold for either normal arterial wall or atherosclerotic plaque.[11] It is difficult to predict whether this approach will be superior to the patency rate achieved by immediate balloon angioplasty for acute myocardial infarction, which has success rates as high as 97%.[12,13] On the other hand, no interventional technique is associated with uniformly high success rates when filling defects are present. Pulsed dye laser thrombolysis should thus be targeted for lesions associated with filling defects.

Fluorescence Feedback

Emission spectroscopy based on laser-induced fluorescence has been developed as a method to discriminate between normal tissue and atherosclerotic plaque. The purpose of laser-induced fluorescence is to allow the selective ablation of atherosclerotic plaque and thus avoid vessel perforation. Low-power radiation is transmitted through a fiber-optic probe to induce fluorescence at the target site without damaging the tissue. The same fiber collects the fluorescence radiation and transmits it to a spectrometer. If the spectroscopic pattern is recognized as abnormal, high-power laser energy is transmitted through the same fiber-optic probe to ablate the plaque. If the pattern is recognized as normal, high-energy laser output is inhibited. In spite of the appeal of the fluorescence-feedback laser system, several limitations have become apparent. The algorithms that discriminate normal from atherosclerotic tissue have been limited by relatively slow response times and lack of specificity. The latter problem was encountered in one study with a pulsed dye laser operating at 480 nm, in which vessel perforation was encountered in 8 of 66 patients (12%) with ileofemoral occlusion.[14]

Holmium

The mid-infrared pulsed lasers, such as holmium:yttrium-aluminum-garnet lasers, are solid-state systems that operate at a wavelength of 2.1 μm. The holmium laser system delivers a pulse of 250 μsec at a repetition rate of 5.0 Hz, generating an energy level of 250 to 600 mJ/pulse and a fluence of 125 to 375 mJ/mm².

In the early clinical experience with holmium laser coronary angioplasty, 331 patients have been treated.[15] Procedural success was achieved in 94% of patients. The perforation rate was 1.9%.[15]

Excimer

The excimer lasers are pulsed laser systems, operating in the ultraviolet range of the electromagnetic spectrum. The XeCl excimer laser emits light at 308 nm in a pulse of 135 to 210 ns at a repetition rate of 20 to 25 Hz, generating an energy level of 15 to 32 mJ/pulse and a fluence of 40 to 70 mJ/mm².

Several large studies have reported the clinical results with excimer laser coronary angioplasty.[16,17] In almost 4000 patients, the overall clinical success was 89% to 90% (defined as ≤50% residual stenosis and no in-hospital complication such as Q-wave myocardial infarction, coronary artery bypass surgery, or death). Vessel perforation occurred in 1.9% of patients and was related to the size difference between laser catheter and the diameter of the target vessel,[18] and to operator experience.[19]

CURRENT CLINICAL APPLICATION OF LASER ANGIOPLASTY

Indications

The current indications for excimer laser angioplasty include saphenous vein graft lesions, aortoostial stenoses, total occlusions, lesions greater than 20 mm in length, and balloon dilatation failures.

Saphenous Vein Graft Stenoses

The success rate for excimer laser angioplasty of saphenous vein graft lesions is 92%.[16,17] Complications include death in 1.0%, emergency bypass surgery in 0.6%, and Q-wave myocardial infarction in 2.4%. Angiographic complications include embolization in 3.3%, perforations in 1.3%, dissections in 8.8%, and angiographic restenosis in 55%.[20]

Aortoostial Stenoses

The success rate for excimer laser angioplasty of aortoostial stenoses is 90% to 94%.[21,22] Complications include death in 0.6%, emergency bypass surgery in 2.3%, and non-Q- or Q-wave myocardial infarction in 2.3%. The rates of angiographic restenosis are 39% to 41%.

Total Occlusions

Total occlusions that can be crossed with a guidewire have a procedural success rate of 84% to 90% with excimer laser angioplasty.[16,23] In one report, the rate of angiographic restenosis after excimer laser angioplasty of total occlusions is 46%.[16]

Long Lesions

The success of excimer laser angioplasty is independent of lesion length, as demonstrated consistently in several studies.[16,17,24] The drawback of laser angioplasty, which is similar to that for all interventional techniques, is a high rate of angioplasty restenosis in the range of 60% to 70%.[16] When restenosis occurs in a long lesion, however, it usually occurs focally and can easily be treated with repeat angioplasty.

Balloon Dilatation Failures

Calcified fibrotic lesions cannot always be crossed or dilated with balloons. A prospective study found that excimer laser treatment successfully facilitated balloon dilatation in 33 of 36 undilatable lesions (92%). Complications included non-Q-wave myocardial infarction in 2 of 35 patients (6%), but no patient died, required bypass surgery, or experienced Q-wave myocardial infarction.[25]

Contraindications

Thrombus

The presence of filling defects significantly reduces the success rate after excimer laser angioplasty and increases the risk of embolization and myocardial infarction.[26] Most of the episodes of embolization occur during the use of adjunctive balloon angioplasty.

Eccentric Lesions

The use of excimer laser angioplasty to treat highly eccentric lesions is associated with an increase in acute complications.[27]

Bifurcation Lesions

With the use of concentric laser catheters, excimer laser angioplasty consistently is associated with increased complications when it is used to treat lesions at arterial bifurcations.[16,18,24]

Angulated Lesions

The relatively rigid laser catheters should not be used in angulated lesions because of the likelihood that the guidewire can be overdriven and laser energy applied in a radial rather than coaxial direction. Vessel perforation may ensue if excimer laser angioplasty is used to treat angulated lesions.[28]

ANGIOGRAPHIC COMPLICATIONS

Spasm

Background

In-vitro studies have documented that exposure of vascular rings to continuous-wave laser irradiation is associated with an increase in vasomotor tone.[29] On the other hand, treatment of vascular tissue with pulsed-wave systems is not associated with an increase in vasomotor tone. In clinical studies with pulsed excimer laser angioplasty, however, spasm has not been completely eliminated. In certain cases the guidewire and the mechanical effects of the laser catheter may contribute to the spasm.

Clinical Results

In the Percutaneous Excimer Laser Coronary Angioplasty Registry the incidence of spasm was 5%.[16] Empiric treatment with intravenous nytroglycerin is recommended to minimize the likelihood of laser-induced spasm.

Restenosis

Background

Laser angioplasty was initially developed in an effort to reduce restenosis by ablating atheromatous plaque and avoiding injury to the normal components of the arterial wall.

Clinical Results

In the Percutaneous Excimer Laser Coronary Angioplasty Registry report with a clinical follow-up of 94% at 6 months, the incidence of clinical restenosis was 46%.[16] By multivariable analysis the predictors of restenosis were lesion length ≥ 10 mm and stand-alone laser angioplasty. Although the average angiographic restenosis rate after excimer laser angioplasty is about 50%, the likelihood of angiographic restenosis after excimer laser coronary angioplasty was reduced when large vessels were selected for treatment and when a large postprocedure lumen diameter was achieved.[30]

DISSECTION AND PERFORATION: CLINICAL IMPLICATIONS

Dissection

Background

Experimental studies suggested that excimer laser angioplasty may induce lesser degrees of vessel injury than balloon angioplasty, because excimer laser treatment is associated with finely etched margins without dissection or charring. The first clinical reports, however, showed that vessel dissection occurred in about 15% of patients.[24] Unfortunately, the problem of dissection has not been eliminated despite refinements in laser catheter development.[31]

Although an initial report suggested that holmium laser angioplasty was associated with dissections in only 0.8% of patients, the rate of vessel perforation was 1.9%.[15] Because vessel perforation is probably an extreme form of dissection and the rates of perforation are equivalent after excimer or holmium angioplasty, it is unlikely that holmium laser angioplasty has a lower rate of vessel disruption than excimer laser angioplasty. Instead, the apparent differences in rates of dissection between the holmium and excimer studies must be attributed to differences in definitions.

Clinical Importance of Dissection

The clinical impact of dissection during laser angioplasty is very significant. Several laser-induced dissections extend beyond the treated site and result in clinical complications (Figure 18.2). In a previously unpublished analysis of 2071 consecutive patients treated with excimer laser angioplasty at 26 sites participating in the Percutaneous Excimer Laser Coronary Angioplasty Registry, vessel dissection was reported in 309 patients (14.9%). The mean age of the patients was 63 $\pm$ 11 years (range 28 to 91 years), and 1491 of the patients (72%) were men. The 2071 patients had a total of 2286 stenoses intended for treatment with excimer laser coronary angioplasty. The mean age of the patients who experienced coronary artery dissection was 62 $\pm$ 12 years, which was similar to that for the entire 2071 patients. All major complications were higher in the patients who experienced dissection (Table 18.1).

Clinical and Angiographic Determinants of Dissection

Logistic regression methods were used to identify the risk factors for major dissection associated with excimer laser angioplasty (Figure 18.3). Clinical variables associated with an increased risk of dissection included diabetes mellitus and female sex. Angiographic variables associated with an increased risk of dissection included vessel-catheter size difference $\leq$1.0 mm, bifurcation lesions, and calcified lesions. Angiographic variables associated with a decreased likelihood of dissection included discrete lesions, previous angioplasty, saphenous vein graft lesions, and ostial stenoses.

Management of Major Coronary Artery Dissections

The management of a complicated coronary artery dissection during angioplasty requires a systematic approach to treat the vessel disruption successfully. The use of prolonged balloon inflation in the management of a dissection after laser angioplasty has been successful in about one half of the cases, probably by "tacking up" the dissection flap.[32,33] A perfusion cathether, which can almost always be used at any site reached by a stiffer laser catheter, may minimize ischemia from prolonged balloon inflation.[28] Another approach for restoring vessel patency after abrupt closure secondary to major dissection is implantation of the Gianturco-Roubin stent to compress the dissection flap against the arterial wall.[34,35] The limitation of the stents is that the vessel diameter must be larger than 3.0 mm in diameter. Another approach is to use directional coronary atherectomy, which can be used so long as the dissection does not extend beyond the target lesion. Salvage atherectomy should not be used for long, spiral dissections because of the risk of vessel perforation. The ultimate procedure for restoring blood flow in the presence of a major dissection after other measures have failed is coronary artery bypass surgery. In the Registry series, 20% of patients with dissection required bypass surgery (Table 18.1).

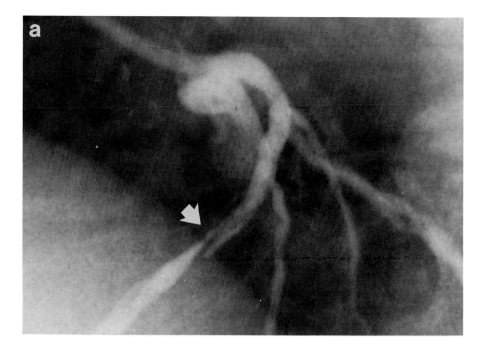

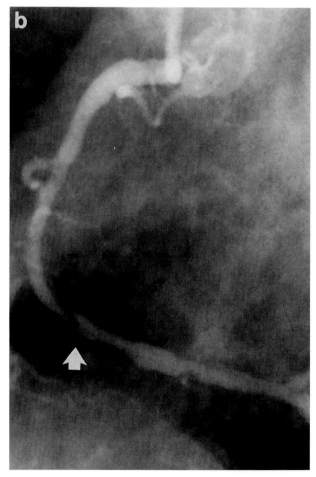

194

TABLE 18.1. Sequelae of Vessel Dissection During Excimer Laser Angioplasty

	Total Population	Any Dissection	P Value
N	2071	309	
Death	27 (1%)	3 (1%)	0.79
Q-wave MI	25 (1%)	26 (8%)	<0.001
Non-Q-wave MI	48 (2%)	24 (8%)	<0.001
Emergency bypass	92 (4%)	62 (20%)	<0.001
Abrupt closure	121 (5%)	77 (25%)	<0.001

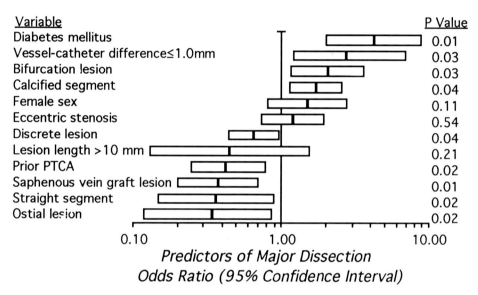

Variable	P Value
Diabetes mellitus	0.01
Vessel-catheter difference≤1.0mm	0.03
Bifurcation lesion	0.03
Calcified segment	0.04
Female sex	0.11
Eccentric stenosis	0.54
Discrete lesion	0.04
Lesion length >10 mm	0.21
Prior PTCA	0.02
Saphenous vein graft lesion	0.01
Straight segment	0.02
Ostial lesion	0.02

Predictors of Major Dissection
Odds Ratio (95% Confidence Interval)

Figure 18.3. Predictors of major dissection. Relative risk analysis for dissection during excimer laser coronary angioplasty in 2071 consecutive patients. Odds ratios indicate the likelihood of dissection among patients with the specified variable, as compared with all other patients. The statistical reliability of the odds ratio is given by the 95% confidence interval.

Perforation

Clinical Implications

Coronary artery perforation has been reported to occur in 1% to 3% of patients treated with excimer laser angioplasty.[18,19] Almost half the cases of perforation were associated with a major complication (death, myocardial infarction, bypass surgery, or pericardiocentesis).

Figure 18.2. Dissection. The dissection in the midportion of the left anterior descending artery (a, arrow) in this 55-year-old man occurred after excimer laser angioplasty of a long lesion, persisted after directional atherectomy, and required urgent coronary artery bypass surgery. The dissection in the distal segment of the right coronary artery (b, arrow) in this 75-year-old woman occurred after excimer laser angioplasty of a total occlusion, but responded successfully to prolonged inflation with a perfusion balloon without clinical sequelae.

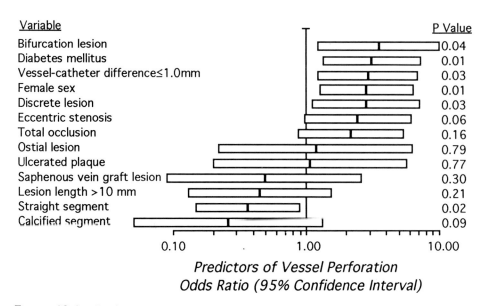

Predictors of Vessel Perforation
Odds Ratio (95% Confidence Interval)

Figure 18.4. Predictors of vessel perforation. Relative risk analysis for dissection during excimer laser coronary angioplasty in 764 consecutive patients. Odds ratios indicate the likelihood of perforation among patients with the specified variable, as compared with all other patients. The statistical reliability of the odds ratio is given by the 95% confidence interval. Reproduced with permission of Bittl et al.[18]

Clinical and Angiographic Determinants of Perforation

Logistic regression methods have been used to identify the risk factors for perforation associated with excimer laser angioplasty (Figure 18.4). By multivariable analysis, the risk of perforation was increased in cases where the size of the laser catheter approached the reference diameter of the target vessel, and in patients with bifurcation lesions or diabetes mellitus.[18] Clinical variables associated with an increased risk of dissection included diabetes mellitus and female sex. Angiographic variables associated with an increased risk of dissection included bifurcation lesions.

Management of Coronary Artery Perforation

The treatment of coronary artery perforation requires that a balloon catheter be rapidly advanced over the guidewire and inflated at the site of the leak in the vessel (Figure 18.5). Small perforations manifest as focal extravasation are successfully treated with prolonged balloon inflation alone. Larger perforations communicating with the pericardial space require more aggressive therapy. If hemopericardium develops, the border of the cardiac silhouette stops moving under fluoroscopy, suggesting that pericardiocentesis might be required to treat cardiac tamponade. A free perfora-

---

Figure 18.5. Vessel perforation. Excimer laser treatment of a lesion in the angulated segment of the midportion of the right coronary artery (a, arrow), resulted in perforation (b, arrow), which was treated with prolonged inflation of a perfusion balloon

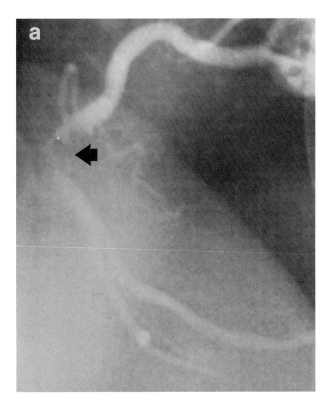

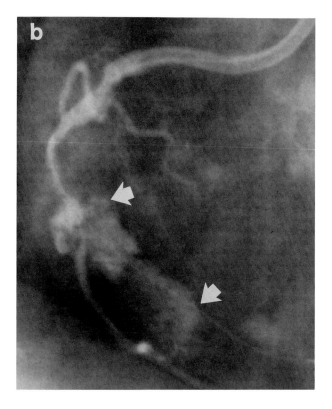

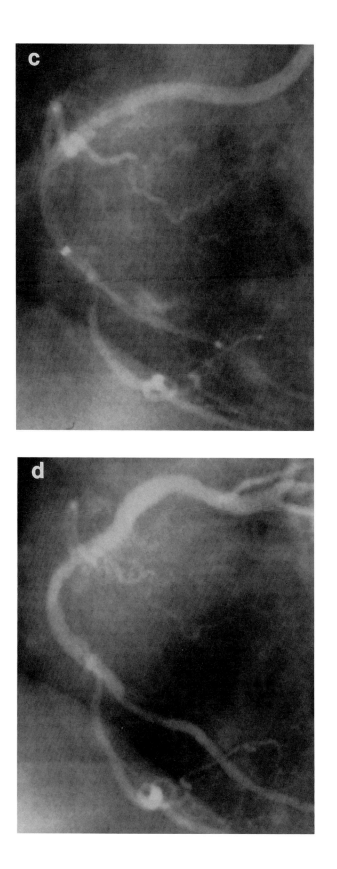

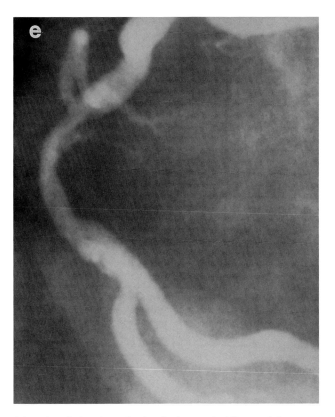

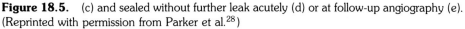

Figure 18.5. (c) and sealed without further leak acutely (d) or at follow-up angiography (e). (Reprinted with permission from Parker et al.[28])

tion communicating with the pericardial space that does not seal with prolonged balloon inflation requires reversal of anticoagulation, emergency bypass surgery, and surgical repair of the perforation site.

MECHANISMS OF VESSEL DISRUPTION IN LASER ANGIOPLASTY

Basic Mechanisms

In balloon angioplasty, dilating force is applied to atheromatous plaque. The heterogeneous biomechanical properties of the plaque govern the nonuniform distribution of tensile and shear stress. The areas within the plaque with the highest tensile and shear stress and less resistance are most susceptible to dissection. Generally, these high-stress regions are located near the junctions of the plaque with the normal vessel.[36] Dissection planes are established along the path of least resistance deep to the plaque that is defined by the cleavage plane between the plaque and the media.[37,38] Plaque geometry (eccentricity, length, curvature), composition (calcium,

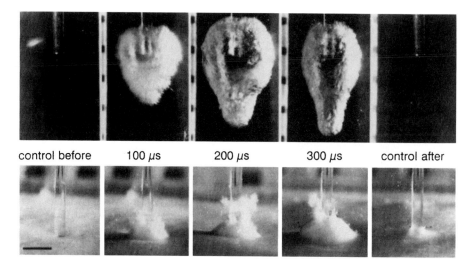

control before   100 µs   200 µs   300 µs   control after

Figure 18.6.   Holmium laser ablation. Tissue ablation with holmium laser irradiation is associated with the rapid formation and collapse of a vapor bubble in saline (upper panels) and abrupt tissue elevation (lower panels). (From van Leeuwen et al with permission [38])

cholesterol, fibrous tissue, cells) and procedural variables (balloon artery ratio, non-compliant balloon, laser energy, and laser catheter size) all play a role in determining the biomechanical properties of the plaque and its interaction with either balloon or laser energy.

Although laser-induced tissue ablation results in both photovaporization and thermal injury,[39] van Leeuwen et al[38] have shown that ultraviolet light at 308 nm produces bubble formation within the treated tissue, and expansion through the pathway of least resistance causes dissection (Figures 18.6 and 18.7). The size of the bubbles and the intensity of the resulting shock wave are further augmented by blood or contrast in the field, causing acoustic injury resulting in cavitations in the surrounding tissues.[40,41] This may explain the apparent differences between the precise excimer laser-induced etching in experimental studies and excimer laser-associated dissections in the presence of blood (Figure 18.8). A thin monolayer of blood between the laser catheter and the target has been associated with markedly different results in experimental studies, leading to evidence of tissue disruption and dissection. The influence of contrast media is thought to be even more important, because the presence of a 1% mixture of any contrast agent and saline leads to explosive effects whereas excimer laser irradiation in saline alone is associated with no shock-wave generation.

Tissue disruption and dissection can be so great as to lead to abrupt vessel closure during laser angioplasty. Although this was initially interpreted as vasospasm, the problem was found to be unresponsive to intracoronary nitroglycerin and usually required balloon angioplasty to restore flow. The results of tissue studies following pulsed laser irradiation have shown that there are extensive dissection planes formed at treatment sites resulting in puffed-up appearance of the tissue surrounding the laser impact site. Because of the resemblance to a multilayered French cake called

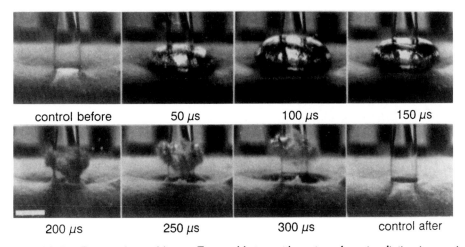

control before   50 μs   100 μs   150 μs

200 μs   250 μs   300 μs   control after

Figure 18.7. Excimer laser ablation. Tissue ablation with excimer laser irradiation is associated with no vapor formation during irradiation of saline (not shown), but with vapor formation during tissue irradiation. (From van Leeuwen et al with permission.[38])

mille-feuilles, meaning "thousand leaves," we used the same term to describe this tissue effect (Figure 18.9).

Dissections and perforations occur with both excimer and holmium laser angioplasty. Several experimental studies have suggested many similarities in the laser-tissue interactions of excimer and holmium laser treatment. Atherectomy specimens obtained immediately after holmium laser angioplasty in eight patients showed an irregular-shaped vacuolar "acoustic injury" surrounded by multiple satellite vacuoles.[42] Histological examination of atherectomy specimens obtained from 12 patients after excimer laser angioplasty showed absence of charring but a pattern of fine, subtle edge disruption in which the involved cells have a "ground glass" appearance. Experimental studies have shown that tissue ablation with holmium and excimer laser angioplasty produces vapor bubbles that expand into the tissue and form microdissections.[38,41]

Lesions that have been treated previously with balloon angioplasty have shown a reduced risk of major coronary dissection. The neointima of the restenotic lesion is generally hypocellular and rich in fibrous tissue, containing predominantly glycosaminoglycans and various forms of collagen differing from the primary lesion.[43] This fibrous cap and the large amount of extracellular tissue may homogeneously absorb the electrical and mechanical forces applied over the lesion in the process of laser angioplasty and thus reduce the risk of major dissection.

Several studies have suggested that women are at increased risk of major dissection or perforation during laser angioplasty. Some studies suggest that atheromatous plaques in women are more cellular-rich tissue but contain less fibrous tissue than those in men.[44] Other studies suggest that dissections occur in regions of atheromatous plaque containing foam cells, suggesting that local factors including enzymatic degradation of the connective tissue matrix may weaken the intimal layer predisposing to fracture.[45]

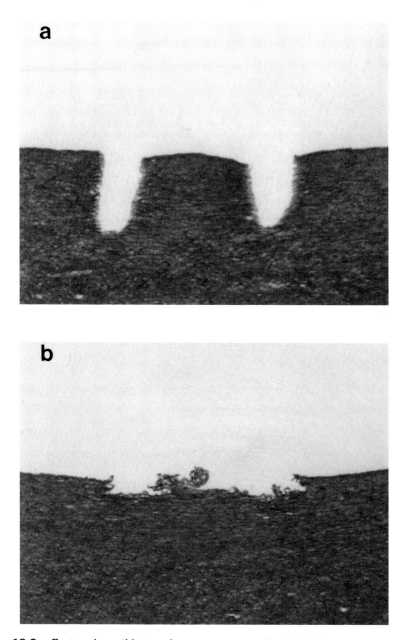

Figure 18.8. Excimer laser ablation of porcine aorta in saline field (a) versus blood field (b). The ablation of underlying tissue in a saline medium results in less disruption of tissue planes than in blood, which is associated with much greater degrees of dissection. (From Bittl et al with permission.[40])

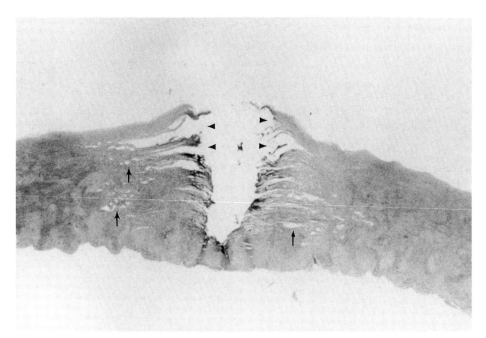

Figure 18.9. "Mille-feuilles" effect. Cross section of normal aorta showing shock-wave injury with dissection following holmium laser irradiation via a 2-mm multifiber catheter. This was performed in a saline medium at a wavelength of 2100 nm, pulse duration of 450 ns, repetition rate of 5 Hz, and energy of 450 mJ per pulse. The artery shows the "mille-feuilles" effect with puffing up at the crater edges and dissection (arrowheads) of the tissue planes along side of the crater with cavitation bubbles (vertical arrows) inside the arterial wall. Thermal necrosis can also be seen lining the edges of the crater. (Published with permission from Abela.[46])

Avoidance of Dissection and Perforation During Excimer Laser Angioplasty

Major vessel dissection might be avoided by selecting patients who have long lesions, saphenous vein graft lesions, ostial lesions, and restenosis lesions. Patients with lesions in a bend >45 degrees are generally not treated with excimer laser angioplasty. Major vessel dissection may occur at lesions in relatively straight proximal vascular segments. If the laser catheter cannot be advanced through a lesion, forceful advancement may overdrive the flexible guidewire and allow laser energy to be directed at the vessel wall instead of the lumen. To avoid this, the laser operator should consider using a small laser catheter or abandon laser angioplasty altogether if 15 seconds of laser time results in no advancement of the laser catheter into the stenosis. The problem of dissection may be avoided by selecting a laser catheter that is more than 1.0 mm smaller than the target vessel. Future developments in catheter design, such as torquable catheter tips or fluorescence feedback, may further reduce the risk of this serious complication. Avoiding an overstretching of the stenosis with the balloon angioplasty after the laser procedure by selecting the best balloon size and material should reduce the risk of major dissection. Finally, decreasing the amount of blood in the field in contact with the laser catheter tip can reduce the risk of dissection. This is achieved by the selection of lesions likely to be in close contact with the tip of the laser catheter by removing all contrast from the target vessel with saline flush.

CONCLUSIONS

Laser coronary angioplasty has become an approved procedure performed in several laboratories. Although the procedure has undergone significant refinements and is now associated with more predictable outcome than early investigations, vessel dissection and perforation continue to occur. These problems can be avoided by careful selection of patients, use of laser catheters >1.0 mm smaller than the target vessel, and elimination of contrast medium from the target lesion before irradiation with laser energy. If dissection or perforation occur, several treatment strategies can be tried. Further study is required, however, to reduce the incidence of vessel disruption during laser angioplasty and to increase the ablation of atheromatous plaque safely.

REFERENCES

1. Geschwind H, Fabre M, Chaitman BR, et al. Histopathology after Nd-YAG laser percutaneous transluminal angioplasty of peripheral arteries. *J Am Coll Cardiol.* 8:1089–1095, 1986.
2. Ginsburg R, Kirr DS, Guthaner P, Tolh J, Mitchell RS. Salvage of an ischemic limb by laser angioplasty: description of a new technique. *Clin Cardiol.* 7:54–58, 1984.
3. Geschwind H, Boussignac G, Teisseire B. Percutaneous transluminal laser angioplasty in man. *Lancet.* 2:844, 1984. Letter.
4. Ginsburg R, Wexler R, Mitchell RS, Profitt D. Percutaneous transluminal laser angioplasty for treatment of peripheral vascular disease: clinical experience in 16 patients. *Radiology.* 156:619–624, 1985.
5. Tobis JM, Conroy R, Deutsch L-S, et al. Laser-assisted versus mechanical recanalization of femoral arterial occlusions. *Am J Cardiol.* 68:1079–1086, 1991.
6. Abela GS, Seeger JM, Barbieri E, Franzini D, Fenech A, Pepine CJ, Conti CR. Laser angioplasty with angioscopic guidance in humans. *J Am Coll Cardiol.* 8:184–192, 1986.
7. Belli AM, Cumberland DC, Procter AE, Welsh CL. Total peripheral artery occlusions: conventional versus laser thermal recanalization with a hybrid probe in percutaneous angioplasty: results of a randomized trial. *Radiology.* 181:57–60, 1991.
8. Reis GJ, Pomerantz RM, Jenkins RD, et al. Laser balloon angioplasty: clinical, angiographic, and histologic results. *J Am Coll Cardiol.* 18:193–202, 1991.
9. Kuntz RE, Safian RD, Levine MJ, Reis GJ, Diver DJ, Baim DS. Novel approach to the analysis of restenosis after the use of three new coronary devices. *J Am Coll Cardiol.* 19:1493–1499, 1992.

10. Foschi A, Myers G, Crick WF, Friedberg HD, Snyder D, Nordstrom LA. Laser angioplasty of totally occluded coronary arteries and vein grafts: preliminary report on a current trial. *Am J Cardiol.* Supplement to v. 63:9F–13F, 1989.

11. Gregory KW, Block P, Knopf W, Buckley LA, Cates CU. Laser thrombolysis in acute myocardial infarction. *Laser Surg Med.* 51 (suppl 5):13, 1993.

12. Grines CL, Browne KF, Marco J, et al. A comparison of immediate angioplasty with thrombolytic therapy for acute myocardial infarction. *N Engl J Med.* 328:673–679, 1993.

13. Zijlstra F, de Boer FJ, Hoorntje JCA, Reiffers S, Reiber JHC, Suyapranata H. A comparison of immediate coronary angioplasty with intravenous streptokinase in acute myocardial infarction. *N Engl J Med.* 328:680–684, 1993.

14. Geschwind HJ, Aptecar E, Boussignac G, Dubois R, Zelinsky R, Poirot G. Results and follow-up after percutaneous pulsed laser-assisted balloon angioplasty guided by spectroscopy. *Circulation.* 83:787–796, 1991.

15. de Marchena EJ, Mallon SM, Knopf WD, et al. Effectiveness of holmium laser-assisted coronary angioplasty, *Am J Cardiol.* 73:117–121, 1994.

16. Bittl JA, Sanborn TA, Tcheng JE, Siegel RM, Ellis SG. Clinical success, complications, and restenosis rates with excimer laser coronary angioplasty. *Am J Cardiol.* 70:1533–1539, 1992.

17. Litvack F, Eigler N, Margolis J, et al. Percutaneous excimer laser coronary angioplasty: results in the first consecutive 3000 patients. *J Am Coll Cardiol.* 23:323–329, 1994.

18. Bittl JA, Ryan TJ Jr, Keaney JF Jr, et al. Coronary artery perforation during excimer laser coronary angioplasty. *J Am Coll Cardiol.* 21:1158–1165, Elsevier Science Publishing Company, 1993.

19. Holmes DR Jr, Reeder GS, Ghazzal ZMB, et al. Coronary perforation after excimer laser coronary angioplasty: the excimer laser coronary angioplasty registry experience. *J Am Coll Cardiol.* 23:330–335, 1994.

20. Bittl JA, Sanborn TA, Yardley DE, et al. Predictions of outcome of percutaneous excimer laser coronary angioplasty of saphenous vein bypass graft lesions. *Am J Cardiol.* 74:144–148, 1994.

21. Eigler N, Weinstock B, Douglas JS Jr, et al. Excimer laser coronary angioplasty of aorto-ostial stenoses: results of excimer laser coronary angioplasty (ELCA) registry in the first 200 patients. *Circulation.* 88:2049–2057, 1993.

22. Tcheng JE, Bittl JA, Sanborn TA, et al. Treatment of aortoostial disease with percutaneous excimer laser coronary angioplasty. *Circulation.* 86:I–512, 1992. Abstract.

23. Holmes DR Jr, Forrester JS, Litvack F, et al. Chronic total obstruction and short-term outcome: the excimer laser angioplasty registry experience. *Mayo Clin Proc.* 68:5–10, 1993.

24. Bittl JA, Sanborn TA. Excimer laser-facilitated coronary angioplasty: relative risk analysis of acute and follow-up results in 200 patients. *Circulation.* 86:71–80, 1992.

25. Bittl JA, Sanborn TA, Tcheng JE, Watson LE. Excimer laser-facilitated angioplasty for undilatable coronary lesions: results of a prospective, controlled study. *Circulation.* 88:I–23, 1993. Abstract.

26. Estella P, Ryan TJ Jr, Landzberg JS, Bittl JA. Excimer laser-assisted angioplasty for lesions containing thrombus. *J Am Coll Cardiol.* 21:1550–1556, 1993.

27. Ghazzal ZMB, Hearn J, Litvack F, et al. Morphological predictors of acute complications after percutaneous excimer laser coronary angioplasty. Results of a comprehensive

angiographic analysis: importance of the eccentricity index. *Circulation.* 86:820–827, 1992.

28. Parker JD, Ganz P, Selwyn AP, Bittl JA. Successful treatment of an excimer laser-associated coronary artery perforation with the Stack perfusion catheter. *Cath Cardiovasc Diagn.* 22:118–123, Wiley-Liss 1991.

29. Cox JL, Chiasson DA, Gotlieb AI. Stranger in a strange land: the pathogenesis of saphenous vein graft stenosis with emphasis on structural and functional differences between veins and arteries. *Prog Cardiovasc Dis.* 34:45–68, 1991.

30. Bittl JA, Kuntz RE, Estella P, Sanborn TA, Baim DS. Analysis of late lumen narrowing after excimer laser-facilitated coronary angioplasty. *J Am Coll Cardiol.* 23:1314–1320, 1994.

31. Bittl JA, Tcheng JE, Sanborn TA. The changing profile of patients and lesions treated with percutaneous excimer laser coronary angioplasty. *Circulation.* 88:I–24, 1993. Abstract.

32. Lincoff A, Popma J, Ellis S, Hacker J, Topol E. Abrupt vessel closure complicating coronary angioplasty: clinical, angiographic, and therapeutic profile. *JACC.* 19:926–935, 1992.

33. Cripps TR, Morgan JM, Rickards AF. Outcome of extensive coronary artery dissection during coronary angioplasty. *Br Heart J.* 66:3–6, 1991.

34. Lincoff AM, Topol EJ, Chapekis AT, et al. Intracoronary stenting compared with conventional therapy for abrupt vessel closure complicating coronary angioplasty: a matched case-control study. *J Am Coll Cardiol.* 21:866–875, 1993.

35. Roubin GS, Cannon AD, Agrawal SK, et al. Intracoronary stenting for acute and threatened closure complicating percutaneous transluminal coronary angioplasty. *Circulation.* 85:916–927, 1992.

36. Lee RT, Loree HM, Cheng GC, Lieberman EH, Jaramillo N, Schoen FJ. Computational structural analysis based on intravascular ultrasound imaging before in vitro angioplasty: prediction of plaque fracture locations. *J Am Coll Cardiol.* 21:777–782, 1993.

37. Fitzgerald PJ, Ports TA, Yock PG. Contribution of localized calcium deposits to dissection after angioplasty: an observational study using intravascular ultrasound. *Circulation.* 86:64–70, 1992.

38. van Leeuwen TG, van Erven L, Meertens JH, Motamedi M, Post MJ, Borst C. Origin of arterial wall dissections induced by pulsed excimer and mid-infrared laser ablation in the pig. *J Am Coll Cardiol.* 19:1610–1618, 1992.

39. Clarke R, Isner JM, Donaldson RF, Jones GI. Gas chromatography light microscopic correlation of excimer laser photoablation of cardiovascular tissues: evidence for a thermal mechanism. *Circulation Res.* 60:429–437, 1987.

40. Bittl JA, Barbeau C, Abela GS. Laser coronary angioplasty: potential effects and current limitations. In: Topol EJ, ed. *Textbook of Interventional Cardiology.* W.B. Saunders Co. Philadelphia, PA. 917–932, 1993.

41. Isner JM, Pickering JG, Mosseri M. Laser-induced dissections: pathogenesis and implications for therapy. *J Am Coll Cardiol.* 19:1619–1621, 1992.

42. Isner JM, Rosenfield K, White CJ, et al. In vivo assessment of vascular pathology resulting from laser irradiation. Analysis of 23 patients studied by directional atherectomy immediately after laser angioplasty. *Circulation.* 85:2185–2196, 1992.

43. Schwartz RS, Holmes DR Jr, Topol EJ. The restenosis paradigm revisited: an alternative proposal for cellular mechanisms. *J Am Coll Cardiol.* 20:1284–1293, 1992.

44. Mautner SL, Lin F, Roberts WC. Composition of atherosclerotic plaques in the epicardial coronary arteries in juvenile (Type I) diabetes mellitus. *Am J Cardiol.* 70:1264–1268, 1992.

45. Richardson PD, Davies MJ, Born GVR. Influence of plaque configuration and stress distribution on fissuring of coronary atherosclerotic plaques. *Lancet.* 2:941–944, October 21, 1989.

46. Abela GS. Abrupt closure after laser angioplasty: spasm or a "mille-feulles" effect? *J Interv Cardiol.* 5:259–262, 1992.

47. Barbeau GR, Abela GS, Seeger JM, et al. Temperature monitoring during peripheral thermooptical laser recanalization in humans. *Clin Cardiol.* 13:690–697, 1990.

— 19 —

Complications of Percutaneous Coronary Atherectomy Devices

Ziyad M. B. Ghazzal, M.D.
Spencer B. King III, M.D.

Over the past few years, several new devices have been approved by the Food and Drug Administration for the percutaneous revascularization of coronary artery lesions. Most of these devices have in general been proven beneficial in the treatment of specific lesion morphologies, but they are certainly not free of complications. This review will address some of the untoward effects of the three percutaneous coronary atherectomy devices in interventional cardiology, namely, the Transluminal Extraction Catheter (TEC device), the Rotablator, and the Directional Coronary Atherectomy (DCA).

TRANSLUMINAL EXTRACTION CATHETER

Description

The TEC device is a core catheter with a conical tip that contains two windows and sharp inner edges that constitute the cutting blades (Figure 19.1). The catheter is threaded over a guidewire and with the help of a motor drive unit is rotated at 750 rpm. As the device is advanced over the guidewire across the lesion, tissue is trapped and shaved on the inner surface of the conical head. Suction is simultaneously applied through the lumen of the catheter and the excised material is withdrawn.

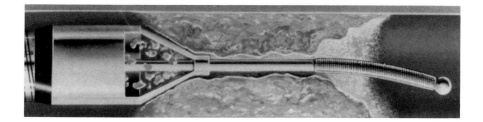

Figure 19.1. Transluminal Extraction Catheter showing the conical head (see text for details) (reproduced with permission of manufacturer—IVT).

Indications and Contraindications

The device is used to debulk atherosclerotic material. It appears to be best suited for lesions complicated by thrombus or in degenerated vein grafts. Absolute contraindications include lesions that cannot be crossed with a guidewire, calcified lesions, internal mammary arteries, and coronary ectasia. Relative contraindications include severe eccentricity or angulation, evidence of dissection, and diffuse disease in native coronary arteries.

Acute Results and Complications

Some of the early experience with the TEC device was recently reported by Safian et al[1]: 158 saphenous vein graft lesions with a mean age of 8.3 ± 3 years attempted with the device were analyzed. Seventeen percent were felt to be diffusely diseased and degenerated. A thrombus was felt to be present in 28% of the vein grafts. The device was successfully advanced through 91% of the lesions and resulted in a significant reduction in the diameter of stenosis. Adjunctive balloon angioplasty was needed in 91.2%. Overall procedural success (TEC ± balloon) was achieved in 84% of the cases (residual stenosis <50% and no major complications). Angiographic complications related to the use of TEC atherectomy were as follows: distal embolization in 11.3%, no reflow phenomenon in 4.4%, and abrupt closure in 5%. Overall clinical complications included death (2%), CABG (0.7%), and Q-wave MI (2%). Another smaller study by Popma et al,[2] analyzed 51 patients. Adjunct balloon angioplasty was also used in a high number of cases (86%), with a procedural success of 82%. Distal embolization occurred in five patients. Major clinical complications were as follows: death 5.8%, Q-wave MI 7.4%, and CABG 3.9%.

Perforation can occur with TEC atherectomy but the incidence is very low. Preliminary unpublished data have indicated a higher risk of perforation in native arteries compared with vein grafts and the overall rate is approximately 1%. A few points are worth keeping in mind to help avoid a perforation: branching vessels on very angulated segments are best avoided. Highly eccentric lesions should also be avoided. The catheter should never be forced forward or advanced against resistance. If a perforation occurs, prolonged balloon inflation, pericardiocentesis, and CABG should be considered pending the hemodynamic condition of the patient.

Luminal tears and dissections are best avoided by following the approach outlined previously in addition to selecting the appropriate catheter size and advancing it very slowly across the lesion, especially during the first pass.

Despite one of the primary indications of this catheter being thrombus-containing lesions, the risk of distal embolization is still significant. This can be due to the fact that such lesions can have a very complex morphology and much friable material, as in degenerated vein grafts. Again, in such instances it is important to emphasize that the catheter should be advanced very slowly to allow the vacuum to suction the tissue more effectively rather than causing mechanical dislodgment of a thrombus and distal propagation. It is also important to ensure the proper functioning of the vacuum system before engaging the lesion. The "no reflow phenomenon" can occur and is best described as an open vessel but with practically no flow. The vessel is filled with dye that often appears to stagnate. The mechanism is believed to be occlusion of the microvascular bed from microembolization or spasm while the epicardial artery or vein is wide open. Treatment strategy can include one or more of the following: intracoronary medications (nitroglycerin/calcium antagonists/urokinase), forceful injection of saline or blood, or intraaortic balloon pump. Coronary bypass surgery is probably of little benefit because it does not address the primary problem of distal microvascular occlusion. The no reflow phenomenon often resolves within a few minutes.

ROTABLATOR

Description

Rotational atherectomy is a mode of percutaneous arterial recanalization that uses a high-speed, rotating, diamond-coated burr.[3–6] The catheter system tracks over a guidewire positioned across the lesion. As the catheter rotates close to 200000 rpm, the burr tip that is front-coated with diamond chips (Figure 19.2) pulverizes the atheromatous plaque into particles generally smaller than red blood cells. These microparticles flow with the blood to the distal circulation. The ablation process follows the principle of differential cutting; the rotating burr theoretically avoids elastic tissue which in most cases is disease-free. Atheromatous tissue is inelastic and therefore does not deflect away from the ablating effect of the rotablator.

Indications and Contraindications

Indications and contraindications are similar to those followed for percutaneous balloon angioplasty. The designated lesion has to be crossed with a special type of guidewire. With evolving experience, calcified lesions have been regarded as a good indication for rotational ablation. Coronary segments that are diffusely diseased and lesions with a bulky plaque are also felt to be acceptable indications; however, the risk of excessive distal embolization should be weighed against the benefit of tissue ablation. Other lesions that are frequently not successfully dilated when attempted with balloon angioplasty, such as the calcified ostial, are achieving favorable results

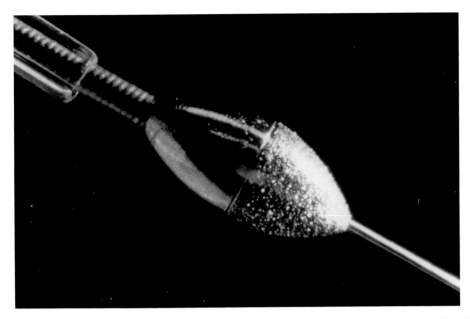

Figure 19.2. Rotablator catheter with the diamond front coating of the burr tip (reproduced with permission of manufacturer—Heart Technology).

with rotational atherectomy. Some of the contraindications to the use of the device include saphenous vein grafts, thrombus-containing lesions, and angiographic evidence of significant dissections. Nevertheless, because this device is relatively new, more experience and analysis of data are needed to better identify the scope of indications and contraindications.

Acute Results and Complications

A number of publications have analyzed the early experience with the rotational atherectomy device. Ellis et al[7] have reported an analysis of 400 stenoses from 316 patients. Lesion complexity according to the ACC/AHA classification was B1, 40%; B2, 30%; C, 6%. Adjunctive balloon angioplasty was used in 82% of the lesions. Procedural success was achieved in 90%. Major ischemic complications were divided as follows: death, 0.3%; Q-wave MI, 2.2%; emergency bypass surgery, 0.9%. Non-Q-wave MI occurred in 5.7% of the patients. This study revealed several independent correlates of ischemic complications: lesion length, right coronary artery lesion, stenosis bend, and female sex. Another smaller study[8] analyzed 116 lesions attempted with rotational atherectomy, of which 17% were calcified and 26% were ostial in location. Significant angiographic complications occurred in 46 lesions (39.6%) and included severe dissections leading to acute closure in 11.2% of the lesions, of which two were persistent and required emergency bypass surgery. Severe coronary spasm was reversed in 13.8%, and guidewire fracture occurred in three lesions. Of the latter, one wire was successfully retrieved by the snare-loop technique and the other two were treated with coumadin. There were three side branch closures and two lesions with distal embolization. There were no perforations. Clinical complications included one death, two emergency bypass surgeries, Q-wave MI in 4.8%, and non-Q-wave MI in 2.9%. Significant vascular injuries requiring repair or blood transfusions occurred in 10.6% of the patients.

The no-reflow phenomenon can occur with rotational ablation. It is felt to be due to poor distal runoff as a result of distal embolization or spasm of the distal microvasculature. Its incidence is reported as 5.1% to 6.1%.[5,7] In the majority of cases flow can be reestablished within a few minutes by using one or more therapeutics modalities (intracoronary nitroglycerin, calcium channel blockers, thrombolytics, balloon inflations, and, rarely, percutaneous mechanical support). The clinical consequences of the slow reflow can be important: 7% suffered a Q-wave MI and 26% a non-Q-wave MI.[7] The study by Ellis also reached independent correlates of the no-reflow phenomenon that included total burring time, right coronary lesions, and, to a lesser extent, recent myocardial infarction in the lesion territory. Other parameters, such as estimates of atheroma burden and runoff bed size, were not independent predictors.

There appears to be a steep learning curve with the use of rotational ablation. A fundamental understanding of the procedure is essential. Attention to details such as choosing the proper burr size and advancing the rotational catheter very gently until the lesion is crossed cannot be overemphasized.

DIRECTIONAL CORONARY ATHERECTOMY

Description

The directional atherectomy catheter is an over-the-wire system that is composed of a housing unit that has a window, 10 mm long on one side and a balloon on the opposite side. The catheter is positioned across the lesion with the window facing the bulk of the plaque. The balloon is inflated at a low pressure so as to anchor the catheter in the desired position and push the housing window firmly against the plaque. A cylindrical cutter inside the housing unit is advanced slowly while it spins at 2500 rpm with the help of a battery-operated motor drive unit. Tissue that is trapped inside the housing will be shaved during this process and will be packed inside a flexible nose cone attached to the distal end of the housing unit. The balloon is then deflated, the catheter is rotated in quadrants where atheromatous disease is appreciated angiographically, and the process is repeated.

Indications and Contraindications[9]

Directional coronary atherectomy can be used in lesions that are crossed with a guidewire in proximal to midsegments of coronary arteries or in saphenous vein grafts. Its best indication is in bulky and discrete lesions in nontortuous segments $\geq$ 2.5 mm in diameter. Ostial left anterior descending artery lesions are quite favorable. Heavily calcified lesions should be avoided, and calcified ostial lesions in particular are contraindicated. Directional atherectomy is not recommended in long lesions, diffuse disease, or very tortuous vessels.

Acute Results and Complications

Because directional atherectomy enlarges the vessel lumen by debulking tissue, it was felt that such a modality of percutaneous revascularization may reduce the incidence of dissections and major complication.

However, analysis of acute results has not demonstrated a significantly reduced incidence of complications. The CAVEAT study,[10] which randomized patients to balloon angioplasty versus directional atherectomy, showed a higher rate of early complications with atherectomy. There were 512 patients randomly assigned to atherectomy and 500 to balloon angioplasty. Atherectomy led to a higher immediate gain in the luminal enlargement but there was a higher rate of in-hospital adverse clinical outcome: myocardial infarction (Q and non-Q) was higher in the atherectomy group (6% vs 3%) as was acute vessel closure (7% vs 3%). Early composite events that included death, emergency CABG, acute myocardial infarction, and abrupt vessel closure during hospitalization, were 11% in the atherectomy group versus 5% in the balloon group (P < 0.001). Popma et al[11] have analyzed the outcome of abrupt vessel closure from the early experience with directional atherectomy. Among 1020 procedures performed, the incidence of acute closure was 4.2%. It occurred before the patient left the cath lab in 34 patients and up to 96 hours after the procedure in the remaining nine patients. The incidence was higher in de novo lesions, diffuse lesions, and lesions in the right coronary arteries and native arteries as compared with vein grafts. In 16 lesions there was initial improvement after balloon angioplasty, but one patient died a few days later. Of the 16 patients without initial improvement after balloon angioplasty, 15 required emergency bypass surgery. The 9 remaining patients were taken immediately to surgery.

There is still some debate regarding how aggressive the operator should be in extracting tissue and reaching a very low residual diameter stenosis. This approach is currently being tested to evaluate its influence on restenosis. Studies to this date have shown no substantial increase in the acute complication rates with larger postprocedural lumen diameters.[12–16] However, further analysis is needed to better understand the ideal method to apply directional atherectomy while reducing the complication rate.

REFERENCES

1. Safian RD, Grines CL, May MA, et al. Clinical and angiographic results of transluminal extraction coronary atherectomy in saphenous vein bypass grafts. *Circulation.* 89(1):302–312, 1994.

2. Popma JJ, Leon MB, Mintz GS, et al. Results of coronary angioplasty using the transluminal extraction catheter. *Am J Cardiol.* 70(20):1526–1532, 1992.

3. Bertrand ME, Lablanche JM, Leroy F, et al. Percutaneous transluminal coronary rotary ablation with Rotablator (European experience). *Am J Cardiol.* 69(5):470–474, 1992.

4. Dietz U, Erbel R, Rupprecht HJ, Weidmann S, Meyer J. High-frequency rotational ablation: an alternative in treating coronary artery stenoses and occlusions. *Br Heart J.* 70(4):327–336, 1993.

5. Teirstein PS, Warth DC, Haq N, et al. High-speed rotational coronary atherectomy for patients with diffuse coronary artery disease [see comments]. *J Am Coll Cardiol.* 18(7): 1694–1701, 1991.

6. Zacca NM, Kleiman NS, Rodriguez AR, et al. Rotational ablation of coronary artery lesions using single, large burrs. *Cathet Cardiovasc Diagn.* 26(2):92–97, 1992.

7. Ellis SG, Popma JJ, Buchbinder M, et al. Relation of clinical presentation, stenosis morphology, and operator technique to the procedural results of rotational atherectomy and rotational atherectomy–facilitated angioplasty. *Circulation.* 89(2):882–892, 1994.

8. Safian RD, Niazi KA, Strzelecki M, et al. Detailed angiographic analysis of high-speed mechanical rotational atherectomy in human coronary arteries. *Circulation.* 88(3):961–968, 1993.

9. Whitlow PL, Franco I. Indications for directional coronary atherectomy: 1993. *Am J Cardiol.* 72(13):21–29E, 1993.

10. Topol EJ, Leya F, Pinkerton CA, et al. A comparison of directional atherectomy with coronary angioplasty in patients with coronary artery disease. The CAVEAT Study Group [see comments]. *N Engl J Med.* 329(4):221–227, 1993.

11. Popma JJ, Topol EJ, Hinohara T, et al. Abrupt vessel closure after directional coronary atherectomy. The US Directional Atherectomy Investigator Group. *J Am Coll Cardiol.* 19(7):1372–1379, 1992.

12. Kuntz RE, Safian RD, Carrozza JP, Fishman RF, Mansour M, Baim DS. The importance of acute luminal diameter in determining restenosis after coronary atherectomy or stenting. *Circulation.* 86(6):1827–1835, 1992.

13. Kuntz RE, Hinohara T, Safian RD, Selmon MR, Simpson JB, Baim DS. Restenosis after directional coronary atherectomy: effects of luminal diameter and deep wall excision. *Circulation.* 86(5):1394–1399, 1992.

14. Kuntz RE, Gibson CM, Nobuyoshi M, Baim DS. Generalized model of restenosis after conventional balloon angioplasty, stenting, and directional atherectomy. *J Am Coll Cardiol.* 21(1):15–25, 1993.

15. Popma JJ, De CNB, Pinkerton CA, et al. Quantitative analysis of factors influencing late lumen loss and restenosis after directional coronary atherectomy. *Am J Cardiol.* 71(7):552–557, 1993.

16. Umans VA, Beatt KJ, Rensing BJ, Hermans WR, de FPJ, Serruys PW. Comparative quantitative angiographic analysis of directional coronary atherectomy and balloon coronary angioplasty. *Am J Cardiol.* 68(17):1556–1563, 1992.

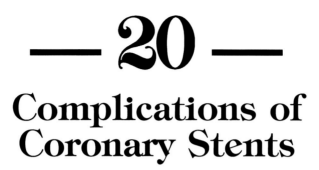

— 20 —

Complications of Coronary Stents

Nowamagbe A. Omoigui, M.D., M.P.H.
Patrick L. Whitlow, M.D.
Stephen G. Ellis, M.D.

HISTORY

As far back as 1912, Alexis Carrel foresaw the future role of arterial stents.[1] In 1964, Charles Dotter proposed intravascular stenting for arterial support. He began implanting tube grafts in peripheral arteries in 1968.

In the late 1970s, Ake Senning developed a double-helix stainless steel alloy spiral device that was successfully tested in the jugular, vena caval, and iliac veins of dogs.[2] Subsequently, Cesare Gianturco and others evaluated less thrombogenic zigzag geometric patterns. Palmaz and associates then developed a balloon-expandable deformable steel stent initially tested in rabbit aortas, followed by limited human testing.[3]

In 1986, Puel, Sigwart, and Serruys implanted the first coronary self-expanding Wallstents.[4] In 1987, Sigwart et al published the European experience with the self-expanding elastic woven wire mesh tube stent (Medivent S.A.) in human coronary and peripheral arteries.[5] These authors recognized the importance of acute angiographic results and suggested 15% stent overexpansion—a concept that has become increasingly appreciated. In the same year, Palmaz et al published results of animal studies suggesting an additive benefit of dextran in limiting stent thrombosis. A Biogold polymer stent coating was subsequently introduced in 1989 to minimize Wallstent thrombogenicity.

The Palmaz balloon-expandable stent is a rigid stainless steel tubular mesh with filaments arrayed in slotted configuration. It deploys as a meshwork of parallelograms. A subsequent design modification by Schatz led to the articulated variant now known as the Palmaz-Schatz stent. Major clinical assessment of the Palmaz-Schatz stent began in 1987, with more than 2000 stents being placed to date in the United States alone.[6]

Problems with an early prototype of the coil stent in 1981 led to its modification in 1985 by Gianturco and Roubin into an incomplete serpentine configuration. The stainless steel device was designed to be commercially wrapped around a deflated balloon, rendering a lower profile than might otherwise be the case with operator assembly. During initial human trials, the stent was used for "bailout" in acute closure. This was extended to "threatened" closure in 1988. FDA approval for the Gianturco-Roubin stent was obtained in 1993.[7]

The Wiktor stent was designed by Dominic Wiktor as a balloon-expandable, single interdigitating 0.125-mm tantalum wire in a sinusoidal helical coil configuration. The idea was to minimize metal-metal and metal-endothelial contact, thus reducing thrombogenicity, while exploiting the radiopacity, biocompatibility, and lack of ferromagnetism of tantalum. Preclinical test results were reported in 1990 and clinical trials began thereafter.[8]

The Strecker stent was designed by Ernst-Peter Strecker as a balloon-expandable tantalum mesh for peripheral vascular use. Because of its knitted design, it retains flexibility when expanded, and has relatively significant recoil and low collapse pressure. It was subsequently introduced to the coronary circulation. Like the Cook stent, it is commercially wrapped around a balloon.[9]

Results of a landmark multicenter study of the Wallstent were published in 1991.[10] High stent thrombosis rates (24%) were ascribed to inadequate and inconsistent anticoagulation, mechanical disadvantages of early prototypes, lack of operator experience, and stent use in thrombotic clinical syndromes. Although the study tempered initial clinical excitement about stents, it identified problems that were to become crucial to the long-term acceptance of stents as a clinical tool, namely, subacute thrombotic closure, bleeding complications, prolonged hospital stay and costs. Concern over early thrombotic complications also overshadowed the reported 13% angiographic in-stent restenosis rate, lower than had hitherto been described with balloon angioplasty. The Wallstent was withdrawn from the market in the fall of 1990.[4]

The search for an ideal stent has led to a variety of other stent designs.[1,11] The Bronco stent (ACS) combines the strengths of the Palmaz-Schatz, Gianturco-Roubin, and Wiktor stents. Temporary stents such as the Heat Activated Recoverable Tissue Support (HARTS) device and the Flow Support Device (ACS, Santa Clara, CA) are being evaluated. Nondegradable and biodegradable polymer matrix systems are also being tested as local drug delivery vehicles.

DESCRIPTION OF THE PROCEDURE

Because the technique of stent placement differs between self-expanding and balloon-expandable stents, general principles will first be described, followed by specific discussion relevant to each stent type and a review of adjunctive pharmacotherapy.

It is important for the operator to understand the uses and abuses of stenting. *When* to intervene is as important as *whether* to intervene.[12] The patient's history, physical examination, and pertinent laboratory data should be synthesized with the coronary angiogram. History of bleeding, risk of bleeding, and social factors such as noncompliance and alcoholism, for example, should be prospectively identified. Considerations that might militate against bypass surgery should also be placed in the balance. Target vessel site and size, myocardial jeopardy score, and relative risk of thrombotic/bleeding complications enter the final decision algorithm. In general, vessels larger than 2.75 mm in diameter offer better benefit-risk ratios for intervention. Vessels supplying low flow demand myocardium and clinical situations associated with preexisting thrombus should be avoided except in the presence of very high diameter flow.

In emergency situations, proximal tortuosity and the ability to visualize the distal end of a dissection are important in determining the risk-benefit ratio of stenting to restore patency.[13] Alternative treatment modalities such as temporary stenting, prolonged inflation at low-pressure with an oversized balloon, and perfusion balloon angioplasty should be considered. If bypass surgery is inevitable, stenting may still be helpful as a bridge to limit ongoing ischemia. However, the potential deleterious effect of subsequent proximal stent thrombosis on nonbypassed side branches should be considered. Metallic stents may also limit adjunctive surgical endarterectomy, or even bypass graft placement.

Adjunctive Pharmacotherapy

Premedication with 325 mg of aspirin is mandatory. Ticlopidine may be considered in aspirin allergic patients and may be superior to aspirin. Additional dipyridamole or sulfinpyrazone is optional. Calcium channel blockers and/or long-acting nitrates may be prescribed. Some centers advocate prophylactic antibiotics (Cefazolin or Vancomycin 1 IV) 1 hour before and 6 to 8 hours afterward. The use of dextran has been challenged, but most investigators agree that if stent placement is certain, 10% dextran-40 infusion should be begun 2 hours before the procedure at 100 to 200 cc/hr for 2 hours, then 15 cc/hr for the next 20 to 24 hours or until aPTT levels are therapeutic after vascular access site sheath removal. It has been advocated that intravenous steroids be administered prophylactically to minimize the risk of allergic reactions to dextran, but reports of late aneurysm formation associated with combinations of steroids and colchicine in stent patients suggest that prudent use of steroids is warranted.[14]

Once vascular access has been established, at least 10000 units of heparin should be given intravenously or intraarterially to achieve an ACT of 425 to 525 seconds throughout the procedure.[15] Intravenous nitroglycerin may be infused continuously for 12 hours after stent delivery.

Equipment selection should always be based on anticipation of problems that can occur at every stage of the procedure. This is particularly important when planning elective interventions with an increased likelihood of acute closure. However, the unpredictability of acute closure mandates such a thought process in nearly all "routine" cases, because expeditious action is often required in the event of complications. Therefore, vascular access sheath size should be adequate for the relevant guiding catheter, and this should in turn be adequate for the appropriate stent diameter. Balloon catheters should be compatible with the guidewire system chosen. Practically speaking, this translates into use of large lumen ($\geq$ 8F) guide catheters, $\geq$ 0.014-in

TABLE 20.1. Design and Deployment of Coronary Stents

Stent	Design	Size Range		Deployment
		Diameter	Length	
Palmaz-Schatz*	Balloon-expandable articulated stainless steel tubular mesh of two 7-mm slots connected by 1-mm bridge mounted on 20 PVC balloon delivered through 5F sheath or stent deployment system	3 to 4 mm	15 mm	large-lumen 8F/9F guide catheter 0.014-in wire; 6 to 8 atm inflation
Peripheral Palmaz-Schatz ('Biliary' stent)*	Balloon-expandable articulated (20-mm) stent expandable to 9-mm diameter. Requires operator crimping. Nonarticulated 10- and 15-mm versions available (Investigational)	4 to 9 mm (note: A 30-mm stent which can be expanded to 18-mm diameter is available for even larger vessels)	10, 15, 20 mm	8F to 9F guide 0.014 to 0.035 in wire; needs peripheral angioplasty balloon > 4.0 mm
Gianturco-Roubin	Balloon-expandable stainless steel coil commercially crimped on 2.5- to 4.5-mm wide, 20-mm long PVC balloon	2 to 4 mm	12* or 20 mm	large lumen 8F/9F guide; 0.018 in extra-support guidewire; 5 to 6 atm inflation
Wiktor*	Balloon-expandable crimped tantalum stent (1.5-mm profile) on 25-mm long PE balloon. Single wire helical design	2.5 to 4.5 mm	14 to 16 mm	8F guide catheter 0.014 in wire 6–8 atm inflation
Strecker*	Knitted Balloon-expandable tantalum mesh commercially wrapped on Slider/Outsider balloon. Silicone end sleeves	3.0 to 4.5 mm	15 and 25 mm	8F/large 7F guide (> 0.072 in) 0.014-in wire; 8 atm inflation for 20 seconds

Key: *Investigational

guidewires, and compatible balloons, in 2.75- to 3.5-mm diameter vessels unless stenting is contraindicated (Table 20.1).

Predilation of the target site as well as approach segments may be necessary, and is particularly important when using the Cook or Strecker stents because of their slightly higher tendency to recoil. This not only enhances subsequent stent deployment, but also identifies noncompliant lesions resistant to dilation. Such lesions are better treated or pretreated with alternative modalities. Predilation for elective stent placement should be 0.5 mm undersized to avoid dissection, except during acute closure when full dilation expedites precise stent placement.

As a result of high profile, 3.0-mm or smaller stents require an 8F guide catheter with an internal diameter of at least 0.079 in, whereas 3.5- and 4.0-mm Cook stents require lumens of at least 0.084- to 0.088-in diameter, which typically implies a large lumen 8F or 9F catheter.[7] A 4-mm Wiktor stent will, however, pass through an 8F guide.[8] Larger stents need larger guiding catheters, in part because they require larger balloons for deployment.[6,9] Although the femoral approach is most common, brachial access to stent deployment with 7F, 8F, and 9F catheters has been described.[16–18] This may become necessary when there is no femoral access, or previous anticoagulation should not be interrupted. Potential advantages include fewer hemorrhagic vascular complications, decreased transfusion requirements, and lower costs. However, patients with small brachial arteries (eg, women) or multiple previous brachial procedures might not be ideal candidates. A radial artery approach using a 6F guiding catheter has also been reported.[19]

Guide catheter support is crucial because of the relative stiffness of the stent-balloon combination, which may be compounded by proximal vessel tortuosity. Distal target sites may, therefore, require deep seating. In general, short-tip left and right Judkins and JCL catheters are adequate for native coronaries, although unusual takeoff angles may necessitate an Amplatz, Hockey stick, or Arani configuration. Multipurpose guides are useful in right coronary saphenous grafts whereas the left Amplatz may be advantageous for left coronary grafts.[13]

An extra-support long wire technique facilitates easy balloon exchange, stent delivery, and stable backup. The 0.018-in ACS extra-support or platinum-plus guidewires are advocated for Strecker and Cook stent deployment, while the coronary Palmaz-Schatz and Wiktor stents are compatible with 0.014-in diameter wires. Newer magnet-based systems may also be used.

Wire placement should be as distal as possible in the target vessel, rather than side branches close to the target site. This allows operator flexibility to deploy additional stents or dilate distally should distal propagation of dissection render it necessary. In addition, the stiffer shaft of the wire is more likely to sit across the lesion, thus straightening out proximal tortuosities, enhancing trackability and deployment.

Stent diameter should be 15% to 20% larger than the diameter of the reference vessel segment.[7,13] It should, however, be noted that expanded stent diameter depends on balloon size and stents may undergo up to 15% to 20% diameter recoil after release. Both the Cook and Strecker stent-balloon systems, for example, should be oversize by 0.5 mm relative to normal vessel diameter because of recoil. Postprocedure residual stenoses were $32 \pm 27\%$ for the Cook, $14 \pm 12\%$ for the Palmaz-Schatz, and $19 \pm 19\%$ for the Wiktor ($p < 0.001$) in a recent study.[20] The Palmaz-Schatz stent appears to be less prone to recoil than either the Cook or Wiktor stents, perhaps because of its slotted-tubular design. The Cook stent is mounted on a balloon with nominal diameter 0.5 mm greater than the nominal stent size. An oversize stent, therefore, implies a markedly oversized balloon, which may in turn cause complications.[21] If it is necessary to deploy a stent distally through a very tortuous vessel, a proximal stent, short or disarticulated stents,[22] and 5F sheath systems like the Teleguide (Schneider) or SDS (Johnson and Johnson) enhance safe delivery, although the last situation is to be avoided as much as possible. Although stents were originally designed for use with over-the-wire systems, monorail catheters have also been used to implant Palmaz-Schatz stents, for example.

The length of the (preferably single) stent should cover the entire dissection-flap in cases of threatened or acute closure. Immediately before balloon inflation, contrast injection helps to ascertain proper positioning. A technique for the simultaneous deployment of two stents on a single long PTCA balloon has been described to minimize overlap, where elective placement of more than one stent is clinically appropriate.[23] Alternatively, disarticulated Palmaz-Schatz stents have been used in situations such as significant vessel tortuosity, need for multiple stents, and risk of major side-branch jeopardy (stent jail).[22,24] If more than one stent is going to be placed, more distal stents should be deployed first except in ostial locations.

The crimped-stent-on-deflated-balloon or commercially available stent-delivery system should be delicately introduced into the Y connector over the guidewire and passed up the guiding catheter. Fluoroscopy is helpful immediately after exiting the Y connector, carefully observing for stent deformation. Before stent-balloon exit from the guide catheter, it is important to ensure that the guide catheter tip is coaxially stable in the coronary ostium. Reengagement of the guide over a prolapsed stent-balloon at its tip risks dislodgment or telescoping. Pushing against resistance at any point is a bad idea.

Intravascular ultrasound-guided stent deployment is feasible, safe, and effective with the Palmaz-Schatz stent, but we have concerns about its use with the Cook and Wiktor stents, having observed both types moved or telescoped by the ultrasound probe. Potential advantages of ultrasonography, however, include accurate reference vessel sizing, stent placement precision, and assessment of adequacy of stent expansion, perhaps even to the point of obviating anticoagulation when stents are "optimally deployed."[25] Angioscopic guidance has also been used.[12,26]

STENT-SPECIFIC TECHNIQUES

Self-Expanding Stents

The Wallstent[4,27] has an unconstrained length of 15 to 30 mm and a fully expanded diameter of 2.5 to 6.0 mm. After predilation, the stent delivery system (outer diameter 1.57 mm) is tracked in an 8F or 9F guiding catheter over a long guidewire to the target site and positioned to cover the entire length of the intended segment. The surrounding constraining membrane around the stent is then pressurized and retracted, resulting in expansion of the stent within the vessel. (The stent shortens during this process). Adjunctive balloon angioplasty can then be performed to optimize stent expansion. It is to be noted that this stent is not commercially available in the United States.

Balloon-Expandable Stents[6,7,8,9]

After predilation and equipment exchange over the guidewire, the stent-balloon with or without a 5F sheath (subselective guide for the coronary Palmaz-Schatz stent) is tracked over wire and placed across the target site. Confirmation of position is carried out with contrast angiography. (Radiopaque stents are helpful in this regard, although radiopacity may interfere with subsequent angiographic assessment after implantation). Stent deployment is then carried out by inflating the balloon 5 to 6 atm for 15 to 60 seconds (after first withdrawing the 5F sheath, if one is used). Full balloon deflation is mandatory, and negative pressure should be applied for up to 60 seconds before the balloon is withdrawn. Before withdrawing the deflated Cook balloon it should be pushed forward slightly. With the Strecker balloon, slight counterclockwise rotation is recommended. Adjunctive balloon angioplasty with a slightly larger (10% to 15%) or high-pressure balloon (1.1 : 1 ratio) to optimally dilate the stented segment may be desirable. Zero percent or less residual stenosis with a smooth lumen is important not only because it is associated with a lower risk of stent thrombosis[13,28] but also because it reduces the probability that late loss will cross the threshold of restenosis.

SUBSEQUENT MANAGEMENT

Sheaths are removed on the same day unless otherwise indicated. To do this, heparin is reduced or withheld until ACT falls to 160 seconds. Firm and prolonged access site digital, Femostop, or C-clamp compression is performed to establish stable hemostasis. Two to six hours later, Heparin infusion is restarted without rebolus. Dextran infusion is maintained until aPTT is therapeutic between 50 and 70 seconds. (An inadequate result may require a higher range). Coumadin is started on the evening of the procedure and adjusted to achieve a PT of 17 to 20 seconds (INR 2.5 to 4.0), although aggressive anticoagulation is probably less necessary when stent deployment and expansion is optimal in larger vessels.[25] Once the PT reaches 17 seconds (INR 2.5), heparin may be stopped. Some investigators advocate that no "loading" dose of Coumadin be given in order to avoid paradoxical protein-C suppression with enhanced thrombosis.[29] Because prothrombin fragments F 1 + 2 assay appears to be a good predictor of anticoagulant efficacy and stent occlusion,[30] it may be preferable to PT assessment in centers that are equipped to perform it expeditiously. This viewpoint has, however, been challenged recently.[31,32] Additional medications advocated by others include H_2-receptor blockers and stool softeners.

Experience over the last few years has emphasized the role of slow mobilization in reducing the incidence of femoral access site bleeding complications.[33] It is currently recommended that patients lie flat until at least 12 hours after sheaths are removed. A 30-degree head elevation and careful upper body turning is then permitted, but bed rest is mandatory. After 36 hours, the patient may sit up in bed. On day 3, the patient is allowed commode privileges and may be out of bed to chair with limited ambulation within the room. Full mobilization is permitted on day 4.

If the brachial approach is used, the sheath can be removed immediately or up to 2 hours after the procedure and the artery can be repaired.[16,17] Intravenous heparin is continued without interruption and Coumadin is initiated to achieve a therapeutic PT or INR. The patient can be ambulatory 6 to 8 hours after coronary intervention. If warfarin is initiated several days before admission, target INR can be achieved quickly and the patient discharged within 2 to 3 days.[18]

After discharge, aspirin is continued indefinitely. Coumadin is maintained for six to twelve weeks at INR 2.5 to 4.0. During this period it is anticipated that endothelialization of the stent surface would have occurred.[34–36] Coronary vasodilators may be continued for six weeks. Some centers advocate prophylactic antibiotics before nonsterile surgery in the 8- to 12-week period after stenting. Data to support or refute this practice are lacking.

TABLE 20.2.   Suggested Indications for Stenting of De Novo Lesions to Prevent Restenosis

Definite
  none
Probable
  Focal LAD or saphenous vein graft lesions in arteries ≧ 3.0 mm
Possible
  Focal LCX or RCA lesions in arteries ≧ 3.0 mm
  Focal LAD or saphenous vein graft disease in arteries 2.6 to 2.9 mm
Definitely not
  Lesions requiring placement of multiple overlapping stents
  Lesions in arteries ≦ 2.5 mm
  Lesions for which closure would be imminently life threatening (eg, unprotected left main
    disease)
  Patients at heightened risk of bleeding

    Abbreviations: LAD = left anterior descending artery; LCX = left circumflex artery;
                 RCA = right coronary artery

Adapted from reference (6). Reproduced with permission.

INDICATIONS

Indications for coronary stenting are evolving because short- and long-term safety, efficacy, and cost data are still being collected and evaluated. Randomized trials comparing coronary devices singly or in combination are ongoing. Results of the "**St**ent **Res**tenosis **S**tudy" (STRESS) and **BE**lgium and **NE**therlands **STENT** (BENESTENT) trial for example, have only recently been reported.[37,38] The **G**ianturco-**R**oubin Stent **A**cute **C**losure **E**valuation (GRACE) trial has recently begun. Adequacy and completeness of data vary between stent designs and sizes. In the United States, only the Cook stent is FDA approved for acute or threatened closure.

    With possible exception of abrupt closure, all apparent "indications" for coronary stenting are "potential indications."[6,39] They include "threatened closure" after complicated PTCA, adjunctive treatment of suboptimal PTCA results, primary prevention of restenosis in de novo lesions, and secondary prevention of restenosis in previously restenotic lesions (Tables 20.2 and 20.3). Special investigational use of large peripheral stents (for example, Biliary stents) in large coronary vessels or grafts constitutes another area of potential utility.[40]

CONTRAINDICATIONS

In general, vessels less than 2.75 mm in diameter should be avoided. Vessels with poor runoff and target sites with significant clot load are also unsuitable for stent deployment. Inability to visualize the distal end of a dissection with absence of anterograde flow and disappearance of angiographic landmarks demands extensive operator experience for successful stent implantation. Other contraindications include a

TABLE 20.3. Suggested Indications for Elective Stenting of Restenotic Lesions to Prevent Restenosis

Definite
None
Probable
Poor initial PTCA result not amenable to treatment with other new devices with lesser risk of bleeding than stents, artery $\geq$ 3.0 mm
Recurrent restenosis in an artery of major importance, artery $\geq$ 3.0 mm
Possible
Any restenosis in artery $\geq$ 3.0 mm
Poor initial PTCA result not amenable to treatment with other new devices with lesser risk of bleeding than stents, artery 2.6 to 2.9 mm
Definitely not
Lesions requiring placement of multiple overlapping stents
Lesions in arteries $\leq$ 2.5 mm
Lesions for which closure would be imminently life threatening (eg, unprotected left main disease)
Patients at heightened risk of bleeding

Abbreviation: PTCA—Percutaneous Transluminal Coronary Angioplasty

Adapted from reference (6). Reproduced with permission.

high risk of bleeding complications and unprotected left main stenosis. Lesions requiring multiple overlapping stents constitute a relative contraindication.

PREVENTION AND TREATMENT OF COMPLICATIONS OF CORONARY STENTING

Complications are more likely in an emergency setting (see Tables 20.4, 20.5, 20.6, and 20.7). Some are common to all percutaneous coronary interventions (eg, arterial trauma, infections, and restenosis), and others are peculiar to stents. They include stent damage (''shortening,'' ''angulation,'' ''unwinding,'' or ''elongation''), failure to deploy, inadvertent deployment, embolization, side-branch occlusion (or stent ''jail''), acute and subacute thrombosis (resulting in myocardial infarction, emergency CABG, or death), coronary bridging and spasm, late coronary aneurysm, and hemorrhagic complications. Dressler's syndrome has also been documented. Complications specific to adjunctive therapies such as dextran-40 include anaphylactoid reactions and ARDS.

Peripheral Vascular Complications

These include hematoma, pseudoaneurysm, arteriovenous fistula, embolization, ischemia, and femoral neuralgia (Table 20.8). Advanced age, female sex, small vessel size, peripheral vascular disease, sheaths larger than 8F, and the periprocedural use

TABLE 20.4. Reported Incidence of Selected Complications of Coronary Stenting (Note: Stent-stent comparisons are not appropriate because of differences in patient selection. Subacute thrombosis in vein grafts may generally be lower than in native vessels)

Complication	Frequency Reported			
	GR	PS	S	W
Clinical setting: Suboptimal PTCA result/acute closure				
Overall Peripheral Vascular (requiring surgery/transfusion)	11.5%	5% to 18%	12%	12%
Groin hematoma	3.5%	3.5%		6.8%
Pseudoaneurysm	3% to 7%	4.7%		3.4%
AVF		1.3%		
Limb Ischemia		0%		
Major bleeding (requiring transfusion or surgery)	14.1%	11.1%	>10%	8.6%
Stent embolization		1.8%		
Subacute Stent Thrombosis	7.7% to 8.6%	5% to 8%	19%	7.6%
emerg. CABS	6.4%	2.6%		10%
Death	2.0%	0.5%	9.4%	5.2%
Restenosis	31% to 52.6%	30%	>22%	30%
Acute MI	3.5%	2.2% to 20%		4.8%

KEY: GR = Gianturco-Roubin; PS = Palmaz-Schatz; S = Strecker; W = Wiktor

References: (21) (6, 7, 8, 9) (50) (72) (73) (45)

of heparin or thrombolytics are associated with these complications in the general angioplasty population. Femoral access sites are more likely to bleed whereas brachial access sites are more likely to have ischemic complications. Because adjunctive antico-agulation is routinely administered during and after stenting, thromboembolic isch-emic complications are much less likely.

Prevention

Prospectively identify patients at risk.[41–45] Single wall vascular access technique, care-fully avoiding high or low entry or tangential penetration, is important. Use the small-est sheath and guide-catheter possible for safe stent delivery. Clean guidewires and flush catheters frequently to prevent thrombosis. Carefully titrate anticoagulation to

TABLE 20.5. Metanalysis of Five Bailout Stent Prototypes in 464 Patients (1986–1991):

In-hospital complications (mean):
Bypass Surgery	8.4%
Acute MI	10.6%
Death	4.1%

Reference: (12)

TABLE 20.6. Reported Incidence of Selected Complications of Coronary Stenting (Note: Stent-stent comparisons are not appropriate because of differences in patient selection.

Complication	Frequency Reported			
	GR	PS	S	W
Clinical setting: Elective placement for restenosis				
Overall Peripheral Vascular		2.5%	1.8%	7%
Groin hematoma				5.8%
Pseudoaneurysm				3.2%
AVF				
Limb Ischemia		0%		
Major bleeding (requiring transfusion or surgery)	12.1%	11.1%		22%
Subacute Stent Thrombosis		3.4%		8.7%
emerg. CABS	1.6%	1.7%		4.5%
Death	2.0%	0.6%		0.8%
Restenosis		29.3%		19.5%
Acute MI	0.4%	2.3%		4.5%

KEY: GR = Gianturco-Roubin; PS = Palmaz-Schatz; S = Strecker; W = Wiktor

References: (74) (8) (75) (6) (9) (7)

minimum need. Adequate sedation and proper immobilization, stool softeners, and antitussives are helpful. If narcotic analgesics are used, antiemetics may be helpful. Extra caution with women, the elderly, and patients with either a previous disposition to bleeding or exposure to multiple catheterizations is necessary. Consideration to bleeding or exposure to multiple catheterizations is necessary. Consideration should be given at the outset to alternative access sites (brachial or radial). Adequate direct compression of the puncture site after same-day ACT-guided sheath removal should be performed.[42] A good rule of thumb is to extend compression for at least 50% longer than with routine angioplasty cases. However, excessive compression can cause thrombosis. Pressure dressings should be used subsequently. Although the use of Vasoseal collagen plugs results in less variable anticoagulation after sheath removal, it does not reduce entry-site related bleeding complications.[46,47] The Kensey-Nash and Perclose systems are also being evaluated. Gradual ambulation after femoral sheath removal, however, is vital in reducing complications.[33] Brachial access also limits bleeding complications.

Treatment

Early identification is helpful (Table 4). Prolonged clinically guided direct puncture site compression, volume expansion with crystalloid or blood, and patient immobilization are important initial steps. Consider reversing (or decreasing) anticoagulation. Obtain ultrasound for diagnostic clarification and possible ultrasound-guided compression. Consider blood transfusion and vascular surgery as indicated. Biodegrad-

TABLE 20.7.   Reported Incidence of Selected Complications of Coronary Stenting

Complication	Frequency Reported	
	Stress	Benestent
Clinical setting: Elective stent for de novo disease in vessels > 3 mm diameter		
Overall Peripheral Vascular	7% (4% surg)	14% (9% surg)
Groin hematoma	NA	6.2%
Pseudoaneurysm	2.44%	5.4%
AVF	0.97%	0.15%
Limb Ischemia	NA	NA
Major bleeding (requiring surgery or transfusion)	7.3%	15%
Subacute Stent Thrombosis	1.9%	NA
emerg. CABS	1.5%	1.6%
Death	0%	0%
Restenosis	29%	18%
Acute MI	1.0%	0.8%

KEY:
STRESS—USA/Canadian/Japanese Stent Restenosis Study with Palmaz-Schatz stent for de novo disease (37) (76)

BENESTENT—European-based (Belgium/Netherlands) multicenter study of Palmaz-Schatz stent for de novo disease (38) (76)

Note: In a nonrandomized Palmaz-Schatz study at 19 sites (n = 1141) in the United States and Germany, the distribution of complications was as follows:

	In-hospital	6 months	12 months
Transfusions	6%	8%	11%
Vascular Surgery	5%	8%	10%
Neither	90%	86%	82%

Ref: (76)

able collagen has been percutaneously introduced into pseudoaneurysms to induce thrombosis, and spring coils have been used to close AV fistulae using an intraarterial delivery system.[48]

Stent Damage

Prevention

Caution should be exercised while crimping the stent onto the deflated balloon (if manual), and transit through Y-adapter should be gentle (special sheath may be provided). Avoid pushing against resistance. Observe the stent at least once as it

TABLE 20.8. Key Features in the Diagnosis and Management of Peripheral Vascular Complications (PVC)

	Diagnosis	Management
Hematoma	Physical Exam: anteroposterior pulsation bruit (nonspecific) CT Scan Pelvis	Volume resuscitation Surgical exploration
Pseudoaneurysm (30% to 60% of PVC)	Physical Exam: radially pulsatile expansion bruit (nonspecific) Color-flow duplex scan	Ultrasound-guided direct com- pression with effective analgesia Conservative follow-up if asymp- tomatic, < 3-cm diameter with- out serial expansion. Repeat ultrasound at one week and as indicated until thrombosis or sur- gery. Consider injected collagen (investigational).
Arteriovenous Fistula (AVF) (5% to 30% of PVC)	Physical Exam: continuous bruit palpable thrill Duplex scan Angiography	Surgical repair (spontaneous resolu- tion has been reported) Ultrasound-guided pressure Coil embolization?
Femoral Neuralgia	Physical Exam: Hematoma Pseudoaneurysm AVF Thigh hyperesthesia Psoas spasm CT Pelvis	Surgical treatment of associated vascular complication Nonsteroidal drugs Tricyclic antidepressants Femoral nerve block Morphine Physical rehabilitation
Limb Ischemia	Physical Exam: pulse loss pallor paralysis paresthesia motor loss (late) Doppler Angiography (may cause delay)	Remove sheath/anticoagulate Upper Limb: resection/anastomosis vein patch angioplasty Lower Limb: embolectomy thrombectomy repair vein patch angioplasty fasciotomy

transits within the guide catheter (radiopaque stents are helpful). Ensure that the guide catheter is well seated and guide support is adequate before exiting guide-tip. Intracoronary "shortening" and "elongation" of the Wiktor stent have been described in detail by Vogt.[49] Shortening can be caused by use of excessive force in response to lack of trackability. Elongation tends to result from balloon-stent impaction during adjunctive balloon angioplasty with a noncompliant balloon. Further inflations should probably be performed with the compliant prime balloon left in place, rather than another balloon.

Treatment

If there is stent damage, and migration on the balloon or herniation between guide-tip and coronary ostium is suspected, withdraw guide/balloon/stent as *one unit* back to groin, but keep coronary wire across lesion if possible. Do not try to withdraw stent *into* the guide catheter. The Palmaz-Schatz stent will tend to shear off the balloon, and the Cook and Wiktor stents may "accordion."

Failure to Deploy

Prevention

Ensure compatibility of stent profile, sheath size, guiding catheter size and shape, and appropriate guidewire for trackability in the context of proximal vessel tortuosity. Adequately predilate the lesion and approach segments. Exclude arterial damage by proper visualization of target vessel. Exclude locking of coronary Palmaz-Schatz stent inside SDS marker. Consider shorter, disarticulated, or more flexible stent (Wiktor or Strecker) in tortuous segments.[50]

Treatment

Stent retrieval. Reevaluate all factors under "prevention" and remedy. Consider bypass surgery.

Inaccurate Deployment (or proximal shift after initial deployment)

Prevention

Meticulous attention to detail is required when stenting ostial lesions in particular. Deploy ostial stent first and cine the stent after delivery when delivering more than one. Use balloon-expandable, radiopaque stents when possible. A double-marker balloon may be useful with some stents.[51] Always recheck location with contrast angiography before final deployment. Because of stent shortening with expansion, anticipate the final stent position relative to target lesion before inflating and ensure adequate initial inflation. Always withdraw *deflated* balloon under negative pressure with a slight twist after initial stent expansion. When using the Cook or PS stent, push deflated balloon forward slightly before withdrawing.

Treatment

For catheter-based retrieval (depending on location—see the following), consider full stent expansion with adjunct PTCA if fully deployed. If coil stent is unwound, with parts of it protruding into left main coronary artery, consider bypass surgery after placement of balloon pump for support. Surgical retrieval may be performed under direct vision. Protruding stents have been retrieved from vein grafts using catheter-based techniques, but such manipulation in the left main coronary artery may not be wise.

Balloon Rupture (leaving an unexpanded or partially expanded stent in situ)

Prevention

Avoid balloon damage when crimping stent unto it. Avoid stenting lesions resistant to predilation, eg, heavily calcified lesions with "spicules." Consider preliminary debulking. Do not deploy or expand stent with balloon that is substantially oversize (>120%). Before passing crimped stent-balloon into Y-adapter (with insufflator in "neutral" position) and before inflation at the target site, apply negative pressure to balloon to confirm integrity. Note: Rupture of an inflated balloon within a stent can cause substantial coronary trauma, including perforation.

Treatment

Stent retrieval or expansion using probing catheter/wire technique[52] or snare (see preconditions following). Do not pull back ruptured balloon until a plan is in place for stent retrieval or definitive expansion. If balloon is entrapped, give intracoronary vasodilators, pass a second guidewire, and attempt release by inflation at the site with another balloon or retrieve with a snare. If balloon is still entrapped (and stent is deployed), consider surgery.

Stent Migration/Embolization

This has been reported in 2% to 3% of PS implants and up to 8% with other stents.[41]

Prevention

Details of technique are crucial. Do not undersize stent (or balloon) relative to vessel. Pay attention to markers. Some authors advocate creating a "dumbbell" effect when crimping PS stent by inflating balloon to 1 atm while holding crimped stent tightly to prevent expansion.[53] Do not force against resistance. Consider sheathed method of delivery or commercially wrapped stent-balloon system. When tracking stent-balloon over coronary guidewire in the coronary tree, pay particular attention to angulated bifurcations with a branch "ledge" on which the stent can be caught and deformed with resultant migration over the balloon. The risk of this is high with a deep-seated guide-tip in patients with short left main trunks. If retrieval of an undeployed stent (within the coronaries) into the guiding catheter is contemplated, caution must also be exercised to prevent the guide-tip from scraping the stent off the balloon by pulling out the guide-balloon-stent in one piece.

Treatment

Snare retrieval (see the following section). If stent is semideployed, consider fixing it by further inflations with larger balloon, followed by appropriate treatment as needed, eg, bypass surgery or prolonged anticoagulation.

Distal Embolization of Thrombus

Prevention

A self-expanding stent without adjunct PTCA may limit the risk.[4] With balloon-expandable systems, select target vessels carefully, eg, avoid degenerate vein grafts. Consider adjunctive thrombolytic therapy or extraction atherectomy before deployment if clot presence is suspected.

Treatment

Intracoronary thrombolysis, balloon angioplasty, or anticoagulation.

Thrombosis

Prevention

Comprehensive adjunctive poly-pharmacotherapy including pre-treatment (see preceding text).[54] Hirudin and c7E3 may become useful adjuncts in the near future.[55] Avoid vessel segments with prestent thrombus or co-treat with thrombolytics. Avoid stent-to-artery ratio < 0.95, vessels less than 3.0 mm diameter, and those with poor distal runoff. Cover dissection completely with stent. Optimal stent expansion can be achieved by postdeployment, high-pressure inflation (16 to 20 atm) with a short balloon followed by confirmation with intravascular ultrasound. Target sites with adjacent aneurysmal segments may pose risks. Avoid underanticoagulation after stent placement, particularly if expansion is suboptimal. Consider using rapid turn-around assays to guide anticoagulant therapy. If patient is aspirin allergic, consider ticlopidine, recognizing that up to 5 days of pretreatment may be necessary for full effect. (Ticlopidine may become more widely used in the future as a primary adjunctive agent.)[56] It is very important to avoid any significant bleeding complication because this tends to require discontinuing anticoagulation which in turn increases the risk of thrombosis. Try to defer elective noncardiac surgery during the 1st month. Better stent materials (or adjunctive endothelial seeding) may become available in the future.[57]

Treatment

Thrombolysis (intracoronary or systemic),[58] direct PTCA[59] or bypass surgery. One useful pearl when attempting to recross an acutely thrombosed stent with a guidewire is to loop the wire when pushing through the clot. This minimizes the risk of "digging" under stent struts. Although some authors advocate the Magnum wire in this situation, we do not recommend it.

Side-Branch Occlusion

This is an infrequent complication that tends to occur when there is baseline branch ostial disease or the branch is compromised by predilation. Long-term patency of side branches is generally well maintained.[60]

Prevention

Avoid stenting across large lesion-related side branches, particularly if they have > 50% ostial disease. However, even if they are free of disease it is important to consider the potential problem of access to the side branch in the event of future distal branch disease (stent-jail). Consider coil stent design because it may be easier to wire and dilate through. Another option is a divided or disarticulated stent.[61]

Treatment

Medical therapy (including short-term anticoagulation) for small branch occlusion. Consider angioplasty/thrombolytic therapy for larger branches and surgery if both the main trunk and its branch are stenosed.

Coronary Spasm

This should be distinguished from residual stenosis and coronary bridging, or "milking."[2]

Prevention

Calcium channel blockers, magnesium, or long acting nitrates. Previous identification of patients at risk for this complication aids in selective use of these agents, eg, in patients with Prinzmetal's angina.

Treatment

Systemic or intracoronary nitrates, calcium channel blockers, oral or intravenous magnesium, intracoronary papaverine, and PTCA (with or without an inflated balloon).

Late Coronary Aneurysm

Prevention

This complication was reported in the setting of adjunctive steroid and colchicine therapy to prevent restenosis.[14] It therefore seems prudent to avoid these drugs unless absolutely necessary.

Treatment

Consider long-term anticoagulation to prevent subsequent thrombosis or distal embolization. Any decision regarding surgical management will depend on the specifics of the individual case.

Infection

Prevention

Standard sterile technique. Consider prophylactic antibiotics (Vancomycin or Cefazoline) particularly when reusing an access site that has recently been punctured (eg, within a week). Minimize hematomas, repeat puncture and prolonged sheath retention.[41] The use of removable stents or alternative modalities of treatment for vessel closure may reduce the risk of intracardiac infection.

Treatment

Consider stent site, vascular access site and occult retroperitoneal collections during fever workup. Antibiotic therapy is based on principles for treating endocarditis (4- to 6-week course for "endothelial" infection) or skin flora in groin abscesses. Consider surgical removal (with or without bypass surgery) or evacuation with vascular reconstruction in the periphery.

Restenosis

Prevention

Complete stent expansion in a large-vessel, zero-residual stenosis or better with smooth and uniform luminal edge. Excessive oversizing, however, is not advisable.[62] Ultrasound guidance may be useful. Do not leave residual stenoses or dissection flaps immediately proximal or distal to the stent. Use a balloon of shorter length than the stent for further expansion (if needed) to avoid traumatizing adjacent unstented segments. Avoid multiple *overlapping* stents as much as possible.[63] One approach that minimizes overlap is to simultaneously deploy two stents on a long angioplasty balloon.[23] Be aware that diabetes, previously treated vessel sites, total occlusions, and ostial and left anterior descending stenoses may be associated with increased risk. When stents are used in a bailout setting, restenosis may also be more likely.

Treatment

Medical therapy for mild cases. Redilation if clinically indicated (objective evidence of myocardial ischemia or angina).[64] In the multicenter Palmaz-Schatz experience, such redilation was universally successful, with a 50% rerestenosis rate at 6 months.[65] Redilation in the Wiktor stent resulted in 25% to 34% restenosis, and a third angioplasty resulted in 39% to 40% restenosis. Atherectomy may not be advisable because of the risk of cutting stent struts, but has been successfully performed.[66] Although data are lacking, most operators do not reanticoagulate if redilation is > 3 months after initial stent deployment. If stent lumen surface looks irregular, seriously consider reanticoagulation. Bypass surgery may be required. Future stents may offer better coating and articulation.[1]

STENT RETRIEVAL

It is important to appreciate the vascular and clinical significance of an errant stent when deciding whether, when, and how to retrieve it from the coronary, cerebral, or peripheral circulations. Stents have been left in situ, particularly when they embolize

TABLE 20.9. Potentially Useful Devices for the Retrieval of Stents

Snare Loops
  Commercially available (Cook Co., Microvena Corp)
Guidewires
  Custom-made into single- and double-wire systems
Baskets
  Dormia stone basket
  Dotter retrieval device
  MediTech multipurpose basket
Forceps
  MediTech Biliary Forceps
Fogarty Balloon Catheter
Bioptome

Adapted from reference (69)

into small branch vessels in the periphery, cause no associated symptoms, threaten no vital organs, and are relatively nonradiopaque, thus presenting a technical challenge that exceeds the utility of retrieval and risks complications. In the coronary bed, the risks of retrieval (endothelial damage/vessel perforation/cerebrosystemic embolization) should be balanced against those of leaving it in situ (thrombosis/vessel occlusion, perforation, arrhythmias, infection, and medicolegal ramifications—*res ipsa loquitor*). It is preferable for the coronary segment over which retrieval is planned to be relatively short and straight. It is also important to ascertain that some stent struts are not buried in the vessel wall. Anticoagulation should be complete and intracoronary nitroglycerin or verapamil administered to minimize spasm. If retrieval is not possible (or too dangerous), full expansion should be attempted. Surgical consultation is advisable.

A number of tools have been used to retrieve intravascular objects in general and stents in particular (Table 20.9). The relevance of each tool varies with operator experience, the location of the stent, and whether it sits astride a guidewire.[67,68] If the stent is within the aorta, baskets and forceps may come in handy. For intracoronary retrieval, snare loop systems are preferable. However, errant stents in this situation are typically seated over the previously deployed guidewire (unless it has been pulled out). Therefore, retrieval usually involves the use of a balloon to splint the stent (without fully expanding it), following which both balloon and stent are withdrawn to the tip of the guiding catheter and the entire assembly extricated intact back to the groin (or brachial) access site.

It is feasible to use the same balloon over which stent deployment had been intended, but loss of low profile, rupture, and loss of trackability (or location of the stent distally) may mandate the use of a new (smaller) balloon that can be advanced (deflated with negative pressure) either until it sits across the stent or is actually beyond it (Fogarty technique). The balloon is then inflated to entrap the stent before withdrawal. This minimizes the risk of cerebral or systemic embolization during retreat but can result in endothelial damage. If possible, the coronary guidewire should be left in the coronary circulation, but this is not always feasible. Once in the iliac tree, it is crucial to ensure that the coronary guidewire is safely positioned as far forward distally as possible to give the stent-balloon complex a reliable saddle on which to sit as efforts are made to retrieve them intact through (or with) the sheath. The balloon catheter can be withdrawn after deflation, and a multipurpose basket or Biliary forceps introduced into the guide catheter to snare the distal coronary wire, thus preventing stent embolization. Alternatively, the guide catheter is withdrawn and the selected retrieval device passed through the sheath beside the coronary wire.

Biliary forceps can retrieve the stent, leaving the coronary wire in place if the wire is not caught and stent geometry is relatively preserved. Because the nitinol gooseneck snare, the Biliary forceps, and multipurpose basket have a diameter range of 0.052 to 0.064 in and are compatible with 8F guiding catheters, a cutdown is rarely necessary to avoid vascular damage as the entire unit is removed through the femoral sheath, unless stent deformation is severe. Even a 7F guide will accommodate them as long as the deployment balloon has been removed—a useful tip for stent retrieval through the brachial artery.[68] Repeat diagnostic angiography of the coronaries is recommended to exclude the possibility of coronary trauma resulting from the maneuver.

If coronary guidewire position has been lost, either a regular prolapsing guidewire or a snare loop can be tried. The 4F nitinol gooseneck snare with 15-mm loop diameter and 120-cm length (Microvena Corp, MN) has the advantage of a 90-degree angulation to the catheter and high tensile strength. Snare loops can also be custom made. An exchange-length guidewire is doubled over, or a knot is tied 1 in from the distal end of a single standard wire, or the flexible ends of two guidewires are tied together. The loop is passed through a probing catheter after putting a subtle (30-degree) bend on it.[69] The probing catheter is advanced through the guiding catheter until near-contact with the stent. An attempt should be made to pass the wire *through* the stent rather than *beside* it. The loop is then evaginated like a lasso to entrap the stent before withdrawal as one unit. (The Wiktor stent can simply be grasped and its single helical coil unwrapped). If the wire is completely *within* the stent tunnel, one option is to track up a balloon and proceed as discussed previously, particularly if the deformed stent is too big to be retracted into the guide catheter using the wire loop.

If the stent is relatively distal or vessel tortuosity is significant, and retrieval still has a favorable benefit-risk profile, a double wire approach may be used. In this case, two independent guidewires (introduced through a single Y-connector) are positioned beyond the stent (one through the stent and the other beside it). The proximal ends of both wires are then passed through a single torque tool and firmly clamped together. A propagating double helix is created by rotating the tool continuously until both wires wrap and thus entrap the stent. In a recent report, such a technique was unsuccessful in one of two patients because the force needed to pull back the trapped stent was thought to be excessive (risking perforation), thus necessitating bypass surgery and open retrieval.[70] A variant of this technique is the placement of a looped guidewire coaxial to the original guidewire, and manipulation of the guidewire through the snare, followed by retrieval of the stent over the original guidewire by pulling tight on the snare.

Because they are stiff, basket devices can potentially perforate the coronaries and may require cutdown for access. An outer layer of steerable wires in parallel helps to move an inner cone that slides in and out of a coronary catheter. The basket is deployed distal to the stent, opened, and then pulled back until the stent is entrapped and "locked" within it, after which the entire apparatus is withdrawn. Alligator jaw forceps are even more rigid and difficult to use around bends. However, as described previously, Medi-Tech Biliary forceps (closed diameter 1.6 mm, opened diameter 25 mm, length 120 cm) have been used to retrieve fragments and stents from large nontortuous coronary vessels and vein grafts, particularly when the proximal end of the stent protrudes into the aorta. Although a 6F bioptome has been advanced through the femoral sheath to capture a deformed stent at the tip of the sheath after removal of the guiding catheter, balloon, and guidewire, it is important to recognize the danger of stent fragmentation with this instrument.[71] In the future, angioscopic guidance may become a useful tool for extracting embolized fragments. As a rule of thumb, full systemic anticoagulation and consultation with an interventional radiologist or vascular surgeon are important when contemplating stent retrieval from the cerebral or systemic circulations.

REFERENCES

1. Sigwart U. An overview of intravascular stents: old and new. In: Topol E, ed. Textbook of Interventional Cardiology. W.B. Saunders Co., Philadelphia, PA 803–815, 1994.

2. Alfonso F, Macaya C, Iniguez A, et al. "Milking" of the left anterior descending coronary artery after stenting. Am J Cardiol. 67:1438–1440, 1991.

3. Palmaz JC, Sibbitt RR, Tio FO, et al. Expandable intraluminal vascular graft: a feasibility study. Surgery. 99:199–205, 1986.

4. Strauss B, Serruys P. The coronary wallstent. In: Topol E, ed. Textbook of Interventional Cardiology. W.B. Saunders Co., Philadelphia, PA 687–701, 1994.

5. Sigwart U, Puel J, Mirkovitch V, Joffre F, Kappenberger L. Intravascular stents to prevent occlusion and restenosis after transluminal angioplasty. N Engl J Med. 316:701–706, 1987.

6. Ellis S. The Palmaz-Schatz stent: clinical applications. In: Topol E, ed. Textbook of Interventional Cardiology. W.B. Saunders Co., Philadelphia, PA 1994:702–711.

7. Cannon A, Roubin G. The Gianturco-Roubin stent. In: Topol E, ed. Textbook of Interventional Cardiology. W.B. Saunders Co., Philadelphia, PA 1994:712–726.

8. Whitlow P, de Jaegere P, Serruys P. The Wiktor stent. In: Topol E, ed. Textbook of Interventional Cardiology. W.B. Saunders Co., Philadelphia, PA 1994:727–741.

9. Hamm C. The Strecker stent. In: Topol E, ed. Textbook of Interventional Cardiology. 1994:742–753.

10. Serruys PW, Strauss BH, Beatt KJ, et al. Angiographic follow-up after placement of a self-expanding coronary-artery stent. N Engl J Med. 324:13–17, 1991.

11. Chapman GD, Gammon RS, Bauman RP, Stack RS. Intravascular stents. Trends Cardiovasc Med. 1:127–131, 1991.

12. Serruys P, Keane D. The bailout stent: is a friend in need always a friend indeed? Circulation. 88(5, part 1):2455–2457, 1993.

13. Hirshfield J, Herrmann H. Stent deployment: technical considerations. In: Hirshfield JaH HC, eds. Clinical Use of the Palmaz-Schatz Intracoronary Stent. Futura Publishing Co., Inc., NY 1993:23–42.

14. Rab ST, King SBI, Roubin GS, Carlin S, Hearn JA, Douglas JSJ. Coronary aneurysms after stent placement: a suggestion of altered vessel wall healing in the presence of anti-inflammatory agents. J Am Coll Cardiol. 18:1524–1528, 1991.

15. Hillegass W, Narins C, Brott B, et al. Activated clotting time predicts bleeding complications from angioplasty. *J Am Coll Cardiol.*   184A, 1994.

16. Jenny DB, Robert GP, Fajadet JC, Cassagneau BG, Marco J. Intracoronary stent implantation: new approach using a monorail system and new large-lumen 7F catheters from the brachial route. *Cathet Cardiovasc Diagn.* 25:297–299, 1992.

17. Heuser RR, Mehta SS, Strumpf RK, Ponder R. Intracoronary stent implantation via the brachial approach: a technique to reduce vascular bleeding complications. *Cathet Cardiovasc Diagn.* 25:300–303, 1992.

18. Rosenschein R, Ellis SG. Preprocedure warfarinization and brachial approach for elective coronary stent placement—a possible strategy to decrease cost and duration of hospitalization. *Cathet Cardiovasc Diagn.* 25:290–292, 1992.

19. Kiemeneij G, Laarman G. Percutaneous transradial artery approach for coronary stent implantation. *Cathet Cardiovasc. Diagn.* 30:173–178, 1993.

20. Maclsaac A, Ellis S, Muller D, Topol E, Whitlow P. Comparison of three coronary stents: clinical and angiographic outcome after elective placement in 134 consecutive patients. *Cathet Cardiovasc. Diagn.* 1994 (in press).

21. Roubin GS, Cannon AD, Agrawal SK, et al. Intracoronary stenting for acute and threatened closure complicating percutaneous transluminal coronary angioplasty. *Circulation.* 85:916–927, 1992.

22. Colombo AN, Hall P, Thomas J, Almagor Y, Finci L. Initial experience with the disarticulated (one-half) Palmaz-Schatz stent: a technical report. *Cathet Cardiovasc Diagn.* 25:304–308, 1992.

23. Nordrehaug J, Priestley K, Rickards A, Buller N, Sigwart U. Simultaneous implantation of two Palmaz-Schatz stents mounted on a long angioplasty balloon. *J Interven Cardiol.* 6:223–225, 1993.

24. Colombo A, Goldberg S, Almagor Y, Maiello L, Finci L. A novel strategy for stent deployment in the treatment of acute or threatened closure complicating balloon coronary angioplasty. *JACC.* 22:1887–1891, 1993.

25. Colombo A, Hall P, Almagor Y, et al. Results of intravascular ultrasound guided coronary stenting without subsequent anticoagulation. *J Am Coll Cardiol.* 335A, 1994.

26. Strumpf R, Heuser R, Eagan J Jr. Angioscopy: a valuable tool in the deployment and evaluation of intracoronary stents. *Am Heart J.* 126:1204–1210, 1993.

27. Serruys PW, Strauss BH, de Feyter P, Urban P. The wallstent: a self-expanding stent. *J Inv Cardiol.* 3:127–134, 1991.

28. Haude M, Erbel R, Straub U, Dietz U, Meyer J. Short and long term results after intracoronary stenting in human coronary arteries: monocentre experience with the balloon-expandable Palmaz-Schatz stent. *Br Heart J.* 66:337–345, 1991.

29. Vigano, D'Angelo S, Comp P, Esmon C, D'Angelo A. Relationship between proten C antigen and anticoagulant activity during oral anticoagulation and in selected disease states. *J Clin Invest.* 77:416–425, 1986.

30. Swars H, Hafner G, Erbel R, et al. Prothrombin fragment F1 + 2 predicts acute occlusion after intracoronary stenting. *J Am Coll Cardiol.* 17(suppl A):302A, 1991.

31. Strumpf R, Eagan J, Hardigan K, Berg D. Assessment of new coagulation markers for intracoronary stent implantation. *Circulation.* 88(4, pt 2):1199, 1993.

32. Kiemeneij F, Laarman G, Swart H. Is monitoring of prothrombin factor F1 + 2 of additional value in guiding anticoagulation after coronary stenting? *Circulation.* 88(4, pt 2):3447, 1993.

33. George B, Voorhees W III, Roubin G, et al. Multicenter investigation of coronary stenting

to treat acute or threatened closure after percutaneous transluminal coronary angioplasty: clinical and angiographic oucomes. *JACC.* 22:135–143, 1993.

34. Buchwald A, Unterberg C, Werner G, Voth E, Kreuzer H, Wiegand V. Initial clinical results with the Wiktor stent: a new balloon-expandable coronary stent. *Clin Cardiol.* 14:374–379, 1991.

35. Anderson PG, Bajaj RK, Baxley WA, Roubin GS. Vascular pathology of balloon-expandable flexible coil stents in humans. *J Am Coll Cardiol.* 19:372–381, 1992.

36. Ueda Y, Nanto S, Komamura K, Kodama K. Neointimal coverage of stents in human coronary arteries observed by angioscopy. *JACC.* 23:341–346, 1994.

37. Schatz R, Penn I, Baim D, et al. STent REStenosis Study (STRESS): analysis of in-hospital results. *Circulation.* 88(4, pt 2):3194, 1993.

38. Serruys P, Macaya C, de Jaegere P, et al. Interim analysis of the Benestent-Trial. *Circulation.* 88(4, pt 2):3195, 1993.

39. Lincoff M, Topol E, Chapekis A, et al. Intracoronary stenting compared with conventional therapy for abrupt vessel closure complicating coronary angioplasty: a matched case-control study. *JACC.* 21:866–875, 1993.

40. Friedrich S, Davis S, Kuntz R, Carrozza J, Baim D. Investigational use of the Palmaz-Schatz biliary stent in large saphenous vein grafts. *Am J Card.* 71:439–441, 1993.

41. Golden M, Downing S. Peripheral vascular complications of coronary endovascular stent placement. In: Hirshfield JaH HC, eds. *Clinical Use of the Palmaz-Schatz Intracoronary Stent* Futura Publishing Co., Inc., NY 137–150, 1993.

42. Moscucci M, Mansour K, Kuntz R, et al. Vascular complications of Palmaz-Schatz coronary stenting: predictors, management and outcome. *J Am Coll Cardiol.* 134A, 1994.

43. Mansour K, Moscucci M, Kent C, et al. Vascular complications following directional coronary atherectomy or Palmaz-Schatz stenting. *J Am Coll Cardiol.* 136A, 1994.

44. Sutton J, Ellis S, Roubin G, et al. Major clinical events after coronary stenting: the multicenter registry of acute and elective Gianturco-Roubin stent placement. *Circulation.* 89(3): 1126–1137, 1994.

45. Garratt K, Porter P. Wiktor stent clinical trial data for PMA application. Medtronic Wiktor Coronary Stent Investigators Meeting, Atlanta, GA; 1994.

46. Kiemeneij F, Laarman G. Improved anticoagulation management after Palmaz-Schatz coronary stent implantation by sealing the arterial puncture site with a vascular hemostasis device. *Cathet Cardiovasc. Diag.* 30:317–322, 1993.

47. Camenzind E, Grossholz M, Urban P, et al. Mechanical compression (Femostop) alone versus combined collagen application (Vasoseal) and femostop for arterial puncture site closure after coronary stent implantation: a randomized trial. *J Am Coll Cardiol.* 355A, 1994.

48. Ernst S, Mast G, Bal E, et al. Nonsurgical treatment of complications due to arterial puncture. *Circulation.* 88(4, pt 2):1351, 1993.

49. Vogt P, Eeckhout E, Stauffer J, Goy J, Kappenberger L. Stent shortening and elongation: pitfalls with the Wiktor coronary endoprosthesis. *Cathet Cardiovasc Diagn.* 31:233–235, 1994.

50. Reifart N, Langer A, Storger H, Schwarz F, Preusler W, Hofmann M. Strecker stent as a bailout device following percutaneous transluminal coronary angioplasty. *J Interven Cardiol.* 5:79–83, 1992.

51. Brown R, Penn I, Ricci D, Buller C. Double Marker ACX II: A new balloon catheter for coronary stent delivery. *Cathet Cardiovasc Diagn.* 27:82–85, 1992.

52. Pitney M, Cumpston N. A solution to the problem of an unexpanded Palmaz-Schatz stent following balloon rupture. *Cathet Cardiovasc Diagn.* 24:246–247, 1991.

53. White C, Ramee S, Collins T, Escobar A, Jain S. Placement of "Biliary" stents in saphenous vein coronary bypass grafts. *Cathet Cardiovasc Diag.* 30:91–95, 1993.

54. Bucx JJJ, de Scheerder I, Beatt K, et al. The importance of adequate anticoagulation to prevent early thrombosis after stenting of stenosed venous bypass grafts. *Am Heart J.* 121:1389–1396, 1991.

55. Investigators TE. Use of a monoclonal antibody directed against the platelet glycoprotein IIb/IIIa receptor in high-risk angioplasty. *N Engl J Med.* 330:956–961, 1994.

56. Barragan P, Silvestri M, Sainsous J, Bouvier J, Comet B, Simeoni J. Coronary stenting without coumadin. *J Am Coll Cardiol.* 336A, 1994.

57. Dichek DA, Neville RF, Zwiebel JA, Freeman SM, Leon MB, Anderson WF. Seeding of intravascular stents with genetically engineered endothelial cells. *Circulation.* 80:1347–1353, 1989.

58. Bilodeau L, Hearn J, Dean L, Roubin G. Prolonged intracoronary urokinase infusion for acute stent thrombosis. *Cathet Cardiovasc Diagn.* 30:141–146, 1993.

59. Chatelain P, Urban P, Meier B. Balloon angioplasty of a coronary stent occluded for three months. *J Invas Cardiol.* 4:188–190, 1992.

60. Fischman D, Savage M, Leon M, et al. Fate of lesion-related side branches after coronary artery stenting. *JACC.* 22:1641–1646, 1993.

61. Medina A, Hernandez E, de Lezo J, et al. Divided Palmaz-Schatz stent for discrete coronary stenosis. *J Invas Cardiol.* 4:389–392, 1992.

62. Strauss BH, Serruys PW, de Scheerder IK, et al. Relative risk analysis of angiographic predictors of restenosis within the coronary wallstent. *Circulation.* 84:1636–1643, 1991.

63. Ellis S, Savage M, Fischman D, et al. Restenosis after placement of Palmaz-Schatz stents in native coronary arteries: initial results of a multicenter experience. *Circulation.* 86:1836–1844, 1992.

64. Gordon P, Gibson C, Cohen D, Carrozza J, Kuntz R, Baim D. Mechanisms of restenosis and redilation within coronary stents—quantitative angiographic assessment. *JACC.* 1166–1174, 1993.

65. Baim D, Levine M, Leon M, Levine S, Ellis S, Schatz R. Management of restenosis within the Palmaz-Schatz coronary stent (the US multicenter experience). *Am J Cardiol.* 71:364–366, 1993.

66. Strauss B, Umans V, van Suylen R-J, et al. Directional atherectomy for treatment of restenosis within coronary stents: clinical, angiographic, and histologic results. *J Am Coll Cardiol.* 20:1465–1473, 1992.

67. Pan M, Medina A, Romero M, et al. Peripheral stent recovery after failed intracoronary delivery. *Cathet Cardiovasc Diagn.* 27:230–233, 1992.

68. Foster-Smith K, Garratt K, Higano S, Holmes D Jr. Retrieval techniques for managing flexible intracoronary stent misplacement. *Cath Cardiovasc Diagn.* 30:63–68, 1993.

69. Boatman J, Grines C, In Freed M, Grines C, eds. PTCA exotica: unusual problems encountered in the invasive laboratory. *Man Intervent Cardiol.* Physicians Press, Birmingham, 175–194, 1992.

70. Veldhuizen F, Bonnier J, Michels H, El Gamal M, van Gelder B. Retrieval of undeployed stents from the right coronary artery: report of two cases. *Cathet Cardiovasc Diagn.* 30: 245–248, 1993.

72. de Jaegere P, de Feyter P, van der Giessen W, Serruys P. Endovascular stents: preliminary clinical results and future developments. *Clin. Cardiol.* 16:369–378, 1993.

73. Hearn J, King S III, Douglas J Jr, Carlin S, Lembo N, Ghazzal ZM. Clinical and angiographic outcomes after coronary artery stenting for acute or threatened coronary angioplasty. *Circulation.* 88:2086–2096, 1993.

74. de Jaegere PP, Serruys PW, Bertrand M, et al. Wiktor stent implantation in patients with restenosis following balloon angioplasty of a native coronary artery. *Am J Cardiol.* 69:598–602, 1992.

75. Carrozza JP, Kuntz RE, Fishman RF, Friedrich S, Miller MJ, Baim DS. Multivessel coronary intervention with a balloon-expandable intracoronary stent. *Coron Artery Dis.* 3:403–406, 1992.

76. Center for Devices and Radiological Health Review Panel. *Balloon expandable stent and delivery system—premarket approval application.* US Food and Drug Administration; 1994.

Index